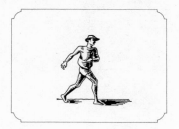

SAVITRI'S WAY TO PERFECT FITNESS THROUGH HATHA YOGA

by Savitri Ahuja

SIMON AND SCHUSTER

NEW YORK

ACKNOWLEDGMENTS

I would like to thank everyone who has been part of the creation of this book: my students, who have worked with me and who have trusted in my methods; my friends, who have advised me throughout the writing of the manuscript; and especially my agent, Bill Adler, who encouraged me to write this book, and the staff of Simon & Schuster, my publisher.

To Narayan Ahuja, my son, and R. K. Menda,
M.B., F.R.C.S., F.A.C.S., F.A.C.G.,
and G. K. Menda, my brothers, and finally, John
Hysom, Ph.D., my friend.

Published by Simon and Schuster
A Division of Gulf & Western Corporation
Simon & Schuster Building
Rockefeller Center
1230 Avenue of the Americas
New York, New York 10020

Designed by Stanley S. Drate
Manufactured in the United States of America

1 2 3 4 5 6 7 8 9 10

Library of Congress Cataloging in Publication Data

Ahuja, Savitri.
    Savitri's way to perfect fitness through hatha yoga.

    Includes index.
    1. Yoga, Hatha.   2. Health.   I. Title.
RA781.7.A38   613.7   78-31984

ISBN 0-671-24023-4

Contents

Introduction to Savitri

In the mirror-walled studio, the wife of a one-time candidate for President pretzels her body into a "twist." Lying beside her, the daughter of a former Chief Justice of the United States swings her legs behind her head in a "plough." A few bodies away, the wife of a Cabinet officer starts guiltily as a stern voice chides: "You with the fat po-po, why are you just lying there? Why aren't you trembling your legs? That'll take some of the jelly-pulley off your thighs."

The voice belongs to Savitri—yoga teacher to Washington's VIPs—the willowy Indian whose warm, dark eyes belie the sometime sharpness of her voice; Savitri, the disciplinarian who refuses to accept "I can't" or "I'll never be able to do that." So the Congressional wives and White House aides, the beautiful people and would-be beautiful people, members of the diplomatic corps and the press corps, professional men and business women learn to translate Savitri's sometimes scrambled English, and meekly obey her edicts.

They bring her their aching backs, their Washington-spawned tensions, their tennis elbows, the fat of too many official dinners, the problems of standing hours in receiving lines. And because they have to keep going, they follow her orders. At first, they're inclined to be skeptical. How can a simple exercise, combined with a change in breathing habits, cure a lingering ache? But the pain disappears and they become believers, returning month after month, year after year, bringing their important friends. They try to impress Savitri with the standing of her new pupils. But half the time, she doesn't even get their names straight. She labels them with the colors of their leotards. Completely apolitical in a political town, Savitri is interested only in the bodies of her pupils. How can she get rid of their tensions, their dowager's hump; how can a sullen, lost look be replaced by an expression of joyous life? She relishes the challenge.

I've been a Savitri-watcher for a dozen years, ever since the night I took my limp to her class for the first time. I was stretching my back as she calls it, trying, and failing, to get the small of my back to touch the floor, when she came to my side and said softly, "I can help you." What conquered the natural skepticism of a reporter was the set of exercises she tailored for me alone. They closely resembled the ones my doctor had been trying to get me to do. I figured if she knew that much about my body after only seeing me once, I'd string along with her for a while. I've been stringing along ever since.

Like many of her other students, I bring her not only my aches and pains, but those of my relatives. My ninety-year-old mother came back from Florida with such a painful attack of arthritis that she couldn't get out of bed. Savitri got her out of bed and down on the floor to do the exercises Savitri had designed to relieve just the pain that bothered Mother. Now, every morning without fail, Mother starts her day with five minutes of lying on the floor, arching her back, rolling from side to side, knees high—faithfully following Savitri's exercise prescription. That was several years ago and arthritis hasn't bothered her again.

An Air Force general's wife, grateful to Savitri for clearing her face of age lines and forcing her to straighten her shoulders, calls Savitri's studio the little red schoolhouse of people problems, where everyone in the class gets something a little different to meet individual needs. There's a waiting list for her classes and for her semiannual seven- or eight-day crash courses because the yoga that Savitri pioneered in Washington has now become a way of life.

Stories about Savitri, her VIPs and her exercise classes appeared in Washington newspapers and across the country, but her classes were closed to television. One day in 1977 television crews finally spent the day and the evening with her and her students. Viewers saw her guiding an evening class of men as well as women in her teaching "uniform" of loose long blouse and tight-fitting pants. Then they watched her with a class composed solely of multiple sclerosis victims. Came the climactic moment when a girl called Norma, who a few months earlier hadn't even been able to sit up without bracing herself, walked unaided across the studio.

The scene shifted to Savitri strolling in Rock Creek Park, a rose tucked in her dark hair, her sari floating behind her, her slim body silhouetted against the trees. The interviewer asked her why she worked such long hours, why she took on the extra burden of teaching even the wheelchair-bound the lesson that yoga could bring new life to muscles they thought had been long dead. She replied simply, "I want to help people."

The lyrical finale, the Indian music strengthening as the camera turned from Savitri to focus on a sky full of puffy clouds, wasn't irrelevant, not to Savitri. For she has confided to close friends the knowledge that she helps people as a gift to her god, Krishna, the Hindu God. She calls him her boyfriend, and her faith is very personal, very alive. Each yoga session begins with palms touching in prayer and every member of her class dutifully makes the prayer gesture. It particularly touched a woman who uses a walker to come to Savitri's multiple sclerosis class. Mother of a Baptist minister, she considers Savitri a woman of faith and listens and accepts her words.

Doctors have applauded what Savitri has done for victims of multiple sclerosis, have marveled at how her exercises, faithfully performed, can control some of the more trying symptoms of MS, such as incontinence. A senator's wife believes Savitri saved her life by showing her how the right exercises and the proper way of standing in receiving lines could prevent blood clots in her legs from killing her. An ambassador's wife says that

Savitri cured the insomnia she thought she could never overcome. A minister whose bible broadcasts reach over six hundred churches and school assemblies across the country, credits Savitri with teaching him how proper breathing would help him pace his sermons better and how her exercises would enable him to meditate without thinking how stiff he was getting.

Her success in waking up sluggish bodies with yoga prompted a recent convocation of Indian doctors to invite her to lecture to them. When her classes got too big for a studio in her home and she opened her mirrored studio on fashionable Connecticut Avenue, the Indian Ambassador to the United States came to dedicate it. He called her India's permanent ambassador to the nation's capital.

This is a woman—she still looks more like a girl—who never went to school, who taught herself whatever English she knows, who broke with the traditions and customs of high-born Indians to live the life she believes her God decreed for her.

Savitri was born in Bombay, India. Her father was a "Sir," a title of distinction. Her four brothers were given formal schooling and distinguished themselves, but she and her sister were supposed to grow up as Indian girls of good family did in those days, unschooled but expected to develop the wifely arts at home.

Her sister, who was older, accepted the life, but six-year-old Savitri rebelled. She wanted to become a dancer. Her family opposed her, but her mother, understanding her beautiful little daughter, told Savitri's father that the child wanted to learn the difficult ceremonial dancing of India to please her God.

Finally, Savitri's father agreed to let her dance on condition that she never appear on the stage. She eagerly agreed, thinking something would happen later to change his mind. But after she was given permission to take lessons, her family tried everything to discourage her. They tried punishment and tempting her with treats to get her mind off practicing the dance. To help her resist and to strengthen her self-discipline, her dance guru suggested she practice yoga. To the eight-year-old child, dancing was her entire life; yoga was her discipline.

As the young years passed, she found the time she devoted to yoga made the demanding figures of the dance far easier. She never forgot that lesson. Today, she tells her students that if they'll practice their yoga before they hit the ski slopes or dive into the pool or play tennis, they'll perform much better.

Savitri's mother had promised her daughter that she wouldn't be a child bride, but when her mother died, the family decided that marriage would put notions of dancing out of her mind. So the motherless child was married at the age of thirteen to a mature, broad-minded man, who quickly gave his consent to let her go on dancing. The birth of a son only stopped her for a year and then she returned to dance all over India. Meanwhile, the yoga which had begun as a discipline continued as a vital part of her life.

When she studied yoga, she never expected to teach it, but as the years passed, people asked her to instruct them in yoga as well as dancing. She was now living with her husband in Calcutta and her studio was in the section where foreigners lived.

She was nineteen or twenty when the foreign wives (the British, Dutch,

German, Swiss, French, and especially the Americans assigned to Calcutta) persuaded her to introduce them to both Indian dancing and yoga. The American diplomats asked her to teach yoga to their wives. Her students called themselves her "foreign troupe."

She was picking up English as she went, teaching herself how to read and write, asking her class to help her master difficult words to express her exact meaning, as she still does. So when her husband was sent to Washington as second and then first secretary of the Indian Embassy, she was ready for American students. But first she had to get the permission of the Indian Government to teach professionally, which was generally forbidden in the diplomatic corps. She got the government's blessing on the ground that she was bringing the beautiful culture of India to the American people.

Her first students in this country came from members of her "foreign troupe" who had come home. When a newspaperwoman interviewed Savitri and she introduced her "foreign troupe," the literal-minded reporter shook her head: "No, no. They're not the foreigners. You are."

Savitri finally corrected that. She goes back to India every year to visit her family and look in on the yoga classes, but she's now an American citizen. Members of her family have changed, too. They're proud of her now and they want her to give them yoga lessons while she's with them. She tries to put them off. "Why don't you go to the gurus here? You've got plenty to choose from." But they want Savitri's yoga.

In Washington, almost imperceptibly, Savitri found her classes changing. She was teaching less dancing and more yoga. Gradually, she realized there was more demand for yoga and no time for dancing.

"I saw what yoga was doing for people," she says. "Yes, dancing was giving pleasure to people but yoga helps their bodies, helps their thinking. It's like you put a seed in the ground and how you feel when the flower grows. You think, 'My gosh, I did this.'"

What she did was create her own adaptations of yoga to meet the needs of the average man or woman. The basic postures like the Twist and the Plough, the Locust, Cobra, and Shoulder Stand are key parts of Savitri's yoga, but so are the ones of her own creation, adaptations of what she learned from the Indian gurus to meet special problems.

The creation of her own yoga goes back to the days when she was still learning and teaching in Calcutta. She would study a posture, as yoga positions are called, and would say to her teacher: "But, Guruji, if someone has a bad back, that will make it worse. If you bend the knees, you can get the same effect without damage." And the girl, still little more than a child, would demonstrate, and the guru would nod his approval and say she was the creative one, born with the gift of yoga.

More and more, she would alter the established postures, not only to prevent strain on untrained bodies but also to repair the damage done by bad posture, tension, strain, or injury. Besides her own eager inventiveness, she had one big advantage. In her family were five doctors, including one of India's top surgeons. She would check out her theories with them. Would this exercise, done this way, improve circulation, would that posture take some of the ache out of the small back (she's never mastered the phrase "small of the back"). Remembering how difficult some of the postures had been for the small Savitri, she began to break them down into what she called little pieces, giving her students a little stretching until they could achieve a maximum stretch, allowing them to do an exercise flat-footedly until they had the balance to lift their heels. She showed them how to visualize what they were doing, to picture in their minds exactly what they wanted to achieve.

She experiments with an exercise on her own body before she introduces it to the group. When she goes to India, she always returns to class with new exercises. Her students assume she got them from the Indian gurus. She didn't. She simply used the time away from class to create new exercises and try them on herself.

She fends off every demand from a student to get just one exercise for a specific problem, such as a fat stomach. She tells them you can't take care of only one part of the body. Every part of your body cries for attention, she tells her students, every part deserves treats. So you bend forward and backward. Like day follows night, you must do opposites. You bend sideways, you twist, you fill and empty your lungs, you increase your circulation.

These are the general rules, the ones her students have long demanded that she incorporate in a book. This she has done. Further, and more important, she warns her readers, just as she does her students, about exercises that should not be done, exercises that might aggravate some problem they already have, as well as the ones that are especially helpful to them. So she has moved Savitri's yoga from her studio to the pages of a book.

Some of Savitri's students have been coming to her for yoga close to fifteen years. Some attend class every day because they need the discipline she gives them. Some sweat out her crash courses to reach the slimmer figure Savitri espouses. She convinces them to have respect for their bodies, not just for this time but for all time. And because they believe in her, they'll do what she says.

That's the real secret of this unschooled woman of India, her ability to get the most sophisticated people in the world to believe in her. Her students say that's her God-given gift. She would say that's her gift to her God.

MIRIAM OTTENBERG
Pulitzer Prize-winning investigative reporter,
formerly with the *Washington Star.*
Author of *The Federal Investigators*
and *The Pursuit of Hope.*

1

The Yoga Experience

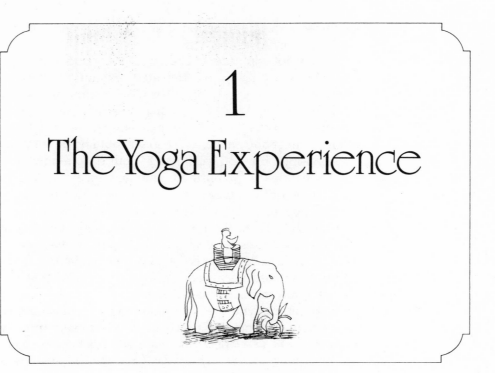

Before I explain how to do the Hatha Yoga exercises, I think it is important to understand, as my students do, exactly what yoga is and how you can use it best. In this chapter, then, I am going to discuss why yoga is *not* any kind of magic from India, but why it *is* a road to self-realization through using your own internal resources.

The yoga I teach is a way of life that offers four freedoms: freedom from assorted aches and pains, freedom from the cravings of a false appetite, freedom from needless strain and tension and, especially, freedom from growing old before your time.

A. *What Yoga Is and Is Not*

Before learning the means of achieving these freedoms, however, you should understand what yoga is not. It's not a religion or something performed only by Indian holy men sitting with eyes closed and legs crossed in the Lotus pose. Although the minute you mention yoga, friends want to know if you stand on your head, yoga is far more than that. In fact, headstands are only for advanced pupils and should not be done by women at all because it gives them a thick, unattractive neck.

There are other misapprehensions about yoga. It's not magic or a form of spiritualism and it's not a competitive sport. You don't compete to see how much better you can do the Cobra than your fellow student. Your incentive is not competition, but your own earnest desire for a mind at peace and an ache-free body.

Yoga is not gymnastics. The yoga in this book is Hatha or exercise yoga, but it does not leave you depleted, exhausted, sweaty, and panting for breath. At the end of a yoga exercise session, you'll know you've had a workout and you may even perspire gently but you'll be the opposite of exhausted. Instead, you'll feel exhilarated, refreshed, renewed, energetic, ready to meet any challenge. You will not find contentment and serenity in a gymnasium, but you will find it in your daily rendezvous with yoga.

Finally, yoga is not for the young and agile only. It's for everyone, and I mean everyone. You may say, as some doubters have said to me before joining my class, "Well, this is all very well for young people, but I'm too old, too stiff, too heavy for all this exercising." Actually, the older you are and the less exercise you've been doing, the more urgently you need yoga. That's true not only because yoga works on every part of your body, inside and out, but also because it's a form of exercise that a person of any age can learn to practice to his advantage.

My pupils range in age from nine to ninety, including men and women. One ninety-year-old gets down on the floor every morning to do her yoga. Women in their seventies and even eighties become increasingly supple in my hour-long classes. They leave the studio pink-cheeked and bouncy. They may only need lipstick.

B. *Hatha Yoga*

If yoga is neither religion nor gymnastics, what is it? Yoga is an ancient science that enables those who practice it to achieve good health, spiritual well-being and mental self-discipline. The word yoga itself derives from the Sanskrit word *yuj* or yoke, meaning a union or joining. Yoga is a joining of body, mind and spirit, a goal reached through many stages, down many paths.

You will be practicing Hatha Yoga, the physical stage, which I have adapted to Western ways and Western needs. It is meant to lead ultimately to union with the Universal Being by whatever name you know Him. Other stages are Karma Yoga, the spiritual path characterized by right action and service to others; Bhakti Yoga, the path of spiritual enlightenment through worship and devotion to the Supreme Being; Jnana Yoga, the intellectual path to self-realization and union with God through knowledge and wisdom; and Raja Yoga, the highest form of yoga, the royal union with the Universal Spirit through meditation.

Anyone who hopes to master yoga meditation or the techniques of total concentration, anyone who seeks the higher, spiritual levels of yoga, must learn to master his or her own body first. Hatha Yoga will help him strengthen his spine to enable him to sit and meditate without allowing his thoughts to stray to his aching back. Yoga breathing, an integral part of Hatha Yoga, will subdue the turbulence of his thoughts to the peace of meditation.

C. *Its Disciplines and Benefits*

Hatha Yoga, however, is far more than simply a preliminary to meditation and the higher levels of yoga. For the hard-working, high-pressured, over-stimulated city dwellers of the last quarter of the twentieth century, Hatha Yoga is an end in itself.

Consider the unhealthful lives most people live today, breathing polluted air, eating too-rich foods, being assaulted by nerve-shattering noise, sitting all the time—in their cars, in their offices, in front of television sets. Almost everyone in my classes complains of a problem spawned by the way they live. It could be high blood pressure, tension headaches, chronic backache, overweight or insomnia. The less we use our bodies and the more we abuse them with poor diets, alcohol, smoking and lack of exercise, the quicker they will deteriorate. We are hastening the aging process, allowing ourselves to grow old prematurely.

Aha, you're thinking, now she's going to tell us that yoga cures all these things, even aging. Yes, I am, because it does. If you practice yoga correctly and faithfully, it will slow down the aging process, you will look younger and healthier, become more relaxed, develop a better figure and feel wonderful!

Just as you can't clap with one hand, as the Indian saying goes, you can't draw the full value from your yoga unless your mind and body work together. Your mind can prey on your body. Stress and tension, anxiety and fear can be translated into ulcers and high blood pressure. So a basic goal of yoga is to bring harmony to mind and body, teaching them to work together rather than in conflict.

Your mind is like a rough sea, often storm-tossed and moody, wandering off-course, restless and uncontrolled. With yoga breathing and yoga discipline, you will learn to control your mind. Yoga gives you mastery over yourself, gives you the discipline to think before you act, to become less impulsive, more in control of your temper, more in command of your actions. Believe that your body belongs to you, you do not belong to your body; in that way you can be its master, instead of being subordinate to it.

In Hatha Yoga, as we learn to coordinate mind and body, we learn to rid ourselves of tension and strain, to relax. You may protest, "But my tension is caused by circumstances over which I have absolutely no control." Even if this is so, and you have to ask yourself honestly if there isn't some way out, yoga will help you live with your problem without destroying yourself in the process.

Just as yoga calms the rough seas of the mind, it follows nature in other ways. Some of its postures are named after the creatures they resemble. Thus, the head, shoulder and chest rising from the floor creates the picture of a cobra lifting its head to strike. That's the Cobra *asana* (the Indian word for pose or posture). And the Locust *asana*, with arms and legs raised simultaneously from the floor, calls to mind the grasshopper with its distinctive antennae. Yoga also follows nature's pattern of opposites and contrasts. In nature, we have heat and cold, day and night, sky and earth, pleasure and pain, life and death, fire and water. In yoga, every movement is followed by its opposite. We stretch and contract our bodies, bend forward and backward, stoop and stand, bend to the right and to the left, twist like a pretzel and straighten like an arrow.

With these opposites, we give what I call treats to all parts of the body. I tell my students that if we neglect any part, it cries like a baby without its milk, meaning that part of our body aches from disuse. Yoga then should follow the concept of the American "package deal," an assortment of goodies.

Some of my students talk to me about spot reducing, getting one exercise to do for a bulging tummy. I always reply that one exercise is never enough. Just as in nature, if you don't water your plants, they die, so in yoga, if you don't nourish your body with a supply of fresh oxygen through breathing exercises, if you don't send the blood racing through your blood vessels, your body will wither too. It takes more than one exercise to achieve these objectives.

Hatha Yoga is one form of exercise that does reach every part of your body inside and out. Although there are eighty-seven principal *asanas,* thousands of *asanas* are part of the yoga repertory. Each one has a different reason for being; fulfills in some way a different bodily need, from a gentle massage to a cure for constipation, from relief of arthritis pains to improving the heart circulation.

Basic to all yoga is the yoga breath—breathing in a way you've never breathed before. You can't do yoga exercises and get any lasting benefit from them until you learn yoga breathing. In my yoga classes, I often maintain the cadence of a repetitive exercise by chanting, "Breathe out to go down, in to come up." I want proper breathing to become an automatic response to contracting and expanding the body.

My students know that when they're contracting their body as they do in bending over, they must get the stale air out of their lungs to make room for the fresh air they breathe in as they stretch upward. Breathing is so vital to yoga that I devote a full chapter to it because breathing has to be learned, by itself and as a necessary accompaniment to the *asanas.*

Another vital element of yoga is the straightening and strengthening of the spine, bringing it back into correct alignment, getting rid of round shoulders and a crooked back. When you don't treat your spine with the respect due it, when you allow yourself to slump or stand with most of your weight on one foot, your poor posture not only invites backache, curvature of the spine and protruding stomach, but you're cheating yourself of your youth. "You are as young as your spine."

Once you become aware of your spine, as you do vertebra by vertebra in yoga, you can stand longer without tiring and escape the back problems of your friends. Since your efforts to stretch your back also affect the spinal cord where the nervous system exists, your yoga stimulates your entire nerve network. Your spine is the powerhouse of your body.

Hatha Yoga is a system of *asanas* or postures. In every posture you should try to hold it as long as possible, usually the length of a breath, to get the maximum effect. Where yoga breathing is not involved, you may hold the pose longer, or you may be instructed to repeat the pose six times. On occasion, when the aim of the exercise is to make your heart pump faster or stimulate your circulation, you may be told to keep it up for a minute or two before slowing or stopping.

Every *asana* has one principal benefit and two or more additional re-wards. No yoga exercise is good for only one thing. The Shoulder Stand is a prime example of the many different benefits of one *asana*. Because your chin is locked against your chest, the thyroid gland is stimulated. An active thyroid burns off the flab; gets rid of rolls of unwanted flesh as your weight is being redistributed.

That, however, is just one of the Shoulder Stand's good deeds. The Shoulder Stand with its inverted posture acts as a counterbalance to the aging process. As we age, we become more susceptible to the pull of gravity. The skin of our face sags, breasts start to hang, shoulders droop, the stomach sticks out and internal organs become displaced. With the body upside down in the Shoulder Stand, blood rushes to the head, stim-ulating the brain to mental alertness and giving the face the youthful flush of yesteryear. Meanwhile, sagging internal organs are gently restored to their original position. Just one exercise does all that!

D. *How People Fit Yoga into Their Lives*

Before considering the many rewards of yoga, however, you'll want to know how to fit yoga into your life-style. First of all, you do not have to withdraw from life or give up everything for yoga. Indeed, yoga makes life more interesting, more challenging.

Just because you ski in winter or swim in summer, you can't say you're getting all the exercise your body needs. As a matter of fact, yoga is a "must" for swimmers, golfers, skiers, tennis players, opera singers, dancers, joggers or runners—for everyone who exercises some muscles and neglects the others. One of the men in my class regularly runs the three miles home from my studio. A skier told me yoga has greatly improved her agility on the slopes and a swimmer reported she has increased both her speed and endurance by treating herself to an hour's yoga before she goes to the pool.

Since no two people are alike, their bodies respond differently to exer-cise. Some exercises, for instance, may be helpful to an arthritic condition but harmful to a heart patient. Some postures can help everyone, young and old, men and women. Others should be altered to individual needs or avoided altogether. That's why my book, unlike most other books on yoga exercises, specifically explains what not to do if the yoga student has certain problems, as well as what he or she can and should do to improve them.

People suffering from high blood pressure or a heart condition should check with their physician before embarking on their yoga program. More often than not, an enlightened physician will encourage them to get into the yoga program but to use common sense and moderation and to follow my instructions on what exercises should be avoided.

You can decide for yourself whether you need yoga to give you wake-up stimulation or bedtime relief from tension. The exercises can be done any-time during the day, but you should give yourself at least a half hour for your Daily Yoga Program in a well-ventilated room, free from mental or physical distractions. Some of my students start their day with an hour's yoga. Others get to it after they send husbands off to work or children off to school. For some, a half hour's yoga before they climb into bed is their recipe for beating insomnia.

E. *Visualizing Yoga for You*

In order to get the most out of your yoga session, you should consider your yoga program not as a chore to be undertaken reluctantly, but as a revitalizing experience, a treat you're giving yourself. Then you should eliminate from your vocabulary the words "I can't." Of course, you can't do it all at once, but my exercise program for you is designed to move gradually from the easiest to the more advanced exercises. You can go at your own pace. Nobody is forcing you to speed up. Actually, that's the last thing you want to do. You want to proceed slowly, to savor, to strive, to enjoy. Forgetting what you can't do, concentrate on gradually improving what you can do. Expect a little more from yourself each day—one more repetition; a breath held a few seconds longer; the back a little straighter; the stretch a bit farther.

The mental exercise guaranteed to make each day's physical exercise more rewarding is to visualize exactly what you want to achieve with your *asana*. Picture yourself in the pose and you'll make it. At first, you may find that difficult to believe, but try it. Put the picture of the *asana* in the front of your mind, blanking out everything else, and suddenly you find yourself in the pose you thought you'd never be able to do.

There are other mental pictures you will find helpful. Think of yourself as a vase of flowers. Your arms are the flowers, moving gracefully, easily, freely. From your waist down, you are the vase—solid, straight, immovable. That picture of yourself enables you to tighten your backside, your thighs, your internal organs, while insuring that you can be straighter with your weight evenly balanced and your stomach pulled in.

While you're visualizing, you should detach each part you're working to improve. By picturing the part of the body involved in the exercise, you learn to leave the rest of your body alone. That way, you can do your stomach lift, without making three chins, you can work on your back muscles without tensing your mouth. You've got to be aware of your whole body to make each part respond to what you're trying to do for it.

Before you start your daily yoga session, you must prepare yourself mentally and physically. You do this by deep breathing, which completely relaxes your muscles. If your muscles are not relaxed, you will not be able to do the postures correctly. Never do a yoga exercise violently. You don't want to risk a slipped disc, a twisted muscle or a wrenched back. Never force your body into a position, always request your body to cooperate. It will, if asked nicely, and you will learn to know your body better than you ever did before. As your body becomes more elastic, it will convey a sense of its own suppleness and your mind will become more alert to what your body is telling you.

Proper and slow breathing, relaxation following stress, nothing hurried—these are the keys to each yoga exercise.

Yoga teaches you to respect your own body, not to mistreat it with fatty foods, late nights, nicotine, narcotics and alcohol. Gradually, you reach such a state of well-being that you no longer crave anything that deadens your senses. You will become proud of your new look and how much more vitality you have.

F. *Rewards of the Yoga Way of Life*

The benefits of yoga are as numerous as the *asanas* themselves, but here are some of the rewards for living the yoga way of life:

Your body stops acting like an antique car and starts performing like a supersonic Jet Liner.

Yoga will increase the efficiency of the heart muscle by improving the circulation. This will prevent heart attacks.

Yoga will also prevent undue fat deposits in some places by proper assimilation and distribution of the fat. It will improve the functions of the liver and the kidneys. For the proper functioning of these and other internal organs, yoga is a must.

You never get out of breath because your lung capacity increases so much from your yoga breathing. You don't tire as quickly. You can stand longer, walk farther, run faster.

When, as you grow older, your spine shrinks and you lose inches in height, yoga prevents that shrinkage and can even restore the inches you lost, or most of them.

As we grow older, poor circulation causes skin to be wrinkled and pigmented. With yoga, our skin is tightened, and pigmentation disappears.

Menopause can bring depression to both men and women. Yoga banishes this depression and frees women from the hot flashes and sick headaches of menopause, too.

Girls escape the monthly cramps of their menstrual periods.

As we age, our gums recede from our teeth. Yoga can prevent this aspect of aging and you can help to preserve your teeth.

Since the Shoulder Stand supplies more oxygen to your head, you don't gray nearly as fast. Instead of falling out, your hair will often continue to grow as fast and fully as it did in your youth.

Older people have to get their prescriptions for eyeglasses changed frequently as their vision alters. With yoga, your vision doesn't change as rapidly and you escape the eye strain, which may be the cause of overall fatigue.

Yoga insures a longer, more satisfying sex life for both men and women.

Yoga helps you to get to know yourself, which is the first step in self-improvement.

Yoga improves concentration and the coordination of your thoughts and actions.

Perhaps you've grown tired of the shallow materialism of life and want something deeper. Drugs won't help you, but yoga will.

Yoga improves your emotional health because emotional health depends in large part on physical health.

Yoga can rid you of two daily or nightly woes: constipation and insomnia.

Yoga is one form of *exercise* you can do without getting muscle-bound or looking like a weight lifter. The muscles build but they don't bulge. Your arms and legs get stronger but they also get more shapely.

With yoga exercises and proper eating, you can have the figure you wish, either twenty pounds lighter or ten pounds heavier. Your figure changes because your weight is redistributed but you can progress from scrawny to slim, from fat to properly proportioned. You will rid yourself of your false appetite, the habit of nibbling all day out of sheer boredom and frustration, even though you're not hungry.

You'll think twice before you take that second helping. Make pushing away from the table a form of exercise, because now that you've got a good figure and a happier outlook you don't want to lose it to a chocolate éclair. You get a self-discipline you wouldn't have believed possible in the fat old days, and along with it you get a true self-confidence; you stand taller.

You keep your temper in check not only because your values have changed, but you know the secret of self-control. Instead of sounding off, you take a yoga breath. That gives you the interval to think before you act, and supplies the oxygen to make your mind more alert so you can prepare the arguments to plead your cause more effectively.

By now, it should be obvious to you that you don't just learn yoga. You experience it.

You will get the most out of your yoga experience if you have a strong motivation to slim down or build up, to learn to relax, to escape daily aches and pains, to feel really fit, to hold back the aging process. Then, you will reach the stage so many of my students reach when they practice their yoga faithfully. Your body will crave daily yoga to the point that if you miss a day of exercise, you will feel unsatisfied all day, deprived, as if you're missing something important. And, of course, you are.

Your health is your fortune—and yoga is health.

2
Yoga Breathing

Before you can embark on your course of yoga, you have to learn to breathe. When I tell that to my new pupils, they're always startled. But, it is true. The breathing they have done up until then has robbed them of nature's principal benefits.

A. *From Normal Shallow Breathing to Full Deep Breathing*

Yoga breathing is a very deep and time-consuming science, which must be learned under the guidance of a knowledgeable teacher. In the absence of an experienced teacher, you can learn some of the fundamentals, at least enough to give your yoga exercises both meaning and benefit. For in yoga, exercise and breathing are intertwined in the same way that mind and body go together. Unless you breathe properly while doing your postures and exercises, you will lose most of the beneficial effects.

Breathing properly stops stress and tension from occupying your mind, and makes you focus your thoughts on taking breath in and out of your body. It is a great first step in putting your mind at ease.

You do not do yoga exercises without yoga breathing. That's one of the important differences between yoga exercises and calisthenics. It is not necessary to think about breathing properly constantly. It becomes natural and automatic if practiced regularly.

Why is correct breathing so important? Well, the breath is a great purifier, flushing the blood with oxygen, which each cell needs for "internal" breathing. So, the tissues and cells are nourished, and the circulation improved. In addition to taking in life-giving oxygen, yoga breathing has a very calming effect on the nervous system. Breathing is an involuntary function, but you can learn to be in control of this function and to use it to your advantage. You learn to breathe deeply and rhythmically, and, just as a baby is calmed by rocking, so you, an adult, are calmed by this rhythmic movement of your body. The yogic science of breathing brings you peace, energy and vitality, and control over your emotions. Without proper breathing, every part of your body suffers, your hair, your eyes, your skin, your heart, your circulation.

The shallow breathing you probably do now, the way you learned in gym classes, will keep you alive, but it can cause tension, irritation, a sunken chest, nervousness, a flabby waist, sallow skin and bad circulation.

Normal breathing movements are mostly involuntary and controlled by the breathing centers in the brain. Although the breathing centers in your brain are fundamentally automatic, and regulated by the need for oxygen in your blood, actions of many parts of your body modify the rate of your breathing. There are interruptions of breathing while speaking, singing, laughing, crying or yawning; when you are in suspense or during periods of fear and excitement.

Yoga breathing can ease moments of crisis and provide better control of breathing at all times. For example, one of my pupils, who was to have minor nose surgery, had heart trouble and could not be given anesthesia. She told her doctor, "I will take a deep yoga breath instead." To the doctor's happy surprise, she went through the operation with very little pain. Several of my pupils have delivered their babies while using this technique and had quite an easy time of it. Other pupils with asthma have been greatly relieved. A clergyman among my pupils works hard on his yoga breathing because he says it helps him to pace his breathing properly when he is delivering a sermon.

Full deep breathing has been helpful during stage performances, important business meetings, active sports, or any other situation where people become excited or nervous or out of breath, even that most hated colon examination in the doctor's office. Believe me, it works!

When you are tired, tense or want to relax, stop and take two full deep breaths. The more oxygen you take into your lungs, the more you benefit. Nature will stop you when you have had enough.

The more oxygen you take, the less food you want, for oxygen and food are enemies. Oxygen is more necessary than food, and is free of calories! For the overweight, escape from calories is certainly the first but not the only benefit of yoga breathing. Wherever oxygen circulates through the body, fat cannot accumulate. Overweight persons, however, cannot take full advantage of the treasures that breathing offers them. The slumped posture, bad muscle tone and weak chest muscles that accompany an excess of fat, makes the overweight person unable to increase the volume of air in his or her chest cavity, thus preventing the full expansion of the lungs and limiting their intake of air. People weighed down by too many pounds should realize, more than the less weighty, that pushing themselves away from the table must accompany pushing the bad air out of their lungs.

Yoga breathing is based on completely exhaling stale air from the body so that inhaling brings a complete change of air. In yoga it is more important to breathe out than to breathe in; thus exhalation in yoga breathing always lasts twice as long as inhalation to empty the lungs as thoroughly as possible each time, making room for fresh air. There's no point in rushing outside to absorb great bursts of air if all you do is push stale air deeper into the lungs.

How can you rid yourself of stale air and fill your lungs with fresh air? Watch a baby breathing. Babies instinctively breathe correctly; their stomachs go up and down rhythmically and regularly. As we grow up, we forget the natural breathing of babyhood. Wrong training combines with careless habits to develop shallow breathing. We are taught to lift our chests, pull in our stomachs and hold our breath. That technique succeeds in blocking the air from reaching the lower part of our lungs and starving them of life-giving oxygen.

We must get rid of our bad breathing habits entirely. The first habit to shun is that of breathing through the mouth. The nose is for breathing; the mouth for talking and eating. The fine hairs in the nose act as a natural filter, which cleanses the impurities from the air as you breathe it in. In the process of going through your nose to your lungs, the temperature of the air is adjusted to that of your body. On the other hand, if you take air in through your mouth, it goes directly to the lungs without being filtered or adjusted to body temperature.

B. *The Role of the Diaphragm in Yoga Breathing*

Now, breathing through the nose, we must replace shallow breathing with deep breathing, yoga breathing. What we are trying to do is reach right down to the lower part of our lungs. Most people breathe from the upper lungs (shallow breathing). Some breathe from the rib cage (middle breathing), and some go deep, to the lower lungs (diaphragmatic breathing). Yoga teaches us to combine all three with a slow, continuous breath that touches all bases.

The diaphragm is the muscular partition between the thorax, or chest cavity, which contains the heart and lungs, and the abdominal cavity, which contains many of the other vital organs. In its normal position, the diaphragm looks like an inverted mixing bowl. When we breathe correctly, the diaphragm is pulled in the opposite direction so that it is almost flat, thus allowing more room for the lower lungs to expand.

In this deep breathing, the diaphragm pushes the abdominal organs down, lengthening the chest cavity, which pushes the abdomen out with each inhalation, like a balloon, allowing the lower lungs to fill with fresh oxygen. This is better than the shallow or middle breathing because it activates the lower and generally unused portion of your lungs.

The secret of breath control is to start by breathing out very slowly, very steadily. That's the technique for increasing your ability to rid your lungs of stale air. When you feel you have squeezed out every dram of air, nature takes over and fills the vacuum that you have created; your lungs are automatically filled with fresh air.

Full yoga breathing gives a treat to the lower area of the lungs, which otherwise would be denied fresh oxygen. Full breathing expels carbon dioxide and activates the sympathetic or involuntary nervous system. In addition, the diaphragm and intercostal muscles, the muscles that are in between your ribs, are strengthened.

C. *Different Styles of Yoga Breathing and How Performed*

To breathe correctly while exercising, keep this principle always in mind. When you breathe in, your body must be in an open position, that is, in a position that allows room for your lungs to expand. So, anytime that you stretch, reach up, stand tall, your body is in an open position; this is the time to take a deep breath. When, in the course of exercising, your body is bent, doubled up, or contracted, it is in a closed position. The organs are compressed, there is no room for the lungs to expand, and this is obviously the time to breathe out. Moreover, some bending, contracting positions actually help to force out the stale air more efficiently.

THE FULL YOGA BREATH

* Stand straight, put your hand on your diaphragm and breathe in slowly. You will feel your breath filling the lungs as though they were balloons. Slowly fill them as full as possible.

* Exhale, bending forward slightly to relax and slowly empty the lungs as much as you can.

Do this exercise a few times a day, but only three times at any one session to avoid hyperventilation. If at first you can't breathe deeply while standing on your feet, another method is to lie down on your back with your feet flat on the floor, knees bent. Put your hand on your diaphragm and feel your lungs filling like balloons as you breathe in, and emptying as you exhale.

This practice of breathing develops mental concentration and control. With it comes the power to visualize every part of your body while doing yoga. In the Daily Yoga Program you will learn when to breathe in and when to breathe out with each exercise, and in no time you will be doing it automatically.

In addition to the yoga full breath and proper breathing while doing exercises and postures, which you have learned, these three breathing exercises offer special benefits: Alternate Breathing, The Cleansing Breath, and Step Breathing.

ALTERNATE BREATHING

* Sit with your back straight and shoulders back.

* Place your right thumb on your right nostril, closing it.

* Inhale through your left nostril slowly until your lungs are completely full, a deep breath.

* With your index finger and second finger between your eyebrows, close the left nostril with your ring finger and hold your breath for a count of four.

* Open the left nostril by releasing your ring finger and exhale slowly and completely.

* Repeat by inhaling through the right nostril this time. Hold for a count of four and exhale through the left nostril. This is one complete round.

* Begin with three rounds, and work up to six. Gradually you will be able to inhale and exhale more slowly and hold your breath longer.

This exercise is designed to remove the stale air from your lungs and to replace it with fresh oxygen, revitalizing the body. It is good for soothing nerves and bringing about a feeling of relaxation and tranquility. Further, it helps to clear congestion of the sinuses.

THE CLEANSING BREATH

* Sit or stand straight in any position that is comfortable.

* Inhale as much as you can, breathing through your nose at all times. As you inhale, expand your abdomen.

* Suck your abdomen in and up under your rib cage with one quick, vigorous movement, forcing the air out of your lungs through your nose. The air should gush out through your nose, making considerable noise as it does. This should be done quickly, taking no more than a half second or one second.

* Inhale the air back into your lungs quickly through your nose. This should take no more time than it took to expel the air before.

* Repeat the sudden and vigorous exhalation and inhalation of air through your nose in quick successive bursts. Each complete cleansing breath should be performed in about one to two seconds. Do this 10 times, once each day.

The Cleansing Breath provides several benefits. It forces impurities from the lungs and it cleans the nasal passages and sinuses. It relieves colds and other respiratory ailments. In addition, it strengthens the abdominal wall and diaphragm. Finally, it is good for awakening in the morning and it clears the mind to start the day.

STEP BREATHING

The Step Breathing exercise is performed while sitting on the floor, with legs crossed, and your hands clasped behind your back. The purpose of this exercise is to gradually expel as much air from the lungs as you can. It is done this way:

* Take a deep breath in.

* Breathe out only in small bursts as you slowly bend forward, almost touching your nose to the floor. Don't cheat by taking air in while you are breathing out.

* Then come up slowly and steadily while breathing in.

* Do this three times.

This exercise replaces the stale air with fresh oxygen and expands your lung capacity for deep breathing. Also, it relieves tension and headaches.

There should never be any strain when you are practicing breathing.

Never do deep breathing on a full stomach, nor take too many deep breaths at one time.

If dizziness occurs, stop for a while before continuing.

Life begins with the first breath and ends with the last and depends on proper breathing.

3
Daily Yoga Program

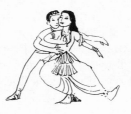

With the breathing you learned in Chapter 2, you're now ready to start your Daily Yoga Program. Exercises and postures, no matter how well you perform them, will be of little benefit without proper breathing. As you start each posture, remember that each is related to the one before it . . . and related to the one that follows it.

The Daily Yoga Program is a science of balance. The exercises and postures are structured to exercise opposite or companion sets of muscle and bone systems. When you bend to the right, then bend to the left. When you bend forward, then go backward. Since we spend most of our time upright, we do inverted postures to reverse the pull of gravity on the body. If you stretch, you contract. The more you breathe out, the more you breathe in.

Some exercises and postures can be done with normal breathing; but most of them, especially those which require you to expand and to contract your body, require proper yoga breathing. Wherever yoga breathing is required, you'll find it in the description of the exercise or posture in the Daily Yoga Program.

Each exercise and posture provides one main benefit and several additional benefits. For best results, it should be part of the total program.

Your full Daily Yoga Program should take three quarters of an hour, assuming that you follow instructions exactly. However, to take you along as I take the students in my yoga classes, I will give you a few exercises to start the first month, gradually increase them in the second month, and finally reach the three quarters of an hour the third month.

As you go through each of the three progressive stages, you will do the numbered exercises for that stage. Each month's program of exercises and postures is designed to reach all parts of your body; so it is essential for you to follow the numbered exercises and postures in each month as you progress, rather than stray to other ones.

When you have mastered stage three, however, you can choose alternative exercises that reach the same parts of the body or achieve the same benefits. For instance, you may substitute the Grand Cobra for the Baby Cobra, or the Bridge for the Fish.

Although you can complete the full Daily Yoga Program in three quarters of an hour, if you have a special problem, as most of us do, you may want to allow extra time to meet your special needs. However do not embark on the special problem programs until you have warmed up your muscles by practicing the First Month Program.

In the following pages, the exercises and postures for each stage are listed by numbers and names followed by detailed instructions.

A. *General Guidance*

These instructions describe what you should do to prepare for your Daily Yoga Program, suggest how to benefit most, and provide some cautions:

* Use a foam rubber mat, one inch thick, about three feet wide and a few inches longer than your height.

* Wear loose garments.

* Practice in an open airy space.

* Abstain from solid foods two hours and liquids thirty minutes before you exercise.

* Do not drink ice water immediately after yoga.

* Take a warm water oil bath after your yoga session. Oil is good for relaxing the muscles.

* Do not do yoga when under the influence of alcohol or you will not know if you are hurting yourself.

* Read each exercise through carefully and try it slowly before you begin. If you have any physical problems, be sure to read the DO NOT DOs before starting the exercise.

* Always go slowly, slowly, and stop if you feel pain. However, a slight ache is no reason to stop. On the contrary, an ache tells you your muscles are working.

* Allow yourself at least forty-five minutes for the full Daily Yoga Program. Give yourself a half minute rest between each exercise and posture to change gears.

* Always think peaceful and beautiful thoughts when you are doing yoga, and smile when you are doing the especially difficult ones.

* Accept the fact that you will not do all of the exercises perfectly. The better you get, the more room there is for improvement. But there is no such word as "never" or "I can't" in yoga. At the beginning, you may think you will never be able to do some of the exercises and postures. But that's not true. If you concentrate on what you are doing and on what each one will do for you, you will succeed.

* Think of the lower part of your body, from the waist down, as a flower vase, which should be stationary. Think of the upper part of your body as a flower, bending easily and gracefully. Hold the lower part very firm so you do not hurt your spine. This applies to all standing exercises and postures.

* Remember to relax your face and neck to keep them from looking tense and tight when you are doing exercises and postures.

* Think of your muscles as children. If you are insistent and firm, but not hard, they will listen and be agreeable with you.

* Don't lie down immediately afterwards. Remember that after a race, they walk the horses before taking them to their stalls.

* Concentrate and think of the part of the body you are working on to get the best results.

* Leave your lips a little open so as not to stretch the skin under your chin whenever an exercise calls for tilting your head backward. But, still breathe through your nose.

* For pregnant women, some can do the Daily Yoga Program throughout their full term, some for most of the first five months, and others not at all. This depends on their health, special conditions and their doctor's recommendation.

* Check with your doctor before starting this program if you have a major medical problem.

Remember, yoga is relaxing, not rushing.

B. *First Month Program*

This is the first of two progressions toward the Daily Yoga Program. Next month your body will be ready for additional exercises. With a little rest between each exercise, you should be spending twenty minutes a day during the first month.

Don't forget to use yoga breathing where it's required. Yoga's main point is to do everything slowly and at your own pace. You are doing this for yourself and not competing with anyone.

DAILY YOGA PROGRAM (First Month)

STANDING

1. PREPARATION
2. FORWARD BEND (3 times)
3. TWIST SIDE BEND (3 times each side)
6. BACK TO THE WALL (1 minute)

CIRCULATION

10. TOUCH AND SIT (6 times)

SITTING

13. SPINAL TWIST (1 minute on each side)
14. HANGING BUTTOCK STRETCH (3 times)

ON BACK

18. FULL BODY STRETCH (1 minute)
19. TREMBLE-TREMBLE (3 times)
20. KNEES TO CHEST (once)
21. HALF WHEEL (BUTTOCKS UP AND DOWN) (3 times)

ON STOMACH

25. HALF LOCUST (3 times)

TRANSITION

28. CAT POSE (once)
35. SIT-UPS (3 times)

STANDING OR SITTING

37. ARMS, NECK AND SHOULDERS (will take you a few minutes)

ON BACK

38. DEAD MAN'S POSE (at your pleasure)

C. Second Month Program

Here we are in the second month. If you have been doing your yoga for about twenty minutes a day for the past month, your body should be ready for the second stage and your muscles should be listening to you. You should be feeling better and looking forward to the second month of your progression toward the Daily Yoga Program.

If you have not practiced every day, give yourself some more days of the first month's program before you move on to this second month program.

Each session this month should take thirty to thirty-five minutes.

DAILY YOGA PROGRAM (Second Month)

STANDING

1. PREPARATION
2. FORWARD BEND (6 times)
3. TWIST SIDE BEND (6 times each side)
4. NOSE TO KNEE (3 times each side)
5. REACH FORWARD (once)
7. DIAPHRAGM LIFT (3 times)

CIRCULATION

10. TOUCH AND SIT (6 times)
11. SIDE BEND, PALMS TO THE FLOOR (6 times each side)

SITTING

13. SPINAL TWIST (1 minute on each side)
14. HANGING BUTTOCK STRETCH (3 times)
15. HAMSTRING STRETCH (3 times)

ON BACK

18. FULL BODY STRETCH (1 minute, twice a day)
19. TREMBLE-TREMBLE (3 times)
20. KNEES TO CHEST (once)
21. HALF WHEEL (BUTTOCKS UP AND DOWN) (3 times)
22. BICYCLE (once—all three levels)

ON STOMACH

24. COBRA VARIATION (BABY COBRA) (once, hold for 1 minute)
25. HALF LOCUST (3 times)

TRANSITION

28. CAT POSE (once)
30. PLOUGH (1 minute)
32. FISH (1 minute)
35. SIT-UPS (6 times)
37. ARMS, NECK AND SHOULDERS (will take you a few minutes)

ON BACK

38. DEAD MAN'S POSE (at your pleasure)

D. *Third Month Program*

This is your whole life program. You must be feeling full of life by now, free from aches and pains, free from false appetite, free from strain and tension, healthier and younger than before. Don't take this "new you" for granted. Make this program a part of your life.

DAILY YOGA PROGRAM (Third Month)

All of these exercises and postures are great to do every day. If your time is limited, however, you may select one of the three circulation exercises (9, 10 or 11); one of the stretching exercises (14, 15, 16 or 17); and one of the exercises on the stomach (24, 25, 26 or 27).

STANDING
1. PREPARATION
2. FORWARD BEND (6 times)
3. TWIST SIDE BEND (6 times each side)
4. NOSE TO KNEE (3 times each side)
5. REACH FORWARD (once)
6. BACK TO THE WALL (1 minute, twice a day)
7. DIAPHRAGM LIFT (3 times)
8. TRIANGLE POSE (3 times each side)

CIRCULATION
9. WINDMILL (6 to 10 times each side)
10. TOUCH AND SIT (6 to 20 times)
11. SIDE BEND, PALMS TO THE FLOOR (6 to 10 times)

TRANSITION
12. MOON POSTURE (½ minute each side—repeat 2 times)

SITTING
13. SPINAL TWIST (1 to 2 minutes on each side)
14. HANGING BUTTOCK STRETCH (3 times)
15. HAMSTRING STRETCH (3 times)
16. PELVIC STRETCH (3 times)
17. SIDE FOLDER STRETCH (3 times)

ON BACK
18. FULL BODY STRETCH (1 minute, twice a day)
19. TREMBLE-TREMBLE (6 times)
20. KNEES TO CHEST (3 times)
21. HALF WHEEL (BUTTOCKS UP AND DOWN) (6 times)
22. BICYCLE (once—all three levels)
23. SHOOTING LEGS OUT (6 times)

ON STOMACH
24. COBRA VARIATION (BABY COBRA) (twice—hold 1 minute)
25. HALF LOCUST (3 times)
26. GRAND COBRA (6 times)
27. FULL LOCUST (6 times)

TRANSITION
28. CAT POSE (once or twice)
29. KNEE TOUCH TO YOUR FOREHEAD (6 times each leg)

ON BACK

    30. PLOUGH (1 minute)

    31. SHOULDER STAND (1 minute, *no more than 3 minutes*)

    32. FISH (1 to 3 minutes)

    33. BOW (3 to 6 times)

    34. BRIDGE (once)

    35. SIT-UPS (6 times)

SITTING

    36. LOTUS (no more than 5 minutes)

    37. ARMS, NECK AND SHOULDERS (6 times once a day)

ON BACK

    38. DEAD MAN'S POSE (at your pleasure)

1. Preparation

> Raising a child is like melting a gold brick.

Remember, in any exercise you do in yoga, as I described in the chapter on breathing, breathe in to expand, breathe out to contract.

Stand absolutely straight with your legs a few inches apart. Breathe in, raise your arms up, keeping your elbows behind your ears. Raise up on your toes to reach for the ceiling. Slowly breathe out while you bring your hands down. Do this twice at the beginning of your Daily Yoga Program to give you balance.

Continue this exercise twice more, without rising on your toes. This time, be sure to breathe out very slowly, sagging a little bit forward to take out all the air you can. This will relax your muscles and make you ready for your program.

THIS PREPARATION IS A MUST FOR EVERYONE.

2. Forward Bend

Luck may sometimes help, work always does.

Stand with your legs apart, put the palms of your hands together, entwine your fingers and invert your hands. Then, while inhaling, raise your hands over your head, palms toward the ceiling, keeping your arms straight and behind your ears. With the load on the lower part of your body, with your knees and back straight, bend from the hip joint and go forward with your chest toward the floor, keeping your arms straight and behind your ears. Exhale slowly while bending forward. Your aim is to press the floor with the palms of your hands. If your hands don't reach the floor at first, they will later as your body becomes more supple. You must keep your back straight even though you cannot touch the floor at first.

It is very important to remember that in any exercise you do which involves bending forward, to the side, or backward, you must keep the bottom half of your body stationary. Hold it tight and contract it to keep from damaging your spine. The upper part of your body is always graceful and free in its movement. Do not stiffen your neck and shoulders when bending from the hips, and do not move your buttocks.

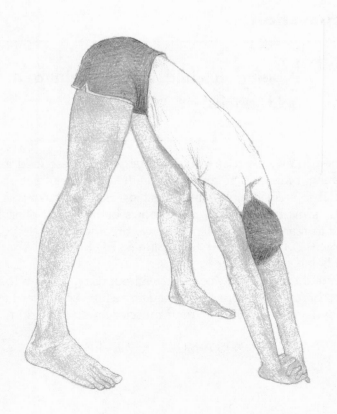

Do this exercise keeping knees straight, unless you have a slipped disc or other back problem. If you have either, then *bend* your knees slightly to come down. If you have a neck problem, do *not* stretch your arms out too vigorously.

Start with three times the first month, progressing to six times after that.
Do the exercise in one continuous movement.

BENEFITS

Helps stretch the spinal column.
Increases the blood flow to the brain.
Most important, relaxes and prepares you for the other postures in this Daily Yoga Program by loosening the back muscles.
Breathes out tension, breathes in serenity and peaceful thoughts.

DO NOT DO

If you have a serious lower back problem.
If you have a middle ear disturbance.

3. Twist Side Bend

> *I don't believe certain people even if they stand on the fire.*

Since each exercise requires that you concentrate particularly on the part of the body you are working on, think now about the sides; the body parts that collect folds of fat because of poor posture.

Remember to hold the lower part of your body steady.

Stand absolutely straight. Separate your legs as far apart as you comfortably can. Clasp your hands together in front of you, entwine your fingers, and invert your hands. Bring your arms up, keeping them behind your

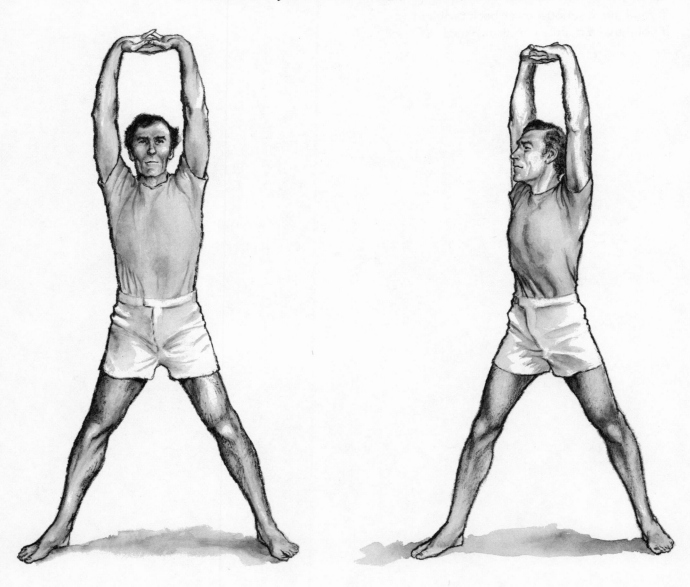

ears, and with palms toward the ceiling. Stretch yourself high from the midriff. Continue breathing in slowly. Don't stretch your arms too much, and do not stiffen your neck. Think about stretching your middle.

Now, take a deep breath.

Breathe out slowly while you bend to the right (remembering that you always start on the right side). Your back is straight and your legs are straight. Bend to the right as far as you can without feeling pain. Twist now to the right as far as possible and bend down, with your arms stretched out. Your aim is to reach down slowly and place your palms, fingers still entwined, to the outside of your right foot, your arms still behind your ears. But if you cannot touch the floor, don't cheat by bending your back or legs.

At first, you will find that you are short of breath. Don't go down any farther. Don't breathe in while you are down; breathe out only. When you have to breathe in, start coming up. After a while you will find that you can hold your breath longer and go down farther.

While you are bending, be sure that only the upper part of your body is moving to the side, not your lower part.

Do this exercise three times each side during the first month, and six times after that.

BENEFITS

Provides suppleness and elasticity and a new kind of stretch to the side muscles through internal pressure.
Gets rid of the extra folders or fat at the side of the waist.

DO NOT DO

If you have a serious lower back problem.

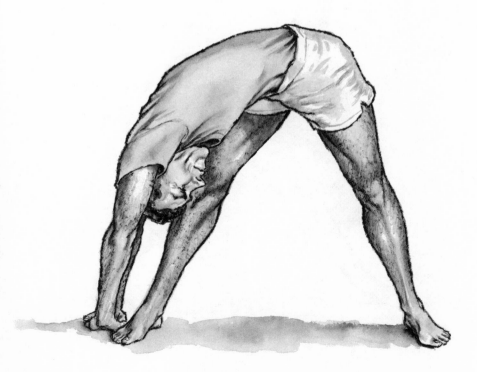

4. Nose to Knee

Falsehood has no feet to stand on.

Stand with your legs as far apart as is comfortable. Interlock your fingers behind your back. Bend your left knee and go forward toward your right leg, which should be straight. Breathe out as you bend. Bring your chest to your thigh first, before you touch your forehead to your leg. Your whole weight and balance are on your left side and you are coming down from your hip joint to your right side, with a straight back. While you are going down, pull your arms back and up, but don't hurt them. Breathe in to come up to stand straight.

Now, bend your right leg and repeat by bending to the left side. Do not forget to breathe out when you go down or you will have a lovely cramp in your stomach. Do not be discouraged if you can't touch your chest to your thigh the first time. One day you will succeed. Do this three times on each side.

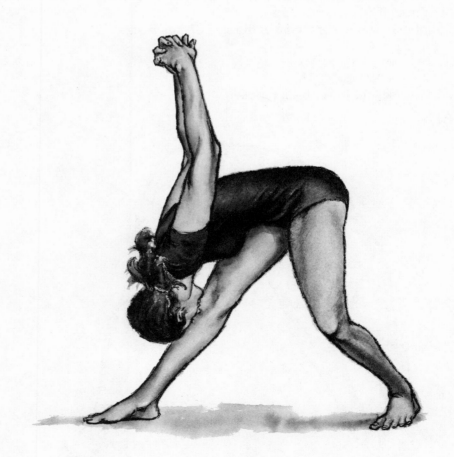

BENEFITS

Brings blood to the face and head, which keeps the skin healthy and helps
retain the hair.
Stretches the lower back.
Good for firming underarms.
Straightens shoulder blades and the dowager's hump.
Slims the waistline.

DO NOT DO

If you have a serious bad lower back problem.

5. Reach Forward

> Do not stretch your feet longer than your blanket, you will catch cold.

Stand with your feet together, arms up, fingertips pointing to the ceiling. Breathe out slowly and bend down, cross your hands behind your legs and get hold of the backs of your legs. Put your nose on your knees and keep your legs and back absolutely straight. That is your aim. Breathe in while coming up.

Now, legs still together, put your hands straight up toward the ceiling, arms behind your ears. Breathe out and bend forward from the hip joints until your back is parallel to the floor. Reach forward as much as you can without making your back round. Hold your stomach tight. Remember, all this time your arms stay behind your ears. Stay there as long as you are breathing out, and don't forget to smile. Start breathing in and come back up. Do this combination once.

BENEFITS

Stretches entire back muscles.
Tones stomach muscles.
Improves posture.
Brings blood to your head.

DO NOT DO

If you have a serious lower back problem.

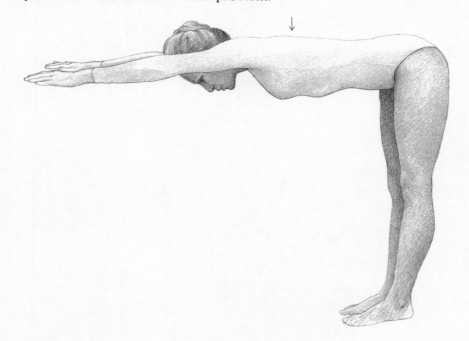

> *A thief's mother will cry in her heart.*

Put your back to the wall. Touch the wall with the back of your heels. Entwine your fingers, invert your hands, stretch your arms over your head with palms toward the ceiling, and press your arms to the wall. Your elbows should be next to your ears. The entire back of your body should be touching the wall.

Your aim is to press the small of your back to the wall without straining your shoulders or making a double chin or bending your knees.

Because your back muscles are stretched now and I know it feels so good, you will continue it. You do not have to worry about a particular time and place; anywhere you find a wall, put your back to it and stretch. This posture is to be performed once a day for one minute the first month and twice a day later.

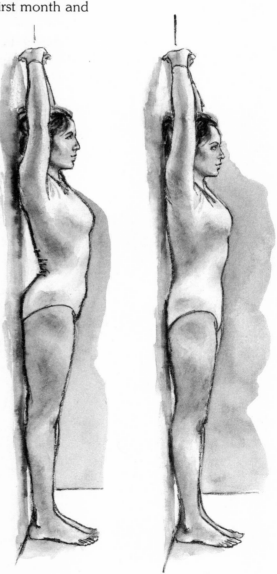

BENEFITS

Straightens your swayback and improves your posture.
Stretches the hamstring muscles.
Helps prevent a double chin.
Helps keep both shoulders on the same level;
    not one up and one down.

DO NOT DO

None.

7. Diaphragm Lift

After the cat eats 100 mice, it goes on a pilgrimage.

Stand straight. Place your legs about twelve inches apart. Breathe in. Very slowly start breathing out, bending forward a few inches, relaxing your muscles, trying to take out the air as much as you can through your nose. Press your hands to the front of your thighs and, when you feel you can no longer breathe out, lift your diaphragm up and under the rib cage, making a hollow space under the rib cage. At the same time, hold empty, lean forward, bending from the hips, making the pose as though you were going to throw up; your chest a little forward, your chin a little forward, your back a little round.

When you can hold empty no longer, start straightening up as you begin breathing in through the nose.

Now, while you are coming up and breathing in, the vacuum inside may make a kind of noise because your lungs are almost empty.

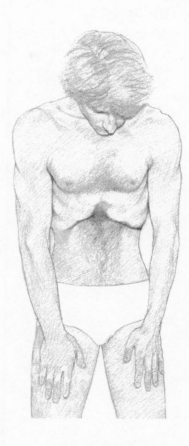

The first time you try this, you will feel that you are not taking out enough air. Wait a minute and try again. The next time you will take out much more. Each time you do this, take a break of a minute before you try again.

Should you feel winded or dizzy, do not lie down, instead walk briskly around the room a bit to get rid of the excess oxygen to which your body is not accustomed. Your aim is to increase the size of the hollow space under the rib cage, which will come with practice.

Practice this three times a day, doing three repetitions each time.

IN AND OUT

An advanced variation of this exercise is the forcing of the abdomen in and out while your air is out. Do this as many times as you can. When you feel that you have to take air in, take it. Whenever you take air in, stand up straight.

SIDE TO SIDE

Another advanced variation of the Diaphragm Lift is that of moving the abdomen from side to side.

You are in the same pose, legs twelve inches apart, breathing out. When you feel empty, bend forward, hands firmly on the front of your thighs. Now, press your right hand hard against your right thigh and move your abdomen from right to left. Then, relax your right hand, press your left hand hard against your left thigh and move your abdomen from left to right. Do this a few times. Now, while you are doing this, visualize your abdomen moving from side to side. Eventually, with practice, it will actually start moving from side to side. No other part of your body should move while your abdomen is moving. When you feel you must take air in, breathe in and come up.

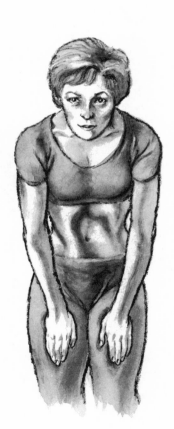

BENEFITS

Massages the internal organs.
Helps digestion; can cure constipation.
Exercises the internal muscles as well as the surface muscles.
Tones the sagging stomach and slims the waistline.
Replaces the old oxygen with new.
Relieves pelvic congestion.
Removes fat inside the body as well as outside.
Straightens the spine.

DO NOT DO

If your bladder or stomach is full.
If you have any kind of ulcers or other stomach problems.
If you have been fitted with an intrauterine device.

8. Triangle Pose (Standing Twist)

Even mad people don't throw stones at their own houses.

Stand with your legs apart and keep your knees straight. Raise both arms, palms down, to shoulder level like airplane wings. Then twist the upper part of your body to your left side and bend down to take hold of your left ankle with your right hand. Your left arm goes back and up until the fingertips are pointing to the ceiling. Your two arms form a straight line. Twist from your waist as much as you can, holding your arms in the same position. Look up to the left hand and feel a good twist in your midriff and shoulders.

Come up to your standing position and slowly turn to the right. Bring your left hand down to take hold of your right ankle, and repeat the exercise to this side. Breathe normally and regularly and stay one half minute each side. Be careful not to pull your neck too much. Repeat both sides three times.

BENEFITS

Chop-chops the waistline.
Helps the entire nervous system.
Makes your drooping shoulders appear younger.
Tones up your thigh muscles.
Expands your chest.
Uses side muscles that have been neglected.
Stretches your hamstring and gluteus maximus muscles.

DO NOT DO

None.

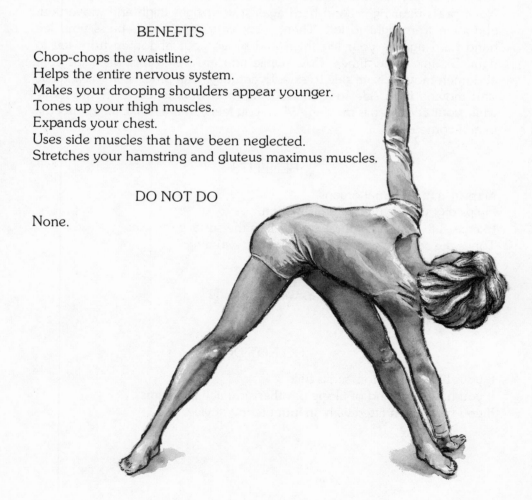

9. Windmill

> The smell of the wealthy is of sweet perfume, the smell of the poor is of sour sweat.

Stand straight, legs as far apart as is comfortable, with your knees straight and arms at your sides. Breathe normally through the whole exercise. Raise your right arm, elbow behind your ear, and bend down to the left side. At the same time, your left arm is swinging back and you look like a windmill. Touch the right hand flat to the floor, next to the outside of your left foot. Your right elbow is still behind your ear.

The right hand comes up and you twist a little to the right and bring your left arm down, and you touch the palm of your left hand to the floor beside the outside of your right foot. At the same time your right hand is swinging back and up. When one hand is pointing to the ceiling, the other is touching the floor, so they never meet.

Your stretch should come from the middle of your stomach, so don't stretch your arms too high. Start slowly and increase the speed and maintain your rhythm. If you have a hard time in the beginning putting your hand to the floor, don't worry. Do this exercise six times on each side and increase to ten each side.

BENEFITS

Helps to get rid of the midriff folders (spare tire).
Expands the capacity of the lungs.
Good for the circulation in your whole body.
Stretches your hamstring muscles.

DO NOT DO

If you have a serious heart condition.

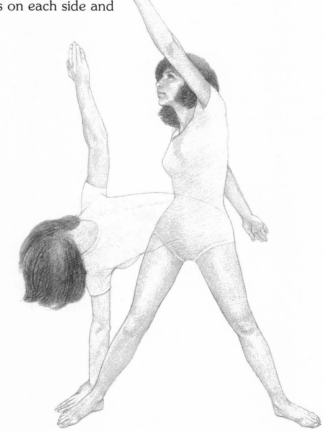

10. Touch and Sit

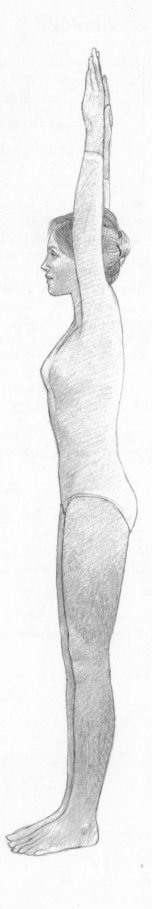

> $\mathcal{M}$ore mouths, more tales.

Stand straight with your feet one inch apart. Breathe normally during the whole exercise.

* Bend forward and try to touch your fingertips to the floor in front of your toes. If you can, go ahead and put your hands flat on the floor. If you cannot, it's all right.

* Stand up.

* Sit on your haunches, keeping heels on the floor, your elbows bent, hands in front of you at shoulder level, and your back straight. If you can't go all the way to your haunches, go as close as you can.

* Stand up.

* Touch the floor again.

* Come up while stretching your arms straight out in front of you to the level your hips would be if you were standing, before bringing your hands up toward the ceiling.

Now, use all the steps together. That means, keeping your heels on the floor throughout the exercise, touch with the knees straight, sit with the knees bent, touch with the knees straight, and stretch with the knees straight. So, touch and sit and touch and stretch and up; touch and sit and touch and stretch and up. Continue this slowly and rhythmically.

Start with six repetitions at a time. Gradually increase to twenty repetitions.

BENEFITS

This is better than jogging—it gives you the same overall circulatory benefits without jarring any part of your body.
Strengthens the heart muscles.
Stretches the hamstring muscles.
Stretches the muscles of the lower back.

DO NOT DO

If you have bad hemorrhoids.

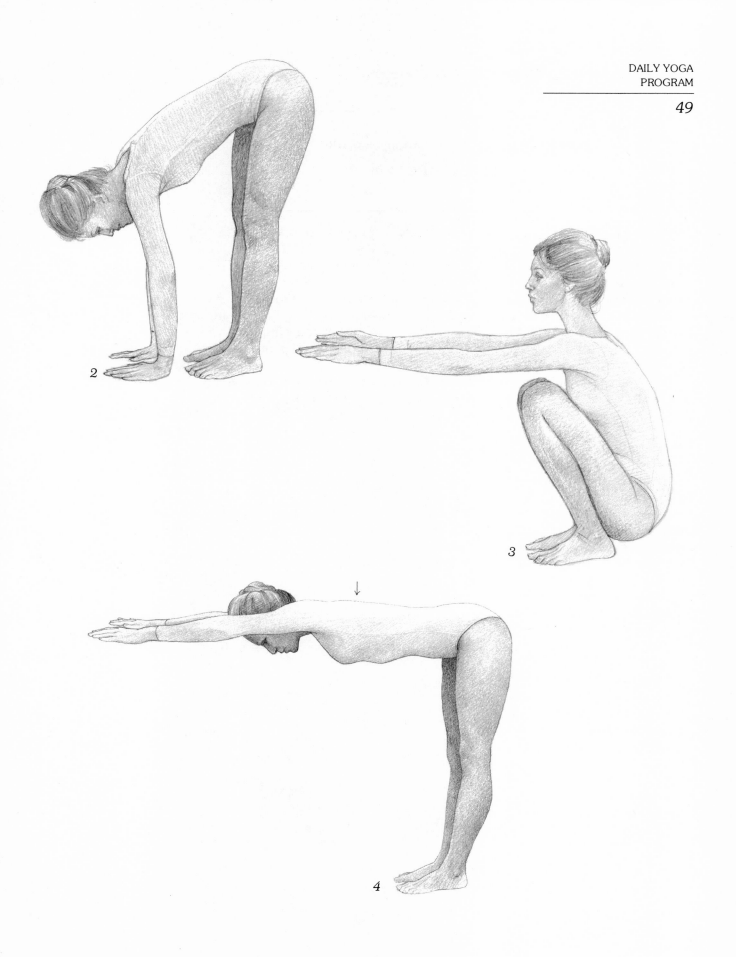

11. Side Bend, Palms to the Floor

Giving alms to a millionaire is like shining a lamp to the sun.

Stand straight, legs as far apart as is comfortable. Lift your arms to shoulder level and bend your elbows a little. Bend your right knee and shift the thigh to your right side. Now, try to put your right hand beside your right foot, palm to the floor, as far to the right of your foot as possible, without straightening your elbow. Come up to your original position. Throughout the whole exercise, your arms stay in the same position, your elbows slightly bent. Repeat this exercise on the left side, bending to the left, touching your left palm to the floor beside your left foot and as far to the left of your foot as possible.

This exercise should be done rhythmically from side to side, not too fast and not too slow. Start with six repetitions and increase to ten each side.

BENEFITS

Firms the inside of thighs.
Firms underarm jelly-pulley.
Improves circulation.
Straightens upper back.
Increases energy.
Keeps knees youthful and flexible.

DO NOT DO

If you have damaged knees.

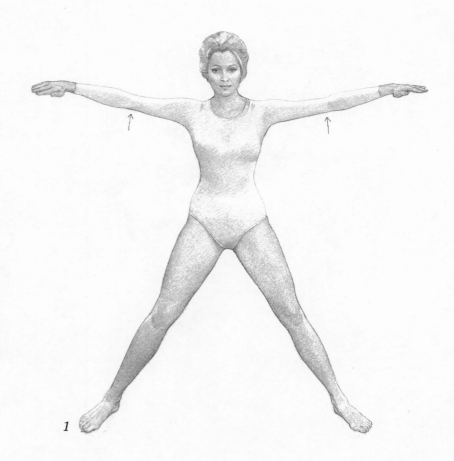

1

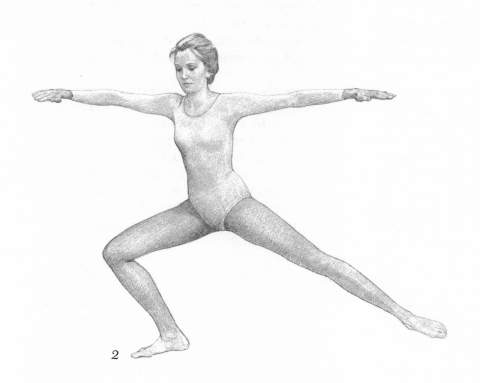

2

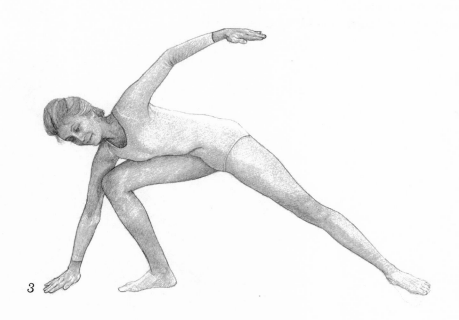

3

12. Moon Posture

A diamond shines, even in the trash.

Stand straight with your legs as far apart as is comfortable, and with your back straight. On the balls of your feet, turn your body to the right. Raise your hands above your head, elbows beside your ears, and put your palms together.

Bend your right knee forward and go down to touch your chest to your right thigh. Your arms are now stretched straight out, elbows still behind your ears, back absolutely straight. Your left foot is in a straight line with your right heel, and your left knee is about two inches off the floor.

As you are, arch backward from your rib cage. Arch as much as you can and hold for one half minute. (The upper part of your body looks like a half moon.) Then come up to the standing position, hands and arms still above your head. Turn to your left, bend your left knee, come down the same way, arch your back, hold for one half minute and return to the upright position. Do one half minute each side; repeat twice.

BENEFITS

Adds flexibility to the spine.
Strengthens the thighs and calves.
Works on the underarms.
Expands your chest.
Stretches the abdomen.

DO NOT DO

If you have a serious lower back problem.
If you have a neck problem, avoid bending your neck.

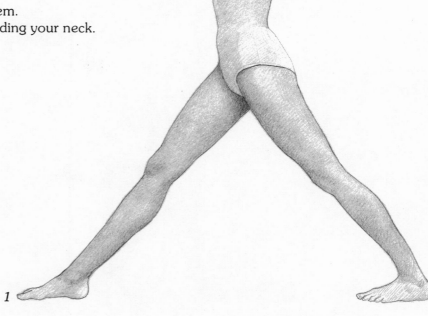

1

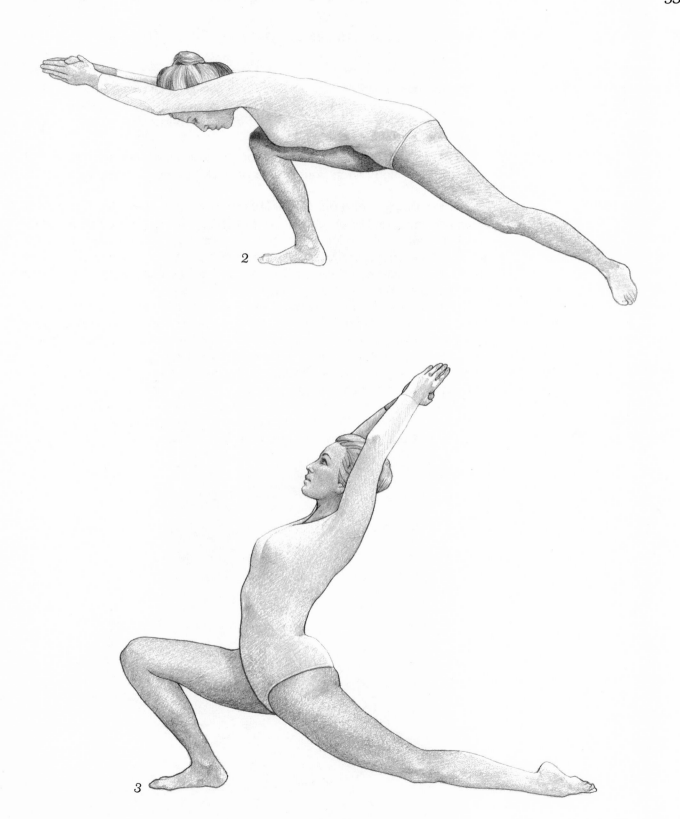

2

3

13. Spinal Twist

> *The tongue cuts deeper than the knife.*

Sit on the mat. From the sitting position, draw your right leg up in front of you until the knee is in line with your nose. Your right foot should be about eighteen to twenty-four inches away from your body, adjusting it to your body height.

Bend your left leg parallel to the floor and touch your left heel to the end of your right thigh. Wrap your right arm back around your waistline, palm turned out.

Twist to the right and bring your left arm over to the outside of your right knee and take hold of your ankle. If, in the beginning, your hand does not reach to your right ankle, take hold of your right calf. While breathing regularly and rhythmically, slowly twist from your midriff to the right side as much as you can comfortably. Turn your shoulders and neck to the right also, but not too much. Your neck should be relaxed.

Twist more and more; as much as you possibly can. Smile and think something beautiful while you are twisting. Keep both sides of your buttocks flat on the floor and try to touch the floor with your left knee. This is not easy! And keep your chins up, your back straight.

After at least a minute on the right side (as time goes on you will increase to two minutes on each side), twist to your left in exactly the same way; left knee up, right heel touching the left thigh, left hand behind your back, palm out, right arm across the left leg, right hand grasping the left ankle (or as close to it as you can get); twist and breathe normally.

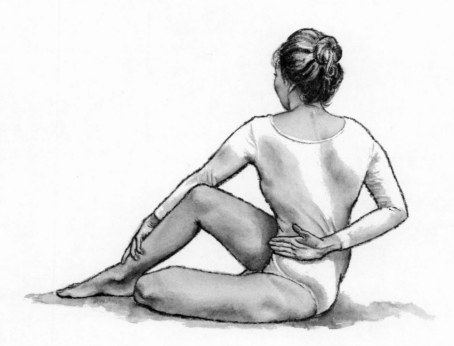

You will be surprised to find how easily you tire. You may not be twisting enough; your back is not straight or your head falls forward; you may forget to keep your buttocks on the floor, or you let the low knee come up from the floor (if it did, indeed, reach the floor).

Do one to two minutes, one time each side.

BENEFITS

Adds flexibility to your spine and to your back muscles.
Improves the function of the liver and kidneys.
Reduces the fat inside the abdomen.
Tightens your waistline and draws in the stomach.
Massages your organs.
Relieves constipation.
Helps your posture and your chin line.
Helps and prevents hemorrhoids.

DO NOT DO

If you have bad ulcers.

14. Hanging Buttock Stretch

> *Miser's wealth is enjoyed only by others.*

Sit on the mat, look straight ahead and smile, and think of something lovely. Place the soles of your feet together as close to your body as you can. Press the sides of your knees to the mat. Your back is absolutely straight. Get hold of your feet or your ankles if you cannot reach your feet, keeping your elbows at your sides. Breathe out and slowly, slowly come forward as much as you can, from your lower back. Be sure that as you come forward, your tailbone stays on the mat. Your aim is to come forward as much as you can. Keep your back as straight as an arrow.

When you have to breathe in, come up without rounding your back. Stretch three times.

BENEFITS

Tightens the gluteus maximus muscles.
Helps the mild hernia.
Very good for firming and slimming the thighs.
Keeps the kidneys, bladder and prostate healthy.
If practiced regularly by men, relieves pain and heaviness in the testicles.

DO NOT DO

None.

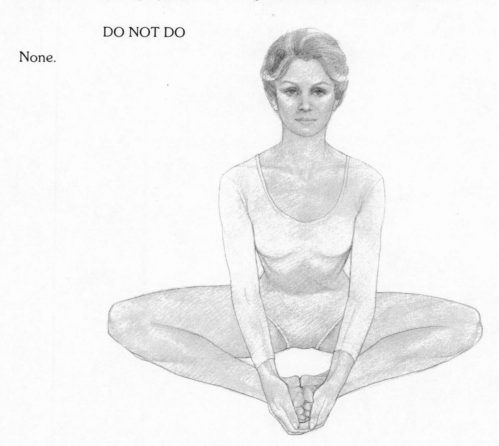

15. Hamstring Stretch

> *Some people are the lion at home,
> the mouse when not.*

Sitting with your legs apart, turn your toes up toward you. Breathe out slowly and reach your hands straight out as far as you can in front of you to place your palms on the mat inside your legs. Your aim is to go forward as much as you can in order to put your chin on the floor. Keep your thighs on the mat and don't bring your knees up. Your back should be straight and you are to bend from your hips only, keeping your tailbone on the floor. When you are ready to breathe in, come up slowly, with your back straight, to resume your sitting position. Stretch three times.

BENEFITS

Stretches the hamstring and lower back muscles.
Keeps the muscles and organs in the pelvic region healthy.
Relieves the pain of sciatica.
Great for women because it increases the circulation of blood in the pelvic region, keeping the menstrual periods regular and the ovaries healthy.

DO NOT DO

None.

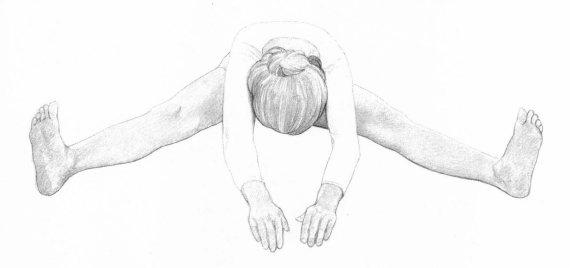

16. Pelvic Stretch

> *People who want to help never ask.*

In the sitting position, back straight, put your legs straight out in front of you, knees together and legs down on the floor. Tightening the muscles at the back of your thighs to pull the trunk forward will help keep the knees down. Breathe out and go forward, sliding your hands along the outside of your legs until you can get hold of your feet from the outside. Remember, your chest has to touch your thighs before you bring your head down. Try to go far enough with your arms outstretched to reach the arches of your feet. If you cannot reach your feet, hold your ankles. The back of your whole body is intensely stretched; do not stretch your arms from your shoulders. Do extend your spine from the hip joint and your back will not hump. Eventually, in this position, your chin will rest on your knees.

Breathe in as you return to the upright position. Going down or coming back up, your back is always straight. Stretch three times.

BENEFITS

Stretches the pelvic area, giving it more oxygenated blood.
Stretches lower back and hamstring muscles.
Strengthens the heart muscles and makes the spinal column more flexible.
Relieves headaches and stretches cervical area of the spine.
Helps and prevents hemorrhoids.

DO NOT DO

If you have a hernia.

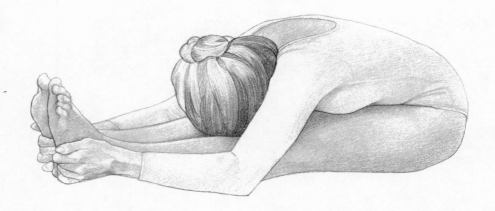

17. Side Folder Stretch

> Good people think everything around them is good.

Sit straight, spread your legs as far apart as is comfortable. Twist and lean to the right and reach your right hand to your right foot, breathing out slowly as you go down, and bring your left arm up over your head and down to clasp both hands around your foot. Your aim is to touch your right side and your ear to your right leg. Remember to bend from your pelvis, not from your upper back. When you have to breathe in, come up slowly.

Now, twist a little to the left and go down the same way to the left side and clasp your left foot with both hands. Stretch three times each side.

BENEFITS

Beautiful for the side folders and for slimming the waistline.
Stretches the hamstrings.
Keeps the muscles in the pelvic region healthy.

DO NOT DO

None.

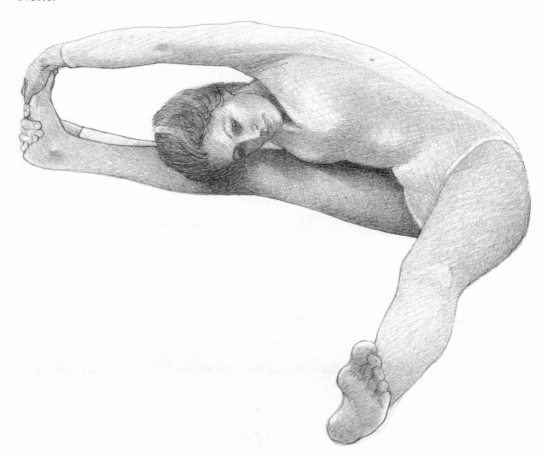

18. Full Body Stretch

> *A foolish friend is worse than a smart enemy.*

Lie down on the mat on your back, feet together, toes straight up, arms beside your head, hands together, fingers interlaced, palms turned up away from your head. Try to touch your elbows and the backs of your knees to the floor. Now, try to press the small of your back to the floor. Breathe normally and hold a few minutes. The first time it may not touch, but with practice, your spine will stretch and you will be able to touch your back to the floor. That is the aim.

   This should be done for at least one minute, twice a day. You are welcome to do it more times.

BENEFITS

Strengthens the spinal muscles and straightens the spine.
Stretches and relaxes the entire body.
Removes dowager's hump.
Relieves shoulder pain, stiffness and arthritic pain of the small back.
Prevents arthritis in fingers and hands.
Stretches stomach muscles.
Promotes good elimination.

DO NOT DO

None. There are no don'ts for this exercise—it is one that anyone can do, and *should* do.

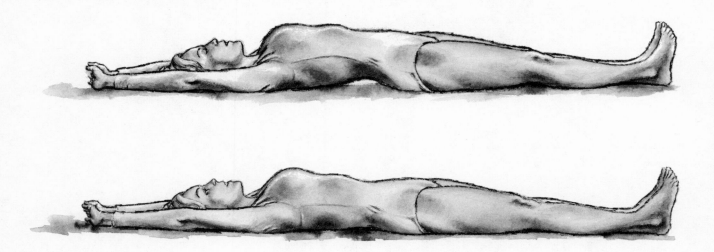

19. Tremble-Tremble

> *The smile you show the world comes back.*

Lie down on your back, raise your legs straight up from the hips. Do not lift your trunk from the floor. Keep the soles of your feet toward the ceiling. Put your arms to your sides, palms down. Tremble your legs, do not shake them. If you watch your thighs, you will notice that your jelly-pulley is trembling. Keep your body still.

With your feet and legs in the same position, open them apart as much as you can without picking up the trunk from the floor or bending the knees. The legs should always be kept at right angles to the body. Bring them together, slowly, and tremble again; then move them apart and bring them together again.

Do this three times to begin with. As you feel more confidence in yourself, increase to six times.

BENEFITS

Keeps you from getting varicose veins.
Firms the stomach muscles and the thighs.
Helps dissolve inner fat.
Stretches the gluteus maximus muscles.

DO NOT DO

None.

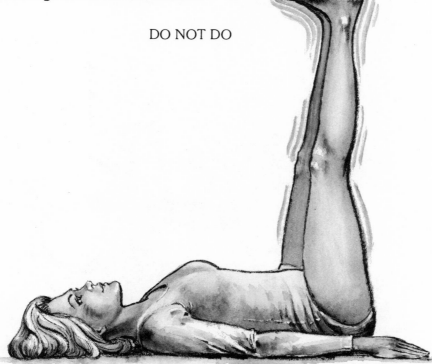

20. Knees to Chest

> He who does not realize one mistake, makes another.

Lie down on your back, take in a deep breath. Hold your knees with your hands. By rolling your trunk, bring your knees to your chest while breathing out. Leave your head on the floor. When you are ready to breathe in, relax the position but do not let go of your knees; you are giving your lungs the space they need for new breath.

Do this once at the beginning and increase to three times.

BENEFITS

Relieves back pain and gives flexibility to the spine.
Takes away tiredness.
Frees you from stomach gas.
Helps you learn deeper breathing.
Relieves pelvic congestion.

DO NOT DO

None.

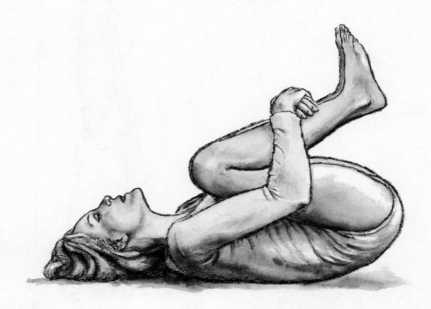

21. Half Wheel (Buttocks Up and Down)

> *What do you expect when you put fire and oil together?*

Lying down on your back, bend your knees, put your feet flat on the floor about fourteen inches away from your buttocks. Your arms are on the floor at your sides. Breathe in, bring your trunk off the floor, as much as you can without picking up your shoulder blades. Feet, shoulder blades, arms, and head stay on the floor.

When you are ready to breathe out, slowly come down as you breathe out. When your back reaches the floor and all the air is out, suck your stomach in and up under the rib cage. Hold empty and at the same time contract your buttocks tight. When it is time to breathe in, it is time to bring your trunk up off the floor, again.

This posture should be done three times at the beginning and six times later on.

BENEFITS

Relieves lower back problems.
Stretches and strengthens the back, and helps the posture.
Massages the internal organs and works to eliminate fat around the thighs and stomach.
Firms thighs, legs, and buttocks.
Relieves pelvic congestion.

DO NOT DO

There is no reason why you should not do this exercise.

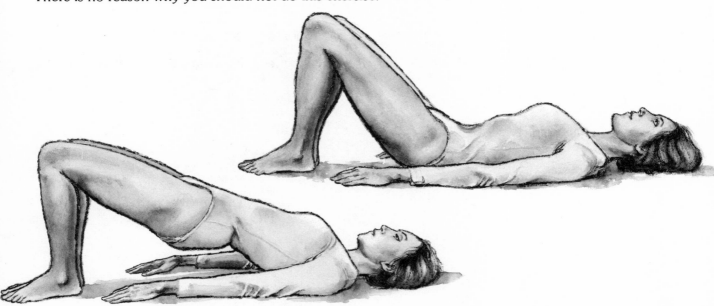

22. Bicycle

Good friends make you, bad friends break you.

This is yoga bicycling and is done on three levels.

First, lie down on your back on the mat. Raise both legs straight up to the ceiling, the soles of your feet parallel to the ceiling, your hands to your sides. Do not roll your tailbone up; instead press the small of your back to the floor. Bring your right leg down to touch the back of your heel to your buttock, leaving your left leg up. Then straighten your right leg up and bring your left leg down. Be sure your knee is always stiff when your leg is up and that each up movement is snappy, without jerking your lower back. Do on that level a few times.

Since this exercise is to be done on three levels, the first with the legs up and the soles of the feet pointing to the ceiling, the second level will be closer to the floor. Do the exercise a few times there. The third level will be even closer to the floor. Do it a few times at this level.

This three-step bicycle exercise is one exercise, with no breaks. The last step is not allowed for people with back problems: the lower you go the more your back is affected.

Do this exercise once a day, all three levels.

BENEFITS

For sagging thighs, droopy knees and flabby stomach.
Good for varicose veins.
Gives your legs a break from carrying you the whole day.
Relieves arthritis in leg joints.
Relieves leg and foot cramps.

DO NOT DO

Everybody should do for healthy legs. However, the last step is not for those with back problems.

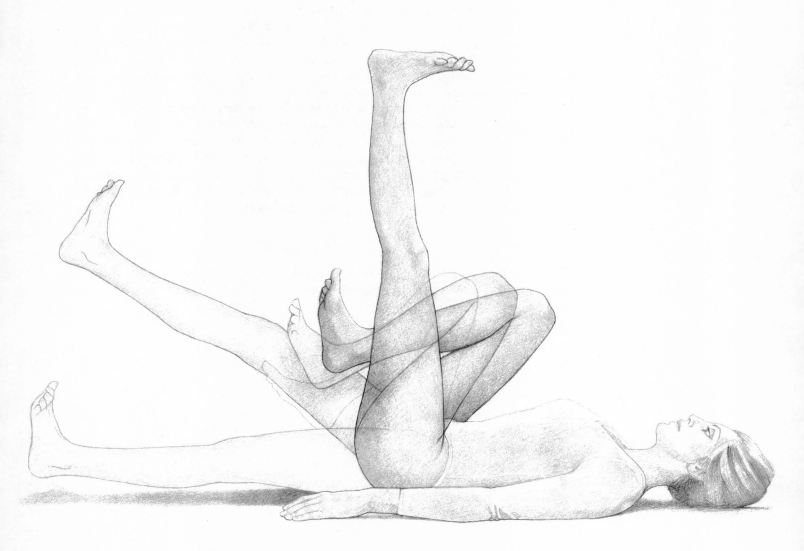

23. Shooting Legs Out

Give them free rein, they come back.

Lie down on your back, arms on the floor at your sides. Bend your knees and bring them toward your stomach while you are breathing out. Start breathing in and stretch your legs straight down, but do not touch the floor. They should be a few inches off the floor. Your toes should be pointed toward the ceiling. While you are in that pose, try to press the small of your back to the floor. If the small of your back does not touch, it will with practice and talking to the muscles. To come back, breathe out, bend your knees and bring them toward your stomach.

You can vary this exercise and benefit your inner thighs as well as your stomach by separating your legs while they are down, a few inches off the floor. Your toes are up but your feet are pointed toward each other, as if you were pigeon-toed. Separate your legs as far as you can, and then bring them back together. When you have to breathe out, bend your knees and bring them toward your stomach. Remember, you are holding your breath in all the time your legs are down. Do this exercise six times.

BENEFITS

Strengthens and flattens the stomach (abdomen) and lower back muscles.
Tightens the inner thigh muscles and helps get rid of fat in that area of the legs.
Stimulates the male sex glands.

DO NOT DO

If you have a serious lower back problem.

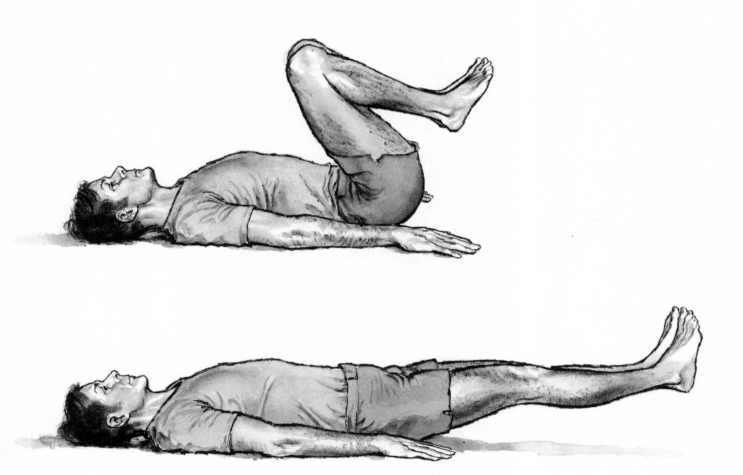

24. Cobra Variation (Baby Cobra)

> *Don't feed a snake, someday it may bite you.*

Cobra is not just one posture, it is a family of postures, so named because the position resembles that of a cobra ready to strike. Because our spines are rigid and we spend so much time bending forward in performing our daily activities, we need to stretch and limber our entire spines by bending them backward.

Sit on your heels from the kneeling position, knees together. Bend forward, stretch your arms out in front of you as much as you can, palms flat on the floor, and try to touch your nose to the floor. Be sure while you are stretching your arms that your buttocks are resting on your heels, whether or not you can touch the floor with your nose. Stay in this position a minute or more, breathing normally, and feel a good stretch in your neck, shoulders and lower back.

Now, raise your body up on your hands and knees so that your back is parallel to the floor. Bring your trunk forward and put your pelvis to the floor. You may have to move your hands forward a little to help you put your pelvis down. Your elbows are turned a little up and out. Stay there and breathe normally a minute or more. Be sure your feet are together, heels touching. Come back and sit on your heels to rest.

Do this posture once at the beginning and twice later.

BENEFITS

Strengthens the stomach muscles and gets rid of the rolls of fat (fat folders) around your middle.
Expands the chest and lung capacity.
Firms the underarms.
Brings flexibility to the vertebrae.
Tightens muscles in the lower part of your buttocks and in your upper thighs.
Keeps menstrual periods regular and eases cramps.

DO NOT DO

If you have a serious lower back problem.
If you have a hiatus hernia.
If you have a hyperactive thyroid.

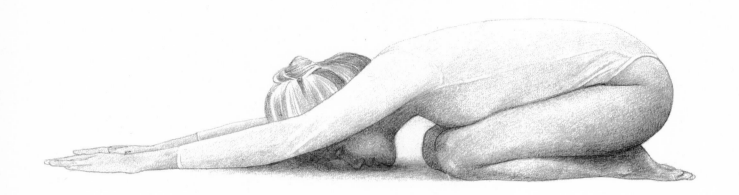

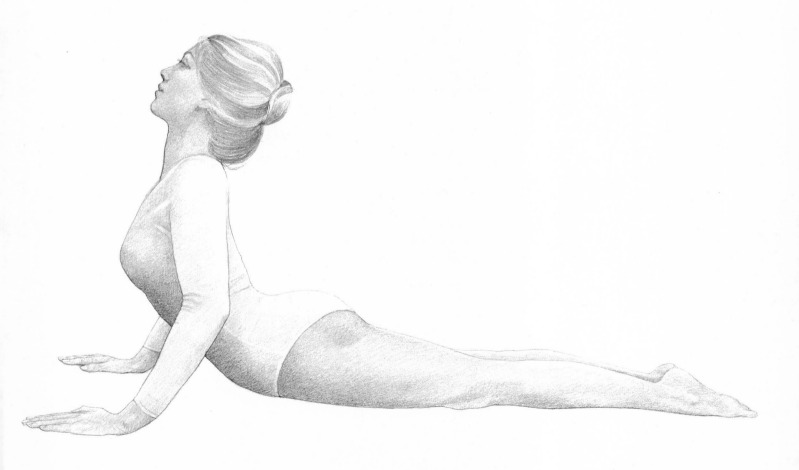

25. Half Locust

> *Marriage is like a lottery.*

The locust consists of two separate exercises or parts, each called the Half Locust. One involves the upper part of the body only, above the waist. The other involves the lower part of the body. Do each part separately first, then both together. This is called the Full Locust.

For the first step of the upper Half Locust, lie flat on your stomach, stretch your arms out, with palms flat on the floor and your upper arms touching your ears. While you breathe in from the nose, raise the upper part of your body, including your head, from the floor as much as you can. Hold your breath about ten seconds. Very slowly and steadily, breathe out and come down. Do not jerk. If you flop down in this exercise, you are flopping the exercise. This is the most important part of the exercise.

The second step is the lower Half Locust. Still on your stomach, chin on the floor, put your hands under your thighs, palms up, elbows in and slightly under your sides. Try to push your lower part up with your hands, pushing up against your thighs and supporting with your forearms. Bring your hands back to the floor. Keep your legs together and knees locked straight. While breathing in, slowly go up as much as you can. Hold for ten seconds. Come down slowly while breathing out. The secret of the Locust is to come down slowly.

Do this posture three times, upper and lower.

BENEFITS

Three times is equivalent to a half mile walk for circulation.
Strengthens lower back.
Tightens hanging thighs.
Straightens round shoulders.
Prevents insomnia.
Prevents hardening of the arteries.
Good for the complexion.

DO NOT DO

If you have high blood pressure, consult your physician before doing it.

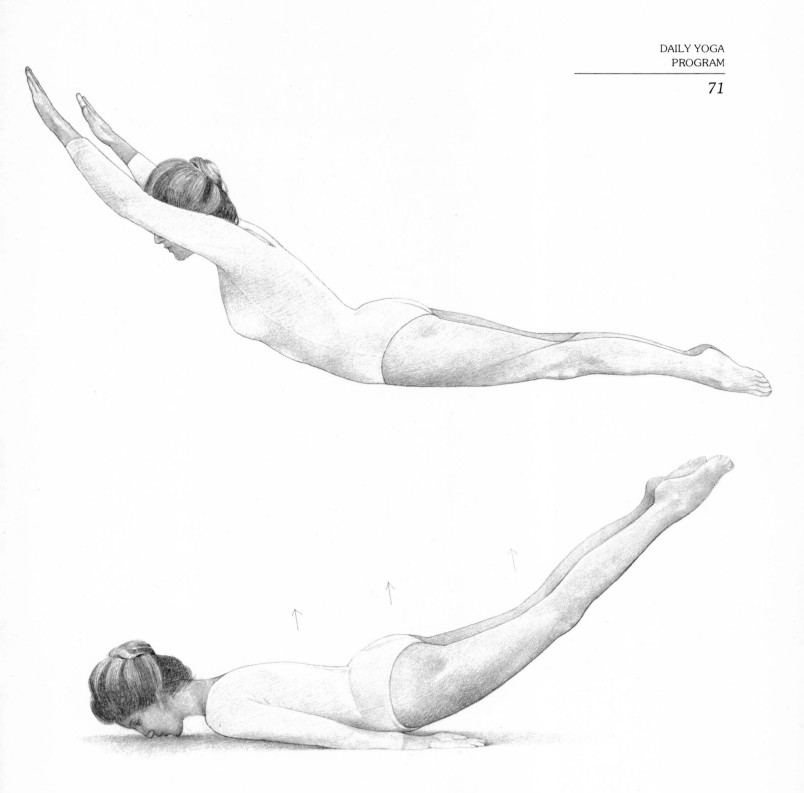

26. Grand Cobra

Kill the snake, but don't break the stick.

Feet together, heels together, knees together lie on your stomach. Put your hands beside your chest, palms on the floor, elbows in tight to your sides. Contract your buttocks.

First, bend your neck back and, while breathing in slowly, continue bending your upper back, vertebra by vertebra. If you have a neck problem, do not bend your neck back. Concentrate on bending your back backward, not on raising your chest.

Your pressure should not be on your hands; you are using the strength of your back, aiming to increase your ability to bend backward, because the major benefit of this posture is for the upper back.

Keep your mouth open a little to prevent stretching the neck and getting a double chin, but breathe through your nose. Hold the posture until you need to breathe out. Then, slowly, breathe out and come down to your original position. The success of this posture depends on coming down slowly.

Start with three times and, over a period of weeks as your spine becomes ready, increase to six times or more.

BENEFITS

Good for the central nervous system because the vertebrae are moved in such a way as to increase the blood supply to the nerves.
Adds flexibility to the middle back.
Firms the chest and bust.
Supplies oxygen to the lower parts of the lungs.
Helps the digestive system.
Dispels fatigue and you sleep well.

DO NOT DO

If you have a hiatus hernia.
If you have a hyperactive thyroid.
If you have a neck problem, do not bend your neck back.

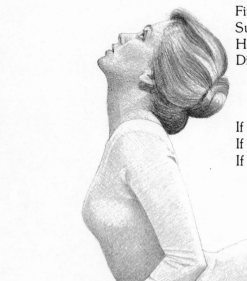

27. Full Locust

> $\mathcal{M}$oney has to be grabbed from the lion's mouth.

For the Full Locust, you are on your stomach, your hands straight out, palms down, above your head, shoulders level with the floor. Raise the upper and lower parts of the body at the same time, breathing in slowly. Hold the breath for ten seconds and then come down slowly while breathing out. If you feel your heart is beating very fast while you're doing this posture, please take a half minute break each time before coming up again.

Do this posture six times.

BENEFITS

Six times is equivalent to a one mile walk for circulation.
Strengthens lower back muscles.
Tightens hanging thighs and lessens varicose veins.
Straightens round shoulders.
Cures insomnia and relieves tension.
Prevents hardening of the arteries.
Good for complexion.

DO NOT DO

If you have high blood pressure or heart trouble, consult your physician before doing this exercise.

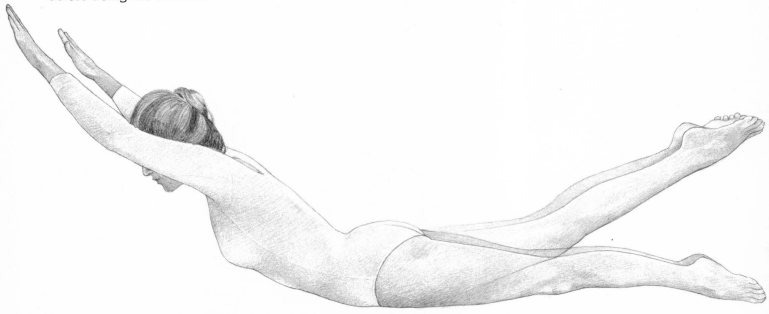

28. Cat Pose

I would rather have a dog friend than a cat friend.

Get on your hands and knees, with your hands directly below your shoulders. Breathe out as much as you can. When you are empty, pull up your diaphragm, contract your abdominal muscles toward your rib cage and hold. Let your head hang down and hump up and arch the middle of your back so you look like an angry cat. Breathe in and s-l-o-w-l-y drop your back down and roll your neck up. Relax.

Do this posture once or twice.

BENEFITS

Good massage and lubrication for your back.
Gets rid of gas.
Flattens your stomach.
Massages your kidneys and helps get rid of the fat around your liver.
Makes your face skin fresh because the blood comes to your face.

DO NOT DO

If you have a hiatus hernia.

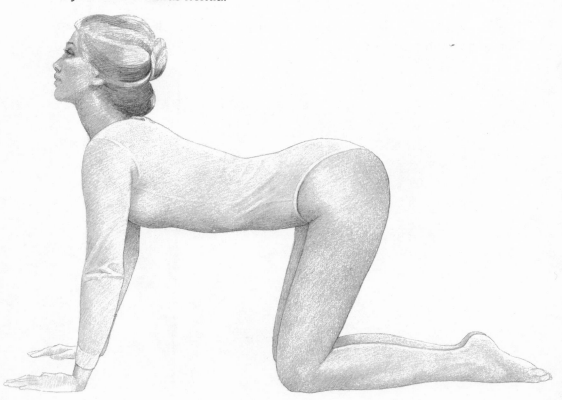

1

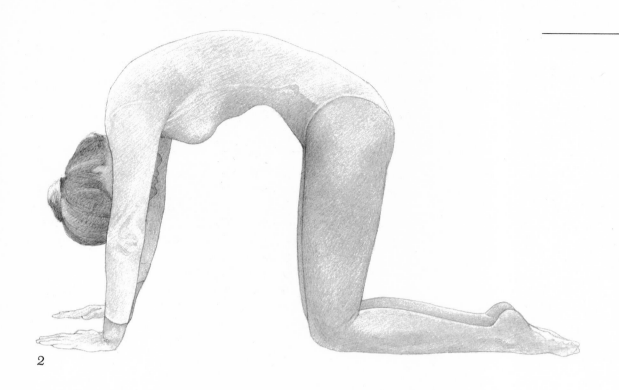

2

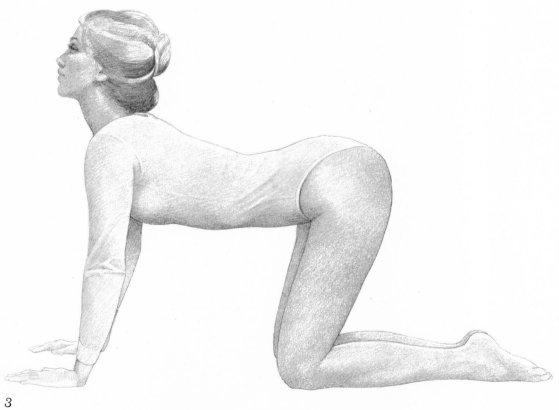

3

29. Knee Touch to your Forehead

> *Salt and pepper go well together,
> not salt and sugar.*

Get on your hands and knees, with your hands directly below the shoulders, about twelve inches in front of your knees, and fingertips straight ahead. Bring your knee up and your head down to touch your knee to your forehead; keep your foot off the floor. Then, extend your leg back and up as far as you can, the knee absolutely straight. At the same time, bring both your neck and your chest up and back and feel the pull on your stomach. Do this twelve times, six times first with the right leg and then repeat the exercise six times with the left leg. If you have a neck problem, do not bend your head too much during the exercise.

Do this exercise six times with each leg.

BENEFITS

Keeps the spine flexible.
Gives a good stretch to the stomach.
Firms the thighs.
Is good for the underarms.
Improves the circulation all over your body, especially around the chest and upper stomach.

DO NOT DO

If you have a hiatus hernia.

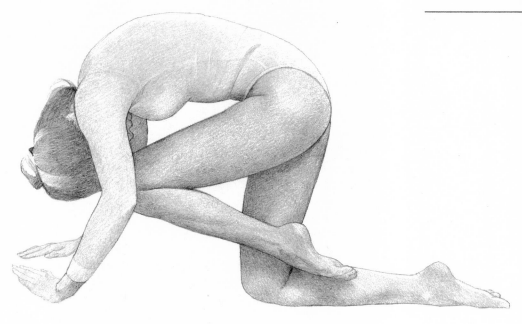

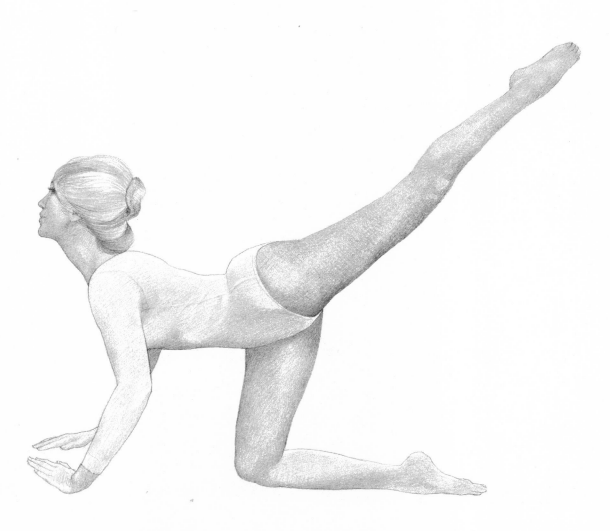

30. Plough

Looking back is like facing a gun.

The Plough is a very helpful posture to do before going into the Shoulder Stand. Even though you may have done preliminary exercises for fifteen or more minutes, you need the Plough to stretch and limber the entire spine, the hips and the legs. This posture should be done a number of times until your spine is flexible enough to touch your toes to the floor and to obtain the chin-lock position.

Feet together, lie flat on your back, arms at your sides, palms pressed against the floor. Exhale and slowly bring your hips and lower back off the floor, aiming to touch your toes to the floor over your head as far from your head as you can. Stay there a minute, breathing regularly and rhythmically. To come out of the Plough, bend your knees to your forehead, roll your hips down, pressing your hands to the floor and keeping your head on the floor, and come down slowly, vertebra by vertebra.

Do this posture for one minute.

BENEFITS

Relieves constipation.
Gives flexibility to the spine.
Stretches the hamstrings.
Rejuvenates the sex glands, liver, kidneys and spleen.
Stimulates the thyroid gland.

DO NOT DO

If you have a very active thyroid gland, do not press the chin to your chest too firmly.
If you have a neck injury.

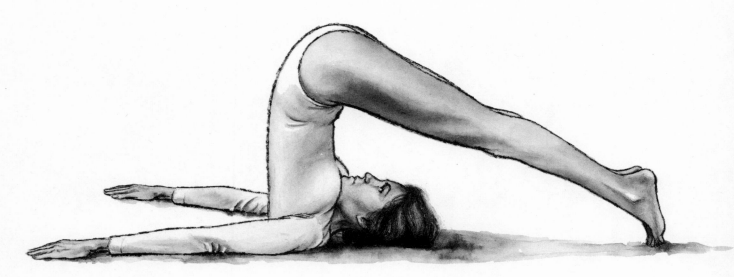

31. Shoulder Stand

Truth prevails, lie withers.

Always do the Plough before doing the Shoulder Stand.

Of the hundreds of postures, or exercises, of Hatha Yoga, the Shoulder Stand is the most important and it must be performed as a part of the Daily Yoga Program.

Before undertaking the Shoulder Stand, you must warm up for fifteen to twenty minutes—tensing, relaxing and stretching the body before inverting it to rest on the shoulders. The reason for this, which is basic, is that the body must be relaxed and the mind prepared to perform the posture so that the muscles of the neck and back will be in readiness.

Bring your body and both legs up with the support of your hands on your back, near the shoulder blades. If you cannot bring both legs up together, then lift one at a time. The weight should be on your shoulders, not on your hands; the hands are there only for support or to help beginners to put their bodies up. You will know you are straight on your shoulders if the load is not on your hands. Stay up there for a minute. Be sure you position your chin up and your chest comes up to meet it, instead of bringing your chin down to meet your chest. If you feel that you are going to fall, do so, but remember to bend your knees at once and roll down like a child. Never fall with a straight spine.

To come down from this position, bend your knees and bring them to the forehead. Put your hands flat at your sides, palms down, head on the floor. Roll down slowly, vertebra by vertebra. Your head should remain on the floor while you are coming down.

If you want to go back up again, please come down and rest for one minute before doing so.

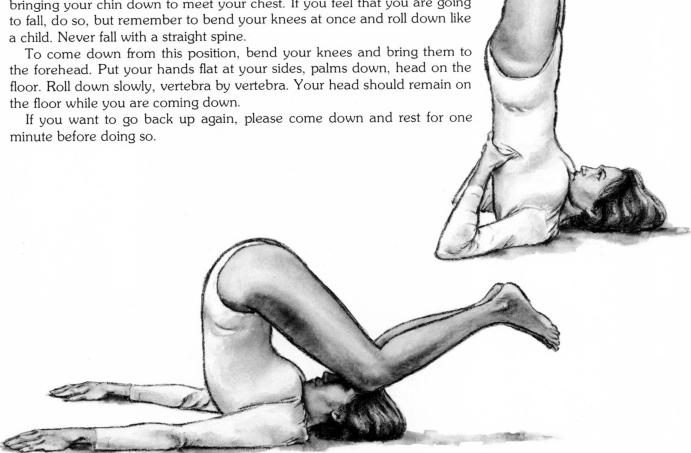

The unique pose of the Shoulder Stand rejuvenates the entire body. Because you have been upside down and breathing properly, you have toned up the endocrine glands, reversed the influence of gravity on your internal organs, stretched your ligaments and the muscles of the cervical region, stimulated your circulation, strengthened your back, and restored your energy.

Among the most important effects achieved is the one upon your thyroid gland, located in the neck. The pressure of your chin against your chest (the chin lock) stimulates the thyroid gland to produce more of the hormone that regulates the metabolism. Since the metabolism determines the rate at which your body uses food and oxygen, an active and properly functioning thyroid will keep your mind alert and your weight under control.

The Shoulder Stand is the most effective posture for streamlining both body and mind, for relieving the minor ailments of everyday life, the tensions, feelings of sluggishness, or the "blahs." You can rely upon the Shoulder Stand to bring you a fresh outlook and a new enthusiasm for living.

You can stay no more than three minutes on your shoulders each time.

BENEFITS

Offers all of the wonderful things mentioned above. So, you should not miss doing this posture.

DO NOT DO

If you are in the first three or four days of your menstrual period.
If you have any serious medical problems, including high blood pressure, low blood pressure, heart trouble, weak eye capillaries, or a middle ear disturbance.

32. Fish

> *A paper boat does not float very long.*

Here are two ways to do the Fish. For the first one, sit on the floor in the Lotus pose, or with your legs folded in front of you. Lean back, rest on your elbows and your head. Remove your elbows from the floor and stretch your arms over your head, which is now on the floor. Bend your elbows and place the palms of your hands near your ears, fingers pointed toward your shoulders. Arch your back, keep your buttocks on the floor and roll your head backward, resting the top of your head (as close to your forehead as possible) on the floor.

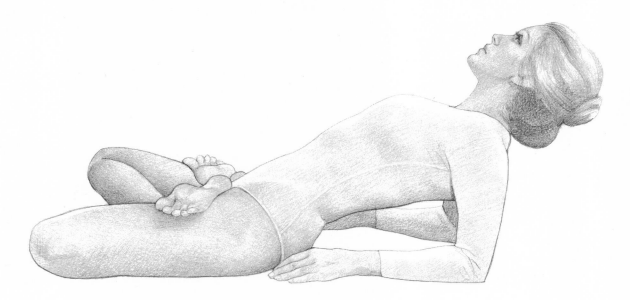

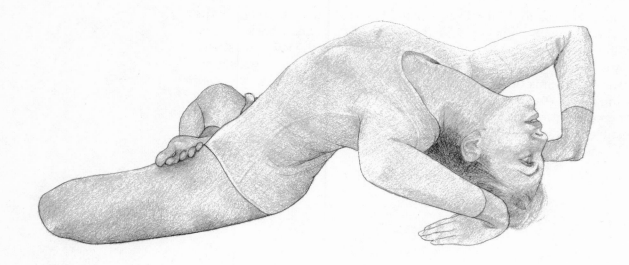

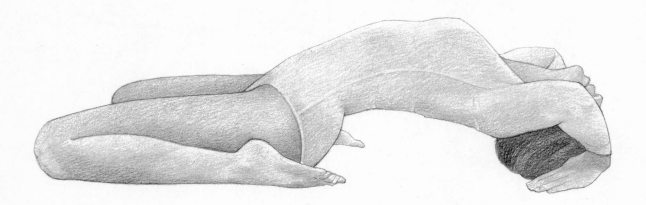

For the second Fish, kneel on the floor and spread your feet apart far enough to sit between them. Then sit on the floor between your feet, and keep the feet beside the thighs. Lean back, rest on your elbows and your head. Remove your elbows from the floor and stretch your arms over your head, bend your elbows and place the palms of your hands near your ears, fingers pointed toward your shoulders. Arch your back, keep your buttocks on the floor and roll your head backward, resting the top of your head (as close to your forehead as possible) on the floor.

Breathe normally during either of these poses and, in each, bring your head up from the floor before returning to the original position.

Since it complements and also has the opposite effect of the Shoulder Stand, you will do the Shoulder Stand and the Fish for exactly the same length of time, one to three minutes.

BENEFITS

Increases flexibility in the vertebrae of the upper and lower back.
Helps straighten round shoulders.
Stimulates the thyroid gland.
Makes free and deep breathing easier.
Improves vocal, bronchial and chest conditions.

DO NOT DO

If you have an ear infection or a middle ear problem.
If you have a neck problem.
If you have any condition affecting the esophagus.

33. Bow

> *Weak man hits 100 times, strong man hits once.*

The Bow, Cobra, and Locust are sister postures.

Lie down on your stomach. Bend your knees and get a firm hold on your ankles or feet. Start breathing in and try to pick up your knees, thighs, chest and head from the floor at the same time. Lift your feet high toward the ceiling, not toward your shoulders. The secret of this pose is to pull upward, not forward. Breathe out, slowly, and come down. If it is too difficult, practice with one foot at a time.

After practice, when the muscles are stretched, you can start rocking back and forth while you are up. When you rock, like a rocking chair, be sure you are using the thigh muscles to rock with, not the neck.

Do this posture three to six times.

BENEFITS

Combines the benefits of the Cobra and Locust postures and adds extra stretch.
Good for blood circulation around abdominal organs, which helps digestion.
Firms bust and arms.
Good for relieving tennis elbow pain.
Relieves stiffness in shoulders and gets rid of dowager's hump.

DO NOT DO

If you have a serious lower back problem.

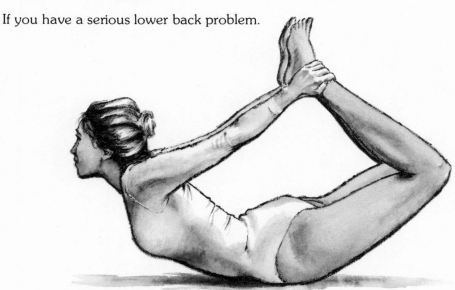

34. Bridge

> *Snakes are hard to train, they have no backbone.*

Lie flat on your back on the floor with your knees up. Bring your heels close to your thighs. With elbows up, now place your hands flat on the floor six inches out from the shoulders, palms down, thumbs in and fingers pointing toward the lower part of your body.

Relaxing your head and neck, arch your body up, pushing with your legs and arms at the same time. Do not push your lower part up first. Try to extend your legs and arms fully. Your head is hanging down but not touching the floor. After you are in the full Bridge position, breathe normally and stay there for only a few seconds the first few times, increasing to one to two minutes with practice.

To come down, bring your head up and lower your back to the floor very slowly, touching the entire back at the same time.

Do this one time.

BENEFITS

Improves your balance.
Stretches the stomach.
Strengthens the arms, shoulders and back muscles.
Increases blood flow to your head.
Expands chest and lung capacity.

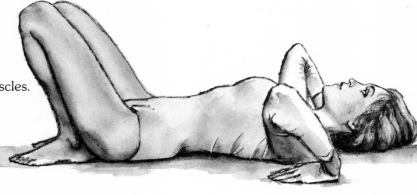

DO NOT DO

If you have a serious lower back problem.

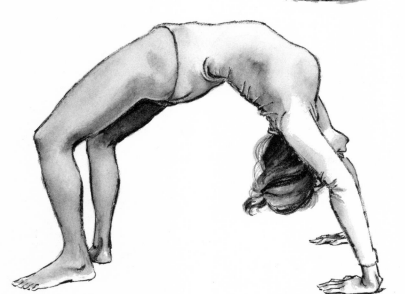

35. Sit-Ups

> **Don't feed a mouse, it will become a lion.**

Lie with your back on the floor, put your arms straight back beside your ears, and keep your feet together. First, breathe in. Then, while breathing out, come up slowly, your arms staying beside your ears, and sit up with your arms and whole back absolutely straight.

Bending forward, put your face on your knees, and your hands to your feet. Hold your feet, if you can, or touch them. Remember, you are still breathing out.

Prepare to return to your original lying-down position. Slowly round your back, pull in your stomach and, as you come up, slide your hands from your feet, along your legs. When your hands reach your knees, start breathing in, slowly. Vertebra by vertebra, from the bottom of the spine, try to touch each vertebra to the floor, one at a time, feeling each as it touches the floor while you are coming down. Stomach should cave in, not stick out. Bring your arms along your body until you are again flat on the floor with your arms above your head.

Do this exercise with somebody holding your feet down for you. If this is not possible, put them under something, a sofa, a bed, or some heavy object that will keep them on the floor. This will give your stomach a good stretch. Persons with back problems should bend the knees a little throughout the exercise.

Start with three to six times at one session.

BENEFITS

Strengthens stomach muscles.
Helps the nervous system.
Stretches the entire spine.
Reverses pressure in the lower back.
Stretches most of the muscles of the body, stimulating the kidneys, liver and pancreas.
Helps you to sleep well.
Aids digestion and elimination.

DO NOT DO

If you have any stomach ailments.

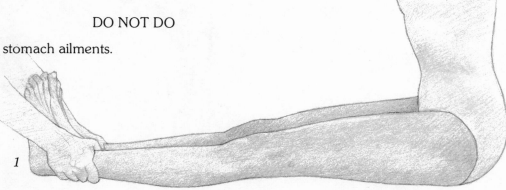

1

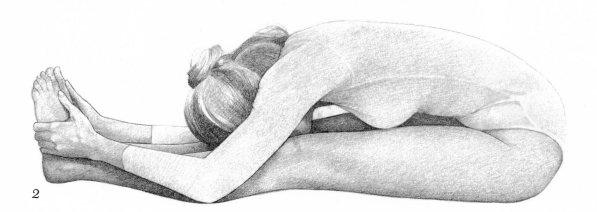

2

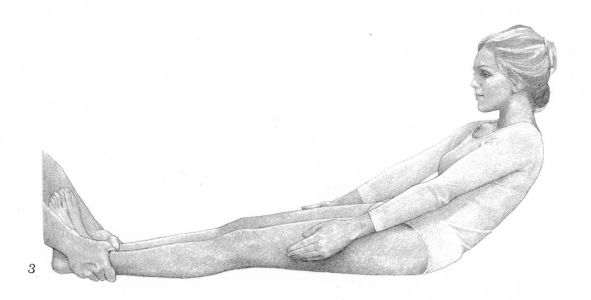

3

36. Lotus

> More haste, less speed.

The Lotus is the classic posture for meditation.

Sit down on the floor with your legs straight. Bend your right knee and bring your foot to the top of your left thigh. Try to touch the end of your heel to your left hipbone. Your right knee should be touching the floor.

Bend your left knee and bring your foot toward your right knee. If your right knee comes up off of the floor, you are not yet ready for the full Lotus. If you right knee *does* touch the floor, pick up your left foot and place it on your right thigh, trying to touch the heel to the hipbone. Now both knees should be on the floor.

You will realize that your back is absolutely straight when you succeed in this posture. This gives you complete balance and security in your body so your mind is thinking as straight as your body is. Put the backs of your hands on your thighs, with the tips of the thumb and forefinger of each hand touching. This *mudra* (symbolic hand gesture) signifies Knowledge.

If you are not able to do both sides, practice one side before you try the other leg. Don't be discouraged. Do not force by pulling your foot—the stretch should come from your thighs to prevent damage to the ligaments of your feet.

Half a minute to five minutes is long enough at any one time.

BENEFITS

Good benefits for everyone.
Preserves elasticity of the muscles connected with the pelvis and legs.
Strengthens your spine.
Develops tranquility and stimulates the mental processes.
Helps you to sit straight without slumping.

DO NOT DO

If you have circulation problems.
If you have knee problems.
If you have varicose veins.

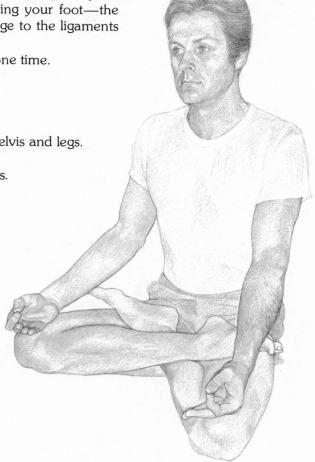

37. Arms, Neck and Shoulders

> When talking, some people throw stones, others spread flowers.

Let us work on tightening up the jelly-pulley under your arms, relaxing your neck, and releasing the tension from your shoulders. All of these will only take a few minues.

ARMS

For this exercise you can either stand or sit. Stretch your arms out like airplane wings, palms down. Then, bend your elbows slightly and lift your arms a few inches higher than your shoulders. Move them back a little and hold. Keep them at the same level, never dropping your arms below your shoulders, and move them up and back, and hold for a second.

Repeat six times, once a day.

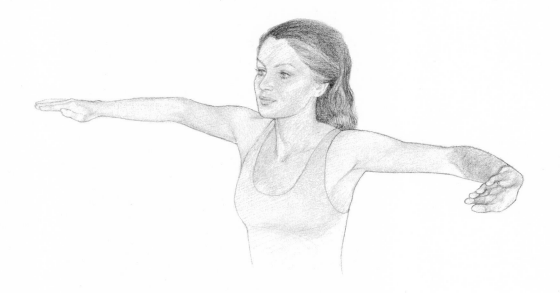

NECK

Sit in the Lotus position if you can. Otherwise, sit straight in any comfortable position. Put your hands on your thighs. Roll your head clockwise two times to twelve counts—six counts for each round. Roll your head from right to back to left; down and to the right. Repeat counterclockwise from the left side, twelve counts, two circles. When the head is moving, the body is steady and the head should feel detached from it.

Repeat these exercises two times, each side.

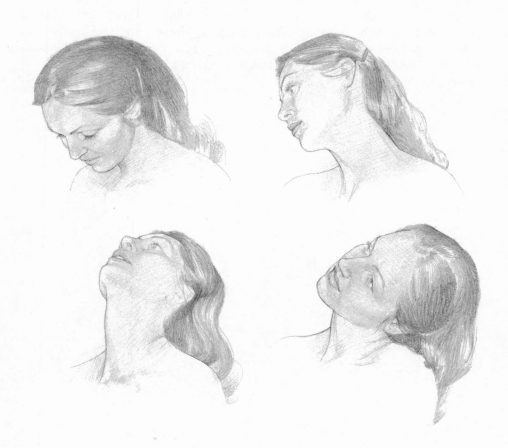

SHOULDERS

Sit in the Lotus position if you can. Otherwise, sit straight in any comfortable position. Put your hands on your thighs. Lift both shoulders up toward your ears while you are breathing in; push back both shoulders, still breathing in, and pull them down while you breathe out. Shoulders go up, back, down. (That means pull, backward down, never forward.)

Do this six times, once a day, or any time you feel tense or tired.

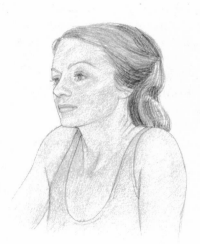

38. Dead Man Pose

> *Patience is bitter, but the fruit is sweet.*

This pose brings relaxation and tranquility and can be assumed anytime your body asks for it.

"Dead man" does not mean just lying down lazy, or sleeping, or doing nothing. This motionless pose requires the mind to be in control of the body and for the two to cooperate. An "easy" pose, it is the most difficult to master.

Lie down on your back as if you were absolutely dead. Turn your toes a little to the outside, your arms are at your sides, palms up.

Start with yoga deep breathing and come to slow, regular breathing. Breathe through the nose only.

You are going to visualize and feel your whole body, one part at a time, and work with it, from your toes to the top of your head. Put your mind on your big toes first. Start thinking your toes are heavy and want to relax.

As your mind moves up your body, one part at a time, you should slowly pick each part off the floor an inch or so, hold for a second, and slowly bring it down, so you feel that part which you are relaxing.

We have thought about the toes; now lift up one foot two inches off the floor, hold, and slowly, bring it down. Next, pick up the other foot and slowly bring it down. One knee at a time off the floor, and down. that's the way to go up the body.

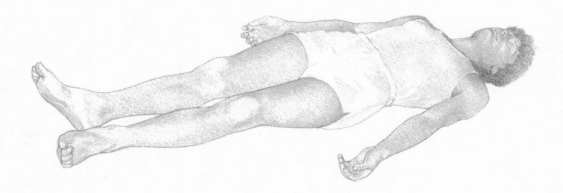

Now the hips, one side at a time, pelvis, upper part of your stomach, chest, each shoulder and each arm. Make a tight fist with each hand and release, blow your cheeks out (mouth closed), open your mouth sharp and relax; open your nostrils and relax them; open your eyes sharp and stare at the ceiling, and slowly close. Leave the eyes closed.

Turn your head from one side to the other, very slowly, while you are breathing. If any part of your body is still tense, pick that part up off the floor once more.

It won't be easy to free your mind from all kinds of thoughts. You have to think, so why not think about your breathing. Just lie there and listen to the sound of it, or to the beating of your heart.

It is much harder to keep the mind in control than it is the body, but you will be able to do it and be glad you did.

BENEFITS

Destroys fatigue.
Calms your nerves.
You will feel comfortable, relaxed and refreshed.
Your energy flows from your head back down to your heels.
Good for poise and serenity.
Renews you and gives you confidence.
Brings perfect balancing of body and mind after the contracting and relaxing of your Daily Yoga Program, and is a beautiful ending to it.

DO NOT DO

Don't miss!

4
Yoga Way of Life

Now that you know the basics of the Daily Yoga Program, you want to fit yoga into your working life, your playing life, your loving life. You want to make yoga such an integral part of your life that your mind and body can meet the challenge for every day with renewed energy and confidence.

The yoga exercises and postures you will meet now should be performed in addition to your Daily Yoga Program (except for pregnant women who have their own special course).They are designed for you to reach your own objectives of a *YOU* of which you can be proud.

In the Yoga Way of Life, you must understand your body before you can help it. You must know why your body responds as it does—or fails to respond. In the following pages, you will find that understanding; as well you will find the exercises and postures you need to reach your individual objectives: those of a person who stands tall, eats correctly, works without strain and gets full value from life.

I am going to look at several major activities and suggest the yoga approach to these basic things you do every day: sex, work, eating, standing, special thoughts for pregnant women, and traveling. Each section explains how yoga fits into these activities and how your yoga program will help.

A. *Meditation—Fifteen Minutes to Renewal*

Your course of Hatha Yoga has given you the physical stamina as well as the mental discipline to do meditation, if you want. You should not attempt meditation until your body and your mind are ready to accept it; indeed to welcome the respite of fifteen minutes out of this world.

As Hatha Yoga strengthens the mind and body, so meditation nourishes the spirit. It provides the great escape from disturbing thoughts and the stress and tensions of daily life. In fact, that quarter hour of meditation may be the only time in the day which is yours alone. You must insist on solitude or forget meditation. It is a oneness with yourself and nobody else, your daily gift to you.

My personal feeling, the attitude accepted by my students, is that it is unnecessary to sit for hours listening to a humming sound, making noises, turning lights on and off, or insisting on total darkness to meditate. The Yogis meditate on a mountain top in daylight.

Instead of sights or sounds which I would find distracting, I offer fifteen minutes of quiet, calm freedom from movement, except for slow, even breathing. My spirit is liberated while my body is at rest.

You may find it helpful to precede your period of meditation by tensing and relaxing every muscle, beginning with your toes and moving upward to your face. Don't permit those muscles to tense again while you meditate.

Each day, after you have already done your Daily Yoga Program, you can choose any time of day or evening to meditate, preferably when you yearn to take a break. Choose a meditation break rather than a coffee break. But don't meditate on an empty stomach when hunger pangs interfere with meditation, or on a full stomach when you would rather lie down than sit straight and when the digestive process interferes with relaxation.

The posture for meditation is a comfortable seated position on a mat, with your spine straight and eyes closed. If you cannot assume the Lotus position, you might find the Tailor position to your liking. A chair would incline you to slump, and if you lie down you might fall asleep.

Throughout your Hatha Yoga course, you have prepared your body to be in a seated position with a straight spine. Now you are ready to put your training to the test of forgetting your body and the difficulty of sitting in one position for fifteen minutes.

Your eyes are shut to avoid distracting sights. You don't want distracting noises either, so find a quiet place to meditate. Since proper breathing will be an integral part of your period of peace, you want a well-ventilated room with subdued lighting.

Breathing will help you sit quietly for your precious quarter hour. Sitting straight, you slowly breathe in. As you slowly breathe out, you bend slightly forward. The longer you take to breathe out, the better.

It will take four or five such slow breaths to get yor mind under control. Your mind has been racing here and there and your body has been tight, strained. Now you must bring mind and body together in the union that yoga promises.

Don't be discouraged if your first efforts at slow breathing fail to ready you for meditation. Wait a few minutes and try again.

To block out distressing thoughts, fasten your mind on the ocean—the long, even swells stretching to the horizon. Or picture gently swaying palm trees; a snowcapped mountain; puffy clouds, or early morning dew. Fill your mind with a vision at once beautiful and at peace. You are on your way to self-realization, but there are no shortcuts.

The first few times you attempt meditation, you will be distracted by an aching muscle or a jumble of thoughts. These invading thoughts might be of the past, the present, or the future, but you must conquer them. Push them away to free your spirit to find peace. After the first few efforts, you will find yourself able to keep worldly thoughts at bay.

You must concentrate on your breathing. As you listen to your breathing or the beating of your heart, you are able to avoid unwanted thoughts.

At the end of your fifteen minutes, you return to the world renewed and refreshed. You will find the fifteen minutes you have stolen from your daily routine more than repaid by hours of fresh energy.

You have gone on an inward journey of the spirit. Yoga meditation has made it possible.

B. *About Sex*

Sex is a beautiful art given to us by nature and by God, and it is up to us to develop and use that art beautifully.

This art, as practiced by two animated bodies, is one of the most creative experiences in the search for happiness. The unbaring of two souls in each other's embrace gives a new meaning to their existence. It is like the fresh April dew that opens spring petals.

Hearts beating in unison create the most celestial music. To reach this crescendo, and to maintain it, both body and mind must be healthy and work together. This is the blessing of yoga.

Yoga exercises and postures lead to good health and mental relaxation. They are the ingredients for a satisfactory sex life. You alone can make it pure, serene and exciting.

Passion is more pleasurable when it is less passionate. Everything about sex should be natural. The key to successful sex is the art of yoga. The body has to be healthy and it has to work with the mind for full pleasure and enjoyment.

The art of loving must be pleasurable for both partners—freely expressed and unhurried.

Sex is not only pleasurable, but it provides other benefits for mental and physical health. It is good for circulation and thus for the heart. It relieves tension. It is good for losing weight. But, remember that an ideal sex life can be greatly improved by regular and controlled yoga exercises.

It should be realized that physical exercises which lead to sound health and mental relaxation are essential to a happy sex life. The muscular activity that takes place in our bodies during sex is hardly restricted to the pelvic region. In a sex act, hundreds of muscles, from the head to the toes, have to function, although the important muscles are those of the buttocks, pelvis, thighs, abdomen, thorax, arms, legs and neck.

Many people have complaints about their sex lives. You may feel that you are a failure as a lover or inadequate in some way; or that your mate cannot "turn you on." While many feelings of inadequacy may stem from emotional problems, better physical conditioning and the discipline that yoga provides can help to solve many of these complaints.

Excessive weight tends to reduce your vitality, your energy, your endurance, perhaps even your interest in sex. But, most important, being overweight impairs your ability to fully participate in and enjoy sex. A good yoga discipline reinforces a person's motivation to lose weight and stay slim. The desire to feel physically attractive is the greatest incentive in any weight control program.

The thyroid and pituitary glands control the sex energies. The Shoulder Stand and the Plough stimulate the thyroid gland and keep it healthy. All the inverted exercises enrich the pituitary. The Stomach Lift relieves congestion in the pelvic region, helps the flow of blood and increases the sexual energy. The Cobra, Half Wheel, Locust, and Fish strengthen the pelvic muscles and tone the sexual organs.

Proper breathing is extremely important during lovemaking. You should breathe through the nose, rhythmically, slowly and with complete control. The satisfaction and the fulfillment of a good sexual act can only be achieved when tensions are eased by exercises and appropriate breathing.

In addition to the exercises mentioned above for stimulating the glands and generally strengthening the muscles in the pelvic area, these special exercises are designed to strengthen specific sets of muscles that are particularly important in performing the sex act.

The following exercise is for men only; a quick variation of Shooting Legs Out. To start this version of Shooting Legs Out, lie down on your back and bring your knees to your stomach. Now, breathe in and quickly shoot your legs straight down, but do not touch the floor. Slowly, bring them back while breathing out and quickly repeat. A man should do this six times, once a day. It strengthens the muscles in the pelvic area and is very good for the male sex glands.

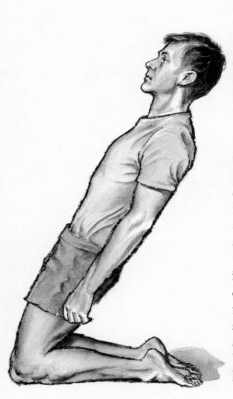

Contracting the buttocks is an excellent exercise for women. It is very important to learn to contract the muscles from hips to knees—contracting and relaxing, contracting and relaxing—frequently, to condition the muscles of the vaginal wall, to tighten them and bring them under control so you can use them at will during intercourse to increase the sensitiveness and give more pleasure to both parties.

These final two exercises are good for both sexes: Lean Back and Pelvic Push. Lean Back is beautiful for strengthening all of the muscles most intimately involved in sexual intercourse. Kneel down on the floor with your feet together. From your knees up, your body should be absolutely straight and stiff. Breathe in and lean back without bending any part of your body, from your knees to your head. Your hands are at your sides. Go backward as far as you can and hold. When you have to breathe out, come forward and return to the original kneeling position. Do this six times, once a day.

Pelvic Push is particularly good for toning the muscles used in sexual intercourse, relieving pelvic congestion and toning the thigh muscles. Lie on your back, bend your knees, put your feet flat on the floor about fourteen inches away from your thigh. Your arms are on the floor at your sides. Breathe in, bring your buttocks and entire back off the floor as high as you can. Your feet, shoulders, arms and head stay on the floor. Hold. While still holding your breath, push your knees forward. Hold. When you have to breathe out, come straight down, slowly.

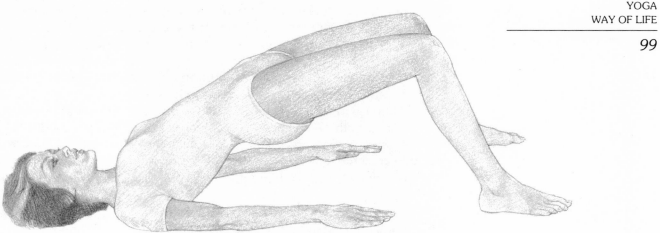

While breathing out, slide your back on the floor up to the original position and suck your diaphragm in, contract your buttocks and hold. When you have to breathe in, do the whole exercise again. Repeat this exercise three times, each with a full breath. With normal breathing, do the exercise ten times, but faster. The rhythm is Up-Push-Down-Pull.

The secret of yoga is to ease the tensions and yet remain strong. To get the most pleasure from your love life, avoid artificial stimulants and depressants such as too much drinking and smoking, do not make love on a full stomach, and do not permit yourself to become overtired.

There is no greater pleasure in life than satisfactory lovemaking.

C. *People At Work*

Does your work require sitting too much, standing too long, bending forward too much or carrying heavy loads? All workers are plagued by the effects of their working habits. Office activities, though necessary, need not be the bane of your existence.

Ask yourself, is your work controlling you? You can learn to control your work. With a few minutes of yoga exercises and deep breathing every hour, you can correct the harmful things you are doing to your body. You will be surprised to find your body and mind working together, smoothly and efficiently. Yoga exercises will become a habit, as natural as breathing or walking.

Is your work more mental than physical? Are you tense because of decisions to make, deadlines to meet? These exercises and postures will help you unwind, to make decisions with a clear mind, meet your deadlines without pressure headaches. You will feel refreshed and relaxed.

Let's begin with the yoga breathing, because deep breathing and yoga exercises and postures are the keys to relaxation. As described in Chapter 2, yoga breathing is done from the diaphragm. Breathe in while you blow your abdomen out like a balloon. Then slowly breathe out and your abdomen will go in, like a balloon beginning to empty. Put your hand on your abdomen below your rib cage to feel that the breath is going in and out. This is the way oxygen reaches the lower part of your lungs, which would otherwise miss it.

Yoga breathing is full, deep breathing from the collarbone to the ribs to the bottom of the lungs. The secret is to breathe slowly and rhythmically, in and out. That will make you refreshed and less tense. Whenever you have a chance, practice this a few times. Later, when your body gets used to this new experience, oxygen reaching all of your lungs, you will breathe this way naturally all the time.

Along with this deep breathing, there are some exercises you can do at the office:

* While standing, stretch both hands up, take a deep breath and reach for the ceiling. Bring your hands down while you are breathing out and completely relax. This will only take a minute. Repeat this twice, a couple of times a day.

* Stand with your back to the wall. Touch the wall with your heels, the back of your arms and the entire back of your body. Try to press the small of your back to the wall, and have fun. You should have that fun two or three times until the small of your back touches without effort. Do this a few times a day, one minute each time.

* After sitting on a chair too long, your neck, shoulders and back begin to hurt. While you are sitting, take a deep breath, lift your shoulders up, back and down. Pull backward only, never bring your shoulders forward. When your shoulders are up, you are breathing in; when they are down, you are breathing out.

* The best way to sit straight is to contract the muscles tight, from the knees to the waistline. That will make your spine straight and also will flatten your stomach. While you are sitting on the chair, put both of your hands beside you on the seat of the chair, palms down. Push down to give yourself support, holding your buttocks a few inches off the chair while you are contracting. Hold a minute and slowly, slowly come down and relax. Do this three times, twice a day.

* You can work on your arms now, whether you are standing or sitting. Stretch them out like airplane wings, palms down. Your elbows should be bent a little. Lift your arms a few inches higher than your shoulders, bring them back, and hold. Keep them at the same level, move them up and back and hold for a second. Don't bring them down or forward at all, or the benefit of this exercise will be lost. Do this exercise six times, once a day. This is beautiful for your chest, underarm jelly-pulley, and tension in the shoulders.

* Are you sitting straight? Is your tailbone touching the seat of your chair? Is your chair the right size for you? Are both feet on the floor? How about stretching one leg out in front of you, level with the seat of the chair? Stretch your toes down and then up toward you, down and up toward you, a few times. Put that leg down and bring your other leg up and do

the same thing with the toes. Then do both legs together. When you do both legs together, be sure your stomach is pulled in. If you do that six times, not only will your stomach tighten up, your back will stop hurting, and your knees and your feet will feel as though they have had a good massage.

* Your neck has had enough bending forward while you have been working. It needs a change. Bring your neck back where it belongs, with your ears in a straight line with your shoulders. Remind yourself to do this, and do it often.

* Now, lubricate your neck by rolling it around. Slowly roll your head to the right, back, to the left, down; then to the left, back, to the right, down. Do this twice to each side, first to one side and then to the other. This will remove the tension. Roll twice, once a day.

* Our hands are hardworking parts of the body and they get tired, too. So while you are sitting or standing, just clench your fists very tight and release them a few times. Do this two or three times a day.

* Whether you are sitting or standing, pay attention to your eyes. Stare straight ahead at one spot, keep your eyes open, don't blink. When your eyes start watering, close them. When you open them again, try to roll your eyeballs from side to side and around while your eyes are still open. Close your eyes again and rest for a second. Do this once a day. The muscles around your eyes will thank you.

If you practice my Daily Yoga Program at home and follow these exercises at the office, you will be more creative and less tired. When you feel better, you work better.

D. *Proper Eating and Weight Control*

Don't say "diet," say "proper eating." When we talk about diet, aren't we really talking about life, about what makes people feel vital, eager for experience, getting the most out of every day? Of course, what we eat determines how we feel, but it only goes halfway toward determining how we look. To look as well as we feel, we have to combine proper eating with shaping our bodies through exercise. I believe the form of exercise that does the most for people is Yoga.

Along with yoga exercises, postures and breathing, there are proper foods and eating habits to be followed. Some people eat the wrong foods or too much because they are emotionally unhealthy; they feel depressed, tense, are sure something is wrong with their lives. Others eat in the wrong way and as a result they become unhealthy. They have eaten their way to tension and depression. For them, too, something is missing.

Excessive eating is a nervous habit and the more relaxed the person, the less compulsive the eating. Emotional frustration and boredom, of course, have a lot to do with overeating.

Calorie counts and the intake of carbohydrates and fats vary with the individual, in size, metabolism, and activity. An ideal diet is one which is different for every person. Skinny people may have to eat a certain quantity of carbohydrates and more fats than the amount found in the normal diet. Extremely overweight people have to eat less fats and carbohydrates than exist in a normal diet. Some people need more proteins or vitamins than others. A doctor will be able to advise you on special diet needs but, in general, these are my principles for proper eating:

* Eat less food, especially fats and carbohydrates, if you want to lose weight.

* Eat more frequently, but each time in small quantity. This will keep the stomach from becoming empty and producing excessive acid.

* Improve the quality of what you eat as you reduce the quantity. Quality means fresh fruits and vegetables instead of the canned or frozen varieties; broiled or boiled food instead of fried; less meat and more vegetables; cheese and fruit instead of candy and junk food.

* Reduce the quantity of salt in your diet.

* Take one less alcoholic drink per day if you must drink.

* If you are a heavy coffee drinker, reduce intake.

* Avoid drastic methods of weight reduction such as a crash diet, crash eating habits like skipping meals or fasting. Be regular in your diet habits. Undereating can be as harmful as overeating.

* Stay away from foods such as fatty steaks, butter and rich desserts because they contain saturated fats, which tend to raise the cholesterol level in the body. Instead, eat foods prepared with polyunsaturated oil.

* Eat a balanced diet. There are five main classes of food: whole grains, vegetables and fruits, dairy products, lean meat, and fish and fowl. Your body requires these and you should eat something from each of these classes every day.

* Drink several glasses of water each day.

* Take proper amounts of fats, carbohydrates, proteins, vitamins and minerals.

* Eat everything. Don't deprive yourself of any food you crave, but eat in moderation. There are right and wrong foods to eat. The wrong foods can be eaten to satisfy your tongue but not your body. They should be eaten infrequently and in small quantities—the smallest quantities. If you feel you must have ice cream and candy, pizzas or french fries to make your soul happy, do so rarely and sparingly. Have one bite, it will make the hostess happy, too.

The older we get, the less food we need. Whatever your age, proper eating requires the following of these rules:

* Do not eat when you are tense. You will swallow air and give yourself cramps. Relax before you eat.

* Do not eat in a hurry. You eat too much. When you eat slowly, you tire of food sooner.

* Do not forget to chew your food well.

* Do not exercise immediately after eating.

* Do not sleep immediately after eating. Instead, take a slow walk.

Yoga and proper eating are close friends. Many of my pupils have not only lost as much weight as they wished by practicing yoga a half hour a day, but they have been able to keep pounds from returning. After losing weight and seeing the attractive things that have happened to their bodies, most yoga pupils are able to keep the weight off because they have developed discipline and are better able to control their eating. Also, after seeing how good they look in the mirror, they develop greater respect for their own bodies and consequently lose the desire to eat the wrong foods. A little success encourages more success.

Yoga performs several specific roles in losing and controlling weight. First, it changes the shape of the body and restores a youthful appearance. It redistributes the pounds. Second, there are certain exercises that stimulate the thyroid gland. This produces more of the hormone that regulates the metabolism, thus increasing the rate at which the body uses the food. Third, yoga has a good effect on your whole system. It improves the circulation, and the free flow of blood prevents the collection of fat. Finally, proper breathing increases the supply of oxygen to the system, which makes you feel healthier and removes the frustrating appetite.

Now that you have mastered your eating habits and are eating the right foods, you will realize how much better you feel the next day; and when you are offered wrong food, you will remember that the food might not be yours, but your stomach is.

E. *Correct Posture*

Posture is important because we live with it the entire day. Exercises such as swimming, running, tennis, calisthenics, or even yoga, we perform only an hour or so at a time. While these activities are important, posture is more important, because it is the way we live, it works more on your body and has more to do with how you feel than any individual exercise can. Posture reflects how you feel and think inside. If you are depressed you will slouch; if you are overtired and distressed, have aches and pains or are sad about something, it will show in your posture. Improving your posture, however, can help improve your attitude, your feeling about yourself. You will look and feel better.

When you are overtired, you have a tendency to push your stomach out and arch your back, round your shoulders, stand on one foot with your hip thrown out. This spoils your posture and hurts your spine. You must have been told: "Stand straight, hold your stomach in, put your shoulders back, chest out." And these words are correct. But, how do we know when we are doing these things correctly?

The first thing you have to do is realize that your body has two parts, lower part and upper part. The lower part, below the waistline, should always be straight and strong. When you contract the muscles of your lower part, your upper part will relax automatically. If your lower part is straight and you contract from your knees to your waist, it will not allow you to throw your stomach forward, buttocks backward, your hips to one side or to stand on one leg. You will stop standing incorrectly. You have taken the first step toward good posture.

Think of your body as consisting of four parts: from ankles to knees, from knees to waist, from waist to shoulders and from shoulders to head. Now, visualize these four parts. Look in the mirror, side view, and see that your ankle, your hip, shoulder and ear are in one line. Be sure that you are not balancing on your toes, but on the balls of your feet and heels.

"Chest straight" does not mean "Push your chest out." "Hold your stomach in" does not mean "Hold your breath and hold in your stomach." "Chin up" does not mean "Throw your head back." "Shoulders back" does not mean "Push your shoulders backward."

Your shoulders must be in line with your anklebones. From ankles to hip you are straight. From hips to shoulders you are straight. Where are your ears? Is your chin forward? Bring your chin back to bring your ears backward to your shoulders, without making a double chin. Your chin should be contracted to go back; never push it hard or bend it backward. Bending your neck backward stretches your skin and that will give you two or three chins.

To be sure that you are keeping that good posture, once a day stand with your back against the wall. Try to press the small of your back to the wall. Now, try to walk in the same posture. Correct posture will help you to use your muscles properly, so you save yourself from muscle spasms and other problems, such as a stomach that sticks out, a swayback, dowager's hump, curved spine, and neck out of line.

Your posture while sitting is important also. Sit straight on the chair, be sure that your tailbone is touching the seat of the chair. Do not cross your legs; that stops circulation. When you have been bending forward, be sure to come back to your correct posture. Whenever you feel tired, contract the muscles of your lower part, release, contract, release, and then keep them contracted as much as you can. Make this a habit when you are sitting and standing; you cannot contract when you are walking. This beautiful habit will be helpful to you. Your spine will have no problems and your neck will feel relieved.

The most important thing when you are standing is to stand with your weight on both feet. Do not shift your balance from side to side.

When you walk, always remember that your feet go before your body. Do not lean forward.

A correct posture is most important to make you feel you are "standing tall." With your good posture and by following the Daily Program, you have it made.

F. For Pregnant Women

Having a baby is a beautiful and joyful experience. Even though she is getting larger, it is still a time in a woman's life when she can look the most beautiful and the most graceful. She cannot appear beautiful in the contemplation of the baby she is carrying unless she feels her best, and this is difficult when her back aches and her food refuses to stay down.

To make yours a trouble-free experience, you must know how to take care of yourself and this other life for which you are responsible. How well you care for yourself and the baby growing inside of you during pregnancy and immediately thereafter can be very important to both of you, then and later. In order to learn about your health and diet needs during this period, you should be under the care of a doctor.

For a happy pregnancy, you should also develop a safe and effective program of exercise. Such a program will give strength and flexibility to your spine to avoid backaches caused by the extra load on the back muscles during the later months of pregnancy. A strong and flexible back is also important during childbirth because the spine and back muscles are under so much strain and stress then. It is important, for example, that the spine and muscles be flexible because the uterus tends to lengthen the ligaments and muscles of the spine as it contracts during labor.

Your exercise program should also focus on the pelvic joints and pelvic area. To provide plenty of room for the baby and to help make the delivery easier, the muscles of the pelvic floor need to be in tone, supple, relaxed and widened. A tight and rigid pelvic floor slows the arrival of the baby.

Your program should stress correct posture, proper breathing and regular practice of the prescribed exercises and postures.

Good posture cannot be neglected if you want to avoid backaches and look and feel better. To achieve and maintain good posture, review the preceding section. Remember to tuck in your buttocks, tilt your pelvis forward to align your spine, keep your shoulders back and your chin up. This posture should be maintained when you are sitting as well as standing. Your posture should not be neglected even when you are lying down. To improve that posture, while lying on your back, contract your hips, hold, then release. Squeeze your legs together, hold, then release. Contract your pelvic floor muscles (urethra, vagina and rectum), hold, then release.

Much of the pain of childbirth stems from fear. A frightened woman in labor may hold her breath or breathe improperly. Then she finds herself more exhausted, tense and out of control. Learning and practicing proper yoga breathing as described in the chapter on breathing will prevent much labor pain.

The pregnant woman, as well as the new mother, needs exercises to tone up and add flexibility to those muscles that are so important before and after childbirth.

Strong and flexible pectoral muscles are needed to support the breasts as they grow during pregnancy and when the baby is being breast-fed. Two exercises to strengthen the pectoral muscles are described in the chapter on Beauty (*see* ''For Supple Hands'' in Chapter 6). They are a key to beauty, but they are equally important for the new mother. The Full Body Stretch from the Daily Yoga Program also keeps the breast muscles strong.

To protect the spine while it is carrying an increasing load, these exercises from the Daily Yoga Program will be helpful: Cat Pose, Back to the Wall and the Half Wheel.

The following exercises are especially designed to widen, strengthen, and add flexibility to the pelvic floor, tone the thigh muscles, and promote circulation to the feet:

* Sit on your heels with your knees together. Separate your knees and feet. Sit solidly on the floor if you can. If this is difficult, don't force yourself. Gradually increase your ability to sit flat on the floor. In this position, spread your knees as wide as possible, then bring them together. Do this six times, once a day.

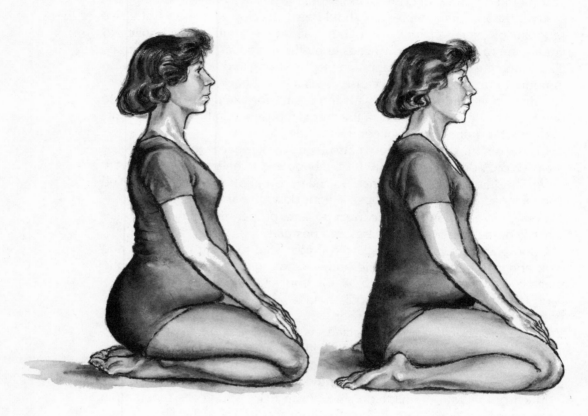

* Lie on your back with your thighs against the wall and your legs straight up against the wall and together. Your toes are turned toward you with the soles of your feet toward the ceiling and hands at your sides. Tilt your pelvis up, push the small of your back against the floor and contract your buttocks. Then release. Contract again and release. Contract six times, once a day.

* Lying on your back against the wall in the same position as above, move your arms over your head straight with your elbows touching the floor. Be sure that the small of your back is touching the floor. Slowly spread your legs apart as far as you can comfortably against the wall. Then bring your legs together slowly. Do this six times, once a day.

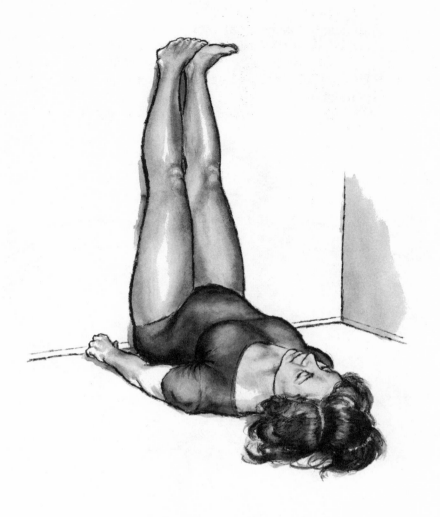

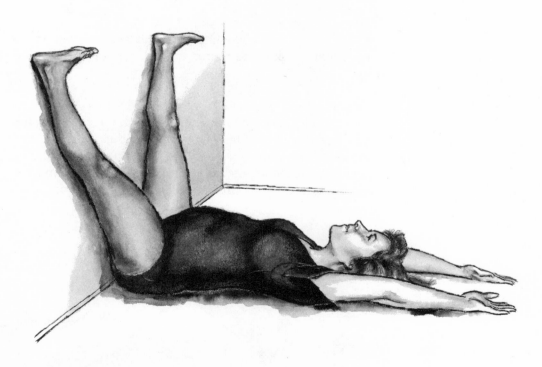

* With your hands braced against a table or a chair to give yourself support, squat down on your toes with knees apart. Now, try to put your heels down flat on the floor. If they do not go down at first, they will with practice. Rise back to your toes and stand up. Do this six times, once a day at first. Increase to ten.

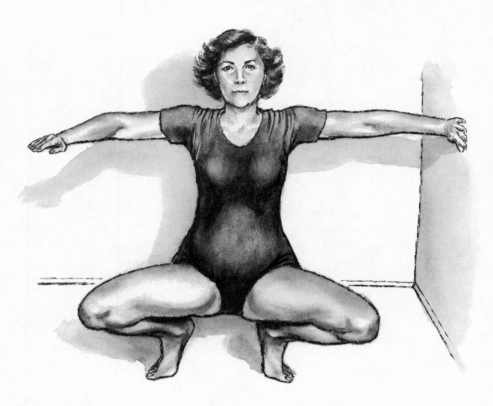

Uterus prolapse, or dropping of the uterus, can occur after the baby is born, as well as with advanced age. This exercise will give strength to the muscles that support the uterus and is *not* to be performed during pregnancy.

* Kneel down on your hands, elbows and knees. Your knees are together and your elbows are at your sides. Touch your chest to the floor and put your head to your side. Contract your buttocks and stay there for two minutes. Now, turn over on your left side and lie there for one minute. Return to the same posture again, stay another two minutes, and then lie on your right side. Do this complete cycle twice a day.

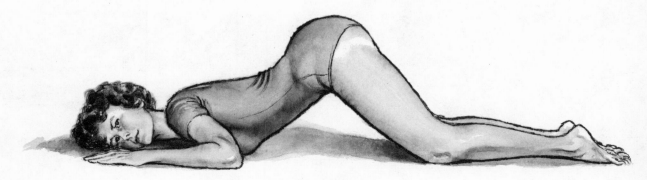

The following are additional hints for pregnant women:

* Absolutely no smoking.

* Limit your drinking of alcoholic beverages to one drink per day, if you have to drink.

* Don't do rigorous exercises.

* Except for the special exercises suggested in this section for pregnant women, postpone my Daily Yoga Program unless your doctor approves and you are under the direction of a qualified yoga teacher. After the baby is born and the doctor says it is all right, resume the Daily Yoga Program.

* Follow a proper diet prescribed by your doctor. Add more foods that supply calcium, such as milk and cheese.

* If you are breast-feeding place a pillow under the baby so you do not stretch your breast.

Your primary goal is a healthy baby and a healthy you.

G. When Traveling

We have become a world of travelers. Wherever we are, we feel impelled to go someplace else. Often, whether we are traveling for business or sheer enjoyment, we may spend at least a day at our destination recovering from the fatigue of getting there.

If you are traveling by plane, you may face the debilitating effects of jet lag. Even if your trip is shorter, you may find your legs stiffened by remaining too long is one position.

If you are traveling by car, again you are in a narrow, enclosed situation where breathing may be less invigorating, legs become cramped, eyes become strained, teeth become clenched and your face becomes more tense by the minute.

Even the freedom of a cruise ship has its problems. We sit more than we exercise, we eat more than we should. A long train trip may find us sluggish, as remaining seated too long always slows down our circulation. The roughness and vibration of the train movement takes its toll on our body, as well.

Whether we fly, drive, sail or go by train, we usually devote more time to thinking about what we are going to take with us than how we are going to look and feel when we arrive at our destination and when we come home.

Ship lovers are the only travelers who can still follow my Daily Yoga Program, and they should faithfully do so to avoid the pounds they are sure to put on from overeating and the condition they will get in from under-exercising.

As for plane, train and auto travelers, here are a few simple exercises and postures you can do to stay limber and refreshed on a long trip. Naturally, you are limited in the exercising you can do in a plane or train. Your back is aching, your shoulders are drooping, your stomach is getting bloated, and your feet and legs are becoming cramped.

* When these things happen to you, but before your food is served, why don't you get up, stand in the aisle, and grab hold of the backrest of your seat. With your feet twelve or more inches away from the seat, and with your body erect and knees stiff, lean forward as far as you can without lifting your heels. Return to the standing position. Do this six times whenever you get a chance. Breathe normally. This will stimulate circulation and take the stiffness out of your body.

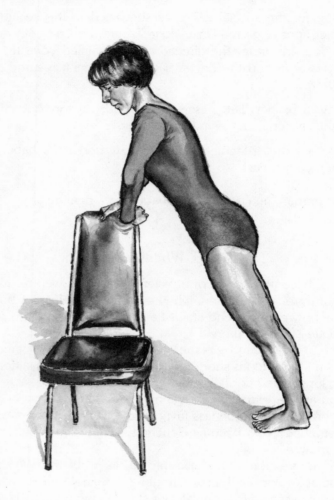

* While sitting, slowly breathe out as much as you can, pull your stomach in, and hold. Breathe in to release your stomach. Do this three times every hour or two.

* Whenever you realize you're slumping in your seat, sit straight and contract your buttocks as many times as you can.

* While still sitting, push your neck back to your shoulder level. Next, pretend that your neck is being lifted by a crane. Hold. Try to sit this way much of the time you are traveling. This will release the tension in your neck and shoulders, and keep your back straight, too.

* When your back is aching, try this posture. You cannot lift both elbows at the same time because you will bother your seat mate. But, you can lift one at a time. Place your right hand on the back of your head, with your elbow straight out. Put the other hand behind your back at your waistline. Twist from your waistline and look at your right elbow. Hold for a half minute. Repeat on the left side. It will give a good twist to your waistline and also will relax your neck. Do this two times each side, every couple of hours.

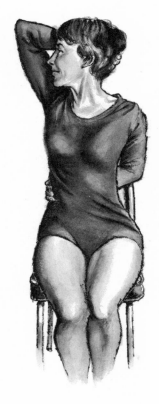

* When you have another chance to stand up, slip your shoes off, hold onto the backrest of your seat again. With your heels together, your toes and knees apart and pointing out, bend down a few inches. Now, lift your heels up. Slowly bring them down, keeping your knees bent, and without moving your body up and down. Do this six times whenever you feel like it. This is good for your arches, calves, knees and thighs.

* After you have been sitting for a while, your feet are crying for circulation. Tense your toes and roll them under toward the arches. Hold. Then release. Press your toes on the floor firmly, heels up. Release. Press your heels on the floor, toes up. Release. Sit absolutely straight while doing this. Repeat this series six times whenever your feet require circulation.

* For a little massage to your hands, lay the back of your hands on your thighs, open your fingers sharply, and then close one finger at a time. When all are closed, take a deep breath, make a tight fist, and hold. Release. Do this six times. Repeat when necessary.

The non-driver, or automobile passenger, should do as many of these exercises listed for plane and train travelers as they possibly can while riding in the car. The driver can do the face exercises described in Chapter 6.

Drivers should avoid wearing coats with heavy collars in order to prevent pressure on their necks and shoulders. They should keep in mind the importance of sitting as straight as possible at all times.

When car travelers stop and get out for meals, they can always put their hands up, stretch fully, and take a deep breath in. Then breathe out and relax completely. They also can rest their eyes by opening them sharp, and then closing them tight; by moving their eyeballs from side to side, up and down, and around in a clockwise and then counterclockwise motion as described in Chapter 6. Do these several times until you feel relaxed and your eyes feel rested.

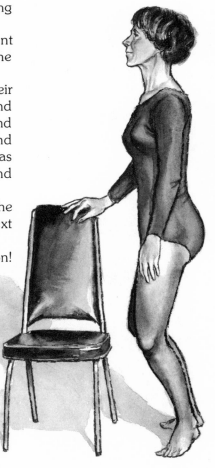

Also, while standing next to the car, you are welcome to do any of the exercises given for the plane and train travelers. When you plan your next trip, don't forget to take this program with you.

Have a good trip and don't come back fat, stiff and soggy from vacation!

5
Special Problems Helped by Yoga

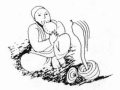

We pay for all the mistakes we make with our bodies in the way we sit, stand and walk as well as in the way we react to the challenges and strains of our daily life.

When our bodies rebel against all the mistreatment we have given them for so long, they proceed to torment us with aches, pains and a variety of bodily ills.

Sometimes, as in the case of disabling illness, the distress is not our fault; but more often than not, we are to blame for what is happening to our bodies and we are the only ones who can reverse it.

Of course, you should follow your Daily Yoga Program and the exercises you need in the Yoga Way of Life, but you should devote special attention to your special problems. Most of them are correctable if you carefully follow the instructions. You will be glad you did when your headaches vanish, when the pain from your arthritis is relieved, when you sleep through the night without pills and when you can forget your aching back.

This chapter, as you will see, starts out with "tension" and then covers such complaints as constipation, headaches, insomnia, and other problems that will be substantially relieved by any kind of exercise program, according to my medical friends. But yoga offers something much more in helping with these problems because so many of them, I am told, are related to *stress*.

Yoga helps everyone deal with stress better because, among other things, it builds up your self-confidence. It reduces your sense of frustration and gives you a better outlook because it helps you believe in your *own* abilities to cope with life as it is. Yoga enables you to take charge of yourself. As you learn to control your body better, you will also learn to discipline your thoughts as well.

A. *Tension*

From the alarm clock that rouses us in the morning to the dreary conflicts on the nightly news, we are bombarded daily by tension makers. The hostess tenses as her guests arrive late and she visualizes the overcooked roast she must serve. The VIP hurries from one meeting to another, and must manage a social life as well. The secretary tenses when the boss tells her the complicated, figure-full letter must be finished by one o'clock, and she has a luncheon date. The college senior drives himself to the edge of exhaustion all the way through his or her finals. The athlete tenses every time his competition gets anywhere near him. The mother is home all day with the children and ready to scream when her husband comes home. All are victims of every day tensions.

Added to the crises of our daily life, increasing our tensions tenfold, are the noises that surround us, the unwanted noises that make us snappish without being conscious of the cause of our ill humor.

What does all this do to our long-suffering bodies? Tension makes us irritable when there is no obvious cause. The back of our neck aches, a nagging pain traces its way across our lower back. Even our fingers feel stiff from unconscious clenching. Our head develops a dull throb. We can feel ourselves frowning, and the corners of our mouths droop.

We feel terribly tired even though the day wasn't too demanding. How can we pull ourselves together to go out for the evening without making everyone miserable, including ourselves? We try a quick nap, but our mind is racing, we can't relax, we toss and turn around on the bed, just getting more tense.

Each and every one of us has his own ways of creating tension; it's human nature. When these tendencies get out of control, unchecked tension penetrates to the very core of the soul; physical and emotional problems take root, and here comes trouble.

We find ourselves seemingly helpless to solve our problems. Mental stress becomes emotional anxiety, which begins to affect the performance of our bodies. And there goes our health.

Among the many causes of stress and tension are marriage, divorce, retirement, aging, loneliness and insecurity. These have an effect on your emotions and can have a direct effect on your health. Too much tension can give you acid stomach, ulcers, migraine, high blood pressure, heart trouble, can cause you to grind your teeth, overeat, and panic. Also, when you are under stress and your muscles are tense, the free flow of your blood is interrupted. And when the flow of the bloodstream is interfered with, the arteries are affected, as are the blood pressure and the rate of breathing: the result can be hypertension. Your adrenal glands, which release hormones through your body, save your life by coping with stress.

As long as you experience stress, the adrenal glands will continue to produce the vital hormones, cortin and adrenalin; if the stress continues too long, these excessive hormones can have a harmful effect on the body.

The most important thing in life is thinking positively. The mind is like a rough sea, however, if you don't control it, your mind won't cooperate with you.

It is a beautiful art to be able to smile and say to yourself again and again that you are happy. Develop this art and, unconsciously, it will control your will and you will succeed. You will be helped internally and externally. This is yogic philosophy; you may find it hard to believe.

In life, time and again, we are tested and have to adjust, just as gold must be tested in the fire again and again to prove that it is gold. Yoga brings serenity to your life; it gives you courage and understanding that you must experience to know. Breathing, one of yoga's main sciences, helps you achieve this. Simple tension, caused by exhaustion and overwork, is different from the mental and physical stress brought on by various outside forces, and can be relieved with a few deep breaths and relaxing.

To help yourself from becoming more tense, take a break mentally and physically by getting away from the tension-producing situation. That's the easiest way to get in touch with yourself and reach out for a guiding light. Get to a quiet place. Stretch, contract, breathe. Half an hour, thirty minutes, of undisturbed exercises from the Daily Yoga Program can give us the mental, physical and emotional appetite for a good evening.

Tension affects each of us in a different part of the body and always strikes the weaker parts: the muscles you use the least are the first to feel the effects of a trying situation. Why don't you throw your tension to your buttocks, where it belongs and is needed?

How about a little Locust or Cobra for your neck and shoulders? Treat your neck, roll it, slowly, with eyes closed, carefully and gracefully.

Be careful in your bendings when you are tense, you really can hurt your neck and back or even displace any part of the body if you move too suddenly. Trying to remember to slow down will help ease your mind. Don't forget to eat slowly, too. If there isn't enough time to eat slowly, don't eat! Drink a glass of juice or milk, instead. And when your mind doesn't want to cooperate with your body, and someone makes you angry, take a deep breath before you respond.

Your day will pace itself according to your will, your evenings will be brighter, and you'll find yourself looking forward to every tomorrow.

B. *Back and Neck Pain*

Back pain is one of the most common complaints among adults, regardless of age, sex or race. Such pain is more likely to strike those who are overweight, overworked and underexercised. Outside of serious medical problems, such as a slipped disc or any other spinal disorder, most backaches can be attributed to the aging process, tension, bad posture and the evils of a sedentary life: flabby muscles and habitual misuse of the body. Such misuse results in muscular distortions, which can have a very painful effect on your back.

Don't panic, tension will only make matters worse, and there is a way to retrain those misguided muscles, by using them in a normal manner: that is, as they should be used!

Back pains can occur in the sacrum, lower back, middle back and the neck. The work you do and the habits you follow affect different parts of your spine, and play a part in determining where pain will strike you if you mistreat yourself. Remember, your spine is your lifeline. As long as it is healthy, your entire body will function well. But if the spine is abnormally bent, inflexible or damaged, any number of problems can result.

Most of the muscles and most of the bones of the body connect directly or indirectly to the spine and back. If any of these muscle or bone systems are out of line, imbalanced or weak, the result can be a pain somewhere in the back or neck. Poor posture, such as a badly shaped spine, an overly swayed lower back or a protruding stomach, can place undue strain on the spine and the back muscles. Weak stomach muscles can force the companion back muscles to hold more than their normal load. Therefore, prevention of back and neck problems and treatment of back and neck pain may very well involve sets of muscles and bone structures other than just the spine.

Many people whose work is lifting and carrying heavy loads usually have lower back problems because they have a tendency to lift with their back instead of with their legs.

Another source of pain in the lower back or sacrum, can be the extra load that comes from a large stomach. A watermelon-shaped stomach in the front forces the lower back to carry an extra load, which either causes or increases the degree of sway or curvature in the back, or puts too much strain on the lower back muscles. Either effect can, and usually does, cause lower back pain. The strength and load-carrying capacity of the stomach muscles are as important as the strength and load-carrying capacity of the lower back muscles. Both are essential for good posture. Both are good friends.

The five lumbar vertebrae and the sacrum, which comprise the lower back, do not act alone but in close relationship with the joints of the hips. If the hip joints are stiff and inflexible, the load of the trunk movement usually falls on the lower back vertebrae. Therefore, to lessen the strain on the lower back, it is necessary to create better movement and flexibility of the hip joints and the muscles that operate them.

The same principles apply to the upper back and neck. Writers and typists, beauticians and dentists, housewives and other people who lean forward much of the time in their work, tend to have upper back and neck problems. It is important to free the shoulder muscles and joints before working with the upper spine and neck.

Furthermore, while it is very important to balance, stretch and strengthen the muscle systems of the body, it is equally important to straighten the spine and other bone structures and to make them flexible to avoid back and neck pain. For example, a rigid hip joint will cause trouble regardless of how strong the muscles are that support it. So, yoga works to straighten and align the bone systems, strengthen the muscles, and add flexibility.

A steady and conscientious program of yoga can put the balance back in your body and your whole life. As so many of my pupils, ranging in age from the teens to the nineties, have found, back problems can be prevented and are often cured by following these few hints and by practicing yoga every day:

* Improve your posture, as described in Chapter 4, "Yoga Way of Life."

* Don't let yourself become too tired or too tense.

* Don't allow yourself to become too cold or too hot.

* When lifting, do not bend your back. Instead, bend your knees and keep your back straight.

* Never bend forward without bending your knees.

* If you have a back pain, always have your knees bent slightly when doing Sit-Ups.

* When sitting or standing, tilt your pelvis forward and contract the muscles from your knees to your waist.

* Sleep on a firm mattress and avoid sleeping on your stomach.

* Since we naturally lean forward so much of the time, do exercises in which you bend backward, and from side to side, so your body moves freely in all directions.

* In the Daily Yoga Program be sure to perform the exercises that are special for the back and neck. These are the Full Body Stretch, Knees to Chest, Knee-Touch to Your Forehead, Sit-Ups, Cat Pose, Back to the Wall, and the Spinal Twist.

Following are exercises that are especially good for the neck, the middle back and the lower back.

FOR THE NECK (cervical spine)

This is a series of exercises in which your head and shoulders do not move. Only your neck and arm muscles are involved. Do not tense your face, keep it serene. Hold each position for fifteen to thirty seconds.

* Sit straight in the Lotus or any comfortable position. Interlace the fingers of your hands and, with your elbows up, put them against your forehead. Without moving your head, push your head forward against your hands and hold.

* With your fingers still interlaced, move your hands to the back of your head, and push your head back against your hands and hold.

* Place your right hand against the right side of your head above your ear, and place your left hand on your left thigh to give you balance and leverage. Push your head against your right hand and hold.

* Place your left hand on the left side of your head above your ear, your right hand on your right thigh. Push your head against your left hand and hold.

* Imagine your head having four corners, with your face, the back, and the sides of your head being the flat sides of a block. Place the palm of your right hand on the upper right front corner of this block (on your forehead). Your left hand is still on your thigh for balance and leverage. Push your head against your right hand and hold.

* Then put your left hand on the left front corner of your head and your right hand on your thigh. Push your head against your hand and hold.

* Do the same exercises for the back corners of your head, right corner with your right hand, left corner with your left hand and hold each time.

Only your head moves in this next series of five exercises. Hold each of these positions for only a few seconds.

* Tilt or bend your head backward, keeping your mouth open to prevent stretching the skin under your chin.

* Return your head to the straight position. Lean your head to the right side and try to touch your ear to your shoulder without bringing your shoulder up toward your ear.

* Return your head to the straight position. Repeat the former exercise, this time to the left shoulder.

* Return your head to the straight position. Then turn your head to your right, looking back over your right shoulder, carefully, as far as you can without straining your neck.

* Return your head to the straight position. Repeat the former exercise, looking back over your left shoulder.

These exercises that you have just completed strengthen and give flexibility to your neck muscles and cervical spine.

FOR THE MIDDLE BACK (thoracic spine)

The Fish and the Full Cobra, which are described in the Daily Yoga Program, are best for the middle back.

FOR THE LOWER BACK (lumbar spine)

An exercise in the Daily Yoga Program that is especially good for the lower back is the Diaphragm Lift. In addition, the following special exercise is tailored for the lower back:

* Sit with the left leg out straight and your left foot under a heavy object to hold your leg is place. Bring the right knee up to your chest with your heel on the floor touching your thigh. Fold both arms around the shin of your right leg. Put your forehead on the right knee. Without moving your forehead from your knee or releasing your arms from your leg, roll back slowly, feeling each vertebra touch the floor until you are lying down flat. Then, release your right leg and lie down flat for half a minute before

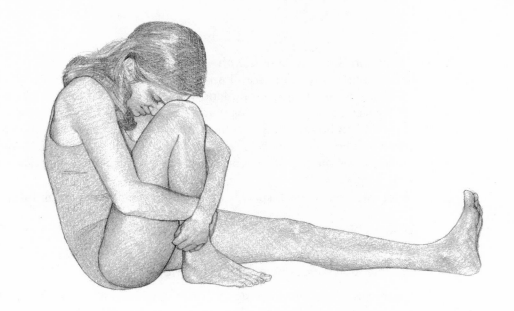

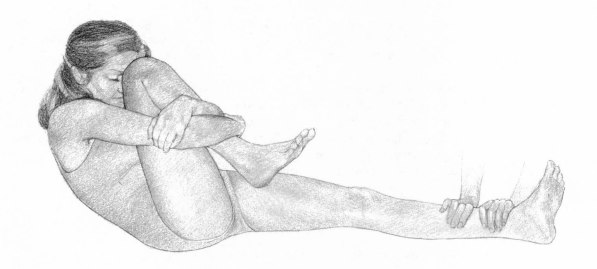

you do the same exercise with your left knee up. Do this exercise twice with each leg, once a day.

C. Constipation

Constipation is not fun to live with.

Constipation can result from bad eating habits, such as eating too much or too little, or eating the wrong kinds of food; tension, or lack of exercise. When constipated, you feel soggy and tired all the time, you can get head-aches, you can have stomach-aches from excess gas, your skin never looks fresh. In addition, constipation can lead to hemorrhoids, colon diseases and other serious ailments. When you are constipated, your whole system is out of order.

If you are constipated, specific advice I have found most helpful is:

* Before going to bed, eat one of these fruits: two figs, a slice of cantaloupe or a slice of papaya.

* Eat one tablespooonful of bran with one of your meals.

* Upon arising in the morning, mix the juice of half a lemon with half a teaspoonful of honey in a glass of warm water and drink it.

* Perform this exercise, a variation of the Diaphragm Lift, fifteen minutes after drinking the water: Standing straight, take a deep breath. Breathe out slowly, leaning a little bit forward. When you are empty, give your stomach this massage: Pull in your stomach and let it out, pull it in and let it out, as many times as you can before you have to breathe in. Breathe in when you can hold no longer. Do this twice.

The following exercises, which should be part of your Daily Yoga Program will be beneficial: Shoulder Stand, Plough and Spinal Twist. The Sit-Up is almost a specific for constipation. These exercises stretch most of the muscles in the abdomen, massage the visceral region and stimulate the liver, kidneys, pancreas and other organs.

When you are free of this problem, you will feel like a new person.

D. Headaches

Headaches can ruin a day faster than anything but a lover's rejection or a cut in pay. The insistent pain, the queazy feeling it produces as the stomach responds to the head's distress, the sense that nothing will come right until the headache goes, makes it imperative to find relief.

Common chronic headaches fall into two main categories: muscle tightening or tension headaches, and migraine headaches. People with sinus or eye problems often get headaches, too, but yoga can provide relief mostly for tension and migraine headaches. Although little is known about the cause of these headaches, tension headaches are thought to be due to contraction of neck and scalp muscles, usually from the stresses and strains of daily life.

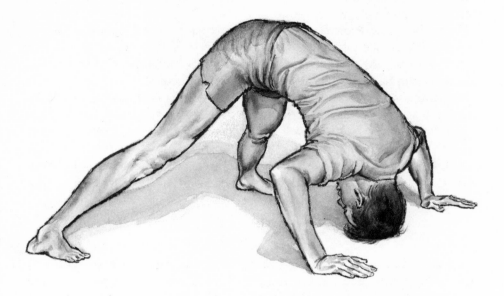

Migraine headaches are often associated with a rigid personality, although stress and tension are frequently the cause, too. It is also believed that heredity is a factor.

When people who have never had headaches before suddenly start getting them, or one's headaches have altered in type, pattern or intensity without a major change in a person's life to explain it, a visit to a doctor is indicated.

Most of the time, though, yoga full breathing and the Daily Yoga Program will relieve the miseries of a headache. From the Daily Yoga Program, emphasize these exercises and postures: Shoulder Stand, Arms, Neck and Shoulders, Reach Forward, and Dead Man's Pose.

In addition, here's a posture specifically designed to free you from tension and migraine headaches:

* Stand with legs as far apart as is comfortable and with feet parallel. Breathe in. Breathe out. Bend your elbows, bend forward to place your hands and head on the floor, with your head between your hands, which are spread as far apart as is comfortable. Your weight should be on your legs and hands, not on your head. Come up when you have to breathe in. Do this posture three times at first, increasing to six later.

E. *Insomnia*

Do you sometimes lie awake at night wondering why you are unable to sleep? Maybe you are too tense, are emotionally upset or overtired. Are you trying to force yourself to sleep or have you taken your work or your worries to bed with you? Has the evening been so exciting that you find it difficult to calm down? Is your stomach full? When did you exercise last? Are you satisfied with your mate?

Even if you are a chronic insomniac, you can learn to control your mind. You have to learn to tell your mind: "Let me sleep now and I will think later," and your mind will respond.

There are a few exercises that will really help you, as they have helped many of my pupils who had not been able to sleep more than a short period at a time for several years. Even my MS (multiple sclerosis) pupils, most of whom have a bladder problem, sleep peacefully all night.

You already, of course, have done your Daily Yoga Program, so fifteen minutes before you go to bed, do the Locust, the Cobra and a few Sit-Ups, several times each. Not only will your body rest, but your mind will relax, too, and you will get up refreshed in the morning.

Aren't you glad that now you can talk your mind into sleeping now and thinking later?

F. *Arthritis*

You don't have to be old to get arthritis. Some people are stricken with arthritis at an early age, others in their middle years, and some late in life. In all cases, yoga provides relief from the pain, suffering and restrictions in movement from arthritis that characterize this common ailment.

Arthritis and rheumatism are words used to describe about a hundred different ailments characterized by pain in the joints or muscles. Most chronic forms of arthritis are of unknown cause, including the two most common types, osteoarthritis and rheumatoid arthritis.

Osteoarthritis is known as a "wear and tear" disease because it frequently affects the weight-bearing joints most severely (ankles, knees, hips and spine). Very often hip joints are attacked, but the most common area is the backbone, especially the lower back, which has a lifetime of stress to support a body that stands upright and which is especially vulnerable when people put extra stress on their backs. The most effective preventative for arthritis of these types is to keep the joints flexible, the body aligned properly and the entire muscle structure in tone and strong to support the joints. Some experts believe that this form of arthritis is part of the normal aging process. Like most forms of chronic arthritis, there is no cure for osteoarthritis, but the symptoms can usually be controlled.

Rheumatoid arthritis is a chronic recurring inflammatory disease that causes swelling and at times deformity of many joints. In this form of arthritis, the hands are frequently involved but it can affect any joint in the body. Treatment of this disease is aimed at not only controlling symptoms, but also preventing deformity. Once again, no cure is known for this form of arthritis.

Yoga has helped many people with arthritis by keeping the joints flexible. While arthritis tends to limit movement, and in many cases is painful, yoga exercises work to expand the range of movement and relieve the pain. With arthritis, joints stiffen; yoga keeps them free.

I have seen dramatic results in many of my pupils. Many have been helped and have gotten their movement back. A woman of ninety could not walk, even had great difficulty getting out of bed in the morning. Now, she gets out of bed without pain. After doing yoga for twenty minutes a day, she walks for three miles.

Yoga relieves arthritic pain because it gives flexibility to the joints by the exercises, postures and deep breathing, and because it increases the flow of blood. Yoga provides relief from the pain of arthritis from any cause; stress, advanced age or any other reason. It also helps prevent arthritis from getting worse from tension or bad circulation.

It is particularly important for people suffering from arthritis to do the entire Daily Yoga Program. This will provide a treatment for all joints and muscles.

Within the Daily Yoga Program are several exercises and postures that are specifically designed to provide relief from arthritic pain and to restore freedom of movement. These are the Spinal Twist, the Full Body Stretch, Knees to Chest, Baby Cobra, Sit-Ups (with knees bent), Half Wheel (Buttocks Up and Down), Bicycle, and Arms, Neck and Shoulders.

In addition, there are two exercises that will help stiff shoulders and aching wrists. The posture called Back Nameste is designed to relieve the wrists from arthritic pain and stiffness. It is called Back Nameste because, when properly formed, it resembles the nameste pose, the Indian greeting in which the palms of the hands are held together in front of the body.

To do this exercise, simply place the palms together behind your back: ends of the fingers first, then the rest of the palms, between the shoulder blades with the fingers pointed up. At first, it may be impossible to place the whole of your palms together because the wrists or muscles of the upper back are too stiff. But, do as much as you can and, as you practice this posture, you will find it possible to bring the palms together. Press the hands together for one half minute, then release. Increase to one minute later. Breathe normally.

The Shoulder Blades Together is an exercise specifically for relieving arthritis in the upper back. It also helps to get rid of the dowager's hump, or round shoulders. To perform this exercise, lie on your stomach, bring your arms back and lift your chest off the floor slightly. Place your hands, palms up, on your buttocks and attempt to touch your shoulder blades together. Hold that position for ten to fifteen seconds, then release and relax. Do this three to six times, once a day. Breathe in while holding up, breathe out when coming down.

You will forget you ever had arthritis.

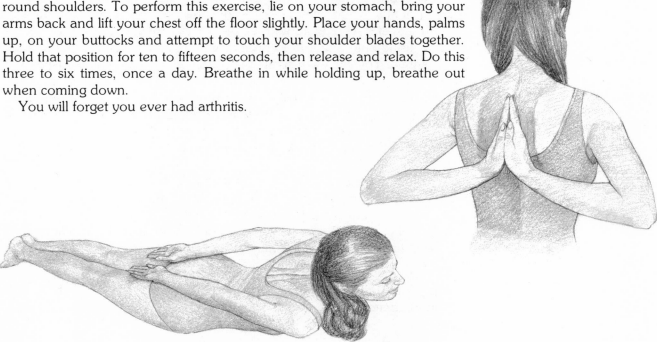

G. *Varicose Veins*

Varicose veins are a very common circulatory disorder, affecting the lower part of the body. Although the cause of the formation of varicose veins is not known, it is thought that they occur when the valves in the veins fail to function and do not permit backflow of the blood. Consequently, the veins become enlarged. Important factors in the cause of varicose veins are pregnancy, heredity, prolonged standing, and phlebitis.

Because people stand upright on two legs, the pressure and load of the entire body is borne by the lower half, following the law of gravity. Particularly susceptible are those who stand too long—behind counters or bars, VIPs standing long hours in receiving lines, and doctors and nurses. Women who have carried and borne children, and many people whose jobs require lifting and carrying heavy loads have the same problem. The older we get, the worse the problem can become.

I have prescribed several special exercises from the Daily Yoga Program for my pupils, and have seen remarkable results. These are the exercises I recommend for this problem. Do each one for two minutes, once a day: Tremble-Tremble, Half Wheel, Bicycle, and Full Locust.

Now you can go swimming and be proud of your legs.

H. *Tennis Elbow*

Most people who have "tennis elbow" do not even play tennis. What is called "tennis elbow" is an inflammation of the tendons or ligaments of the elbow. The cause and the exact nature of this condition are not understood well even by the medical profession.

We hold tension in different parts of our bodies. That restricts our movement and can cause injury and pain.

Other causes include: improper use of weak muscles in such activities as shaking hands in receiving lines for long periods at a time, workouts by amateur athletes who go about their game the wrong way, and workmen's habit of using only one arm to do the same thing all day, like hammering and painting. You can even create the condition while trimming bushes and trees.

Exercises from the full Daily Yoga Program will help relieve the tennis elbow problem, especially the Bow and Bridge. In addition, by practicing these three postures, a lot of my pupils have found relief, and some have gotten rid of that nasty elbow pain, completely.

* Sit with your legs straight out in front of you, the backs of your knees on the floor, arms behind your back, the palm of one hand on the floor near the tailbone, the other hand on top of it. Your fingers point away from your body. Be sure your back and elbows are straight. Hold one minute. Switch hands, and hold one minute.

* Now, sitting in the same position, turn the palms of both hands, one on top of the other, so your fingers face toward your tailbone. Hold one minute, switch hands, and hold one minute.

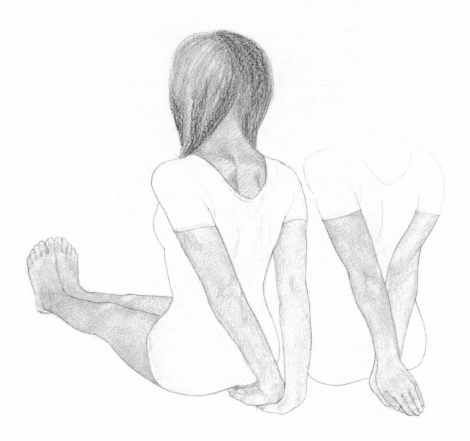

* Choose any sitting position you wish, but be sure your back is straight. Bring your right hand over your right shoulder and place it between your shoulder blades. Bring your left hand under and up behind your back to meet the right hand, and get a good grip on the fingers of both hands behind your back and between your shoulder blades. Hold the posture for a minute. Repeat on the other side, bringing your left hand over the shoulder and the right hand up in back from the waistline. Hold a minute. Do this once on each side at each sitting.

In all three of these positions, proceed slowly and gradually. Increase from one minute to two, and do a few times a day.

As your muscles gain strength, you'll be pleased with the results and happy to be playing tennis without that nasty pain again.

One final note. Yoga provides other benefits for tennis players. It helps them relax and improves coordination. It gives them confidence, speeds up their reflexes and increases their stamina.

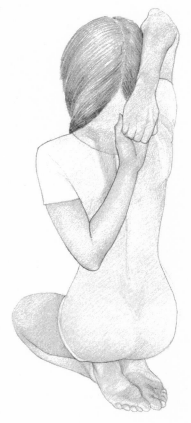

I. *Hemorrhoids*

This is something few people want to talk about.

Most people can endure a considerable amount of physical discomfort, even pain, as long as they can freely complain. With hemorrhoids, often known as piles, they suffer in silence as if some stigma were attached to the ailment. Sitting can become painful, but they are shy about telling anyone that they would be much more comfortable with a soft pillow under them rather than a hard chair. Even television and radio commercials for products to ease hemorrhoids are reluctant to discuss the problem.

Hemorrhoids may make victims as uncomfortable as arthritis or an aching back, but hemorrhoids remain the undiscussed discomfort. Lacking the solace of complaint, the sufferer has a more urgent desire to learn what he can do to be relieved.

The formation of hemorrhoids is the result of the enlargement of the blood vessels in the lower part of the colon. This results from pelvic congestion over a period of time. The congestion is caused by the collection of blood in the pelvic region, which results from the blood not being able to return to the heart as efficiently as it flows from the heart toward the pelvic region. This tends to expand the vessels, creating hemorrhoids.

Hemorrhoids can occur from any one of several causes. The tendency can be inherited. They can result from a tumor inside the abdomen. They can come from straining during bowel movements as a result of constipation. Hemorrhoids can occur from weakness of the muscles in the pelvic area.

People who live an inactive or sedentary life often develop hemorrhoids. People who drink too much alcohol can create hemorrhoids. People who eat too little roughage or too much highly seasoned food, or the wrong food, such as soft food, can develop hemorrhoids.

These few yoga exercises which I recommend for the prevention and relief of hemorrhoids are designed to stimulate the blood flow to relieve pelvic congestion. They also strengthen and tone the muscles in the pelvic area.

The following exercises, which should be part of your Daily Yoga Program, will be beneficial: Diaphragm Lift, Pelvic Stretch, Spinal Twist, Shoulder Stand, Bow and Hamstring Stretch. In addition, this exercise is a specific for hemorrhoids. It should be performed as follows:

* Standing with your feet about twelve inches apart, bend forward and grasp the insteps of your feet with your hands.

    Holding onto your insteps with your feet parallel or toes pointed in slightly, keeping your heels down, slowly lower your buttocks to a position of sitting on your haunches. Keep elbows between your knees. At first, you may not be able to assume a sitting position.

    Slowly raise your buttocks until your legs are straight again, while continuing to hold the insteps of your feet. While raising, contract the muscles in and around the pelvic area.

Repeat this exercise slowly three to six times, once a day, keeping the feet parallel and toes pointed in slightly, or pointed in as much as you can. This is the trick that gives your muscles the best treatment. The important

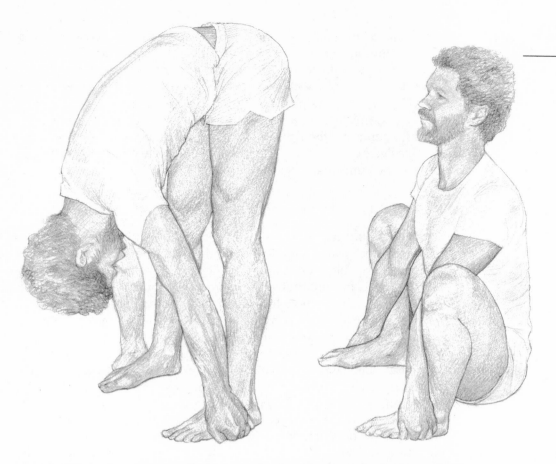

part is the contracting you do as you slowly raise your buttocks each time.
Think how nice it will be to be relieved of this silent suffering.

J. *For Men Only*

Men pay for the strains and tensions of their working lives with a variety of ailments that can put them out of action or slow them down. Often they have a choice. Either they can let their condition deteriorate to the point where only an operation can help them, or they can recognize the early signs and take the steps to help themselves. These are the yoga steps.

Not all male problems are medical. Some are a matter of appearance, at least in the beginning. Just as women have to worry about a bulging lower stomach, men can accumulate a protruding upper stomach that gives them the look of a pouter pigeon. Furthermore, men are even worse off than women when it comes to round shoulders. While women harm their appearance with a dowager's hump, men handicap themselves with stiff shoulders that not only look awkward, but limit their arm movements and their game skills. They have built up their upper back muscles carelessly to the point that they can't even straighten their arms over their heads.

Shortened gluteus maximus muscles and tight hamstrings seem more common among men than women. Where women exercise these muscles by bending over the stove, bed-making or picking up babies, men often lack these natural forms of exercise and thus lose strength and flexibility in their movements.

Other problems that plague some men are the enlarged prostate gland, after age fifty; impotence; hernia, and baldness. No matter how much men fancy themselves as athletes, no matter how faithfully they run or ski or swim, men face some physical problems that women are mostly spared.

For solving any of these problems, the entire body must be healthy. As the body is a complete unit, a series of exercises and postures that stretch the muscles, strengthen the spine, loosen the joints and improve the circulation, such as in the Daily Yoga Program, are essential. In addition, specific exercises and postures are suggested for each problem.

THE PROSTATE GLAND

Some men find after the age of fifty the prostate gland may become enlarged. The prostate gland is located behind the bladder. This enlargement presses against the bladder, causing difficulty in passing urine. Several things are believed to contribute to the prostate problem. Too much sedentary life, too much alcohol, too much highly seasoned food, and too much straining to overcome constipation are all irritating factors that can lead to pelvic congestion and enlargement of the prostate.

Yoga can prevent the enlargement of the prostate and in several ways can reduce the difficulties of passing urine caused by an enlarged prostate. First, practicing yoga will prevent constipation, which may be a contributing factor. Second, practicing yoga will promote good circulation, which will keep the gland healthy. Finally, yoga exercises and postures promote good muscle tone, allowing the muscles in the pelvic area to overcome the obstruction the enlarged prostate gland causes to the passage of urine. The Head Stand and the advanced variations of the Diaphragm Lift, "In and Out" and "Side to Side," in which the abdomen is forced in and out while the air is out, are particularly good for relieving congestion in the pelvic region, which often leads to enlargement of the prostate.

IMPOTENCE

Potency, or the achievement of good sexual function in men, is a complex phenomenon that depends on many factors such as healthy sex glands and good overall physical, emotional and mental health. A few men are impotent because of neurological problems, a lack of hormones or a birth defect. These cases require special medical attention.

However, several factors can contribute to impotence in men who have no serious medical problems. Among them are poor muscle tone, unhealthy sex glands, poor overall health, an overactive bladder, constipation, pelvic congestion, an enlarged prostate, tension, anxiety, and lack of self-confidence.

From the viewpoint of emotional health, an ideal life would be characterized by absolute psychological stability. To achieve this, you should:

* Be aware that your emotional and physical health are one and the same.

* Learn to control your emotions and face the challenges of life.

* Realize that you are your own best teacher. Pay attention to how you react to events and circumstances.

* Never forget that your frame of mind can enormously influence your health and well-being.

To conquer impotence, you must learn to relax, overcome anxiety and develop self-confidence. Yoga provides the necessary discipline to achieve this goal, and many yoga exercises and postures provide relaxation and freedom from anxiety, which is believed to be the number one cause of impotency.

In addition to the Daily Yoga Program, these three exercises are specifics for sexual function: Knees to Chest, Half Wheel and the quick variation of Shooting Legs Out. The first two are included in the Daily Yoga Program, and the quick variation of Shooting Legs Out is covered in the section "About Sex" in Chapter 4.

HERNIA

A hernia is an abnormal protrusion of an organ, or part of an organ, from any cavity of the body to the outside, or from one cavity to another cavity. An example of a hernia between cavities is the hiatus hernia, which occurs between the chest and the abdomen. Hernias can occur in other places in the body also, but the place that a hernia occurs so often in men is in the groin.

Yoga can prevent hernias from occurring and can prevent them from recurring after a hernia operation. Yoga develops and strengthens the muscles and the muscle walls through which hernias can occur, by exercise and by increasing the blood circulation. The Hanging Buttocks Stretch and exercises for the pelvic area in the Daily Yoga Program will help prevent the groin hernia in men.

Another exercise that is very helpful is the contracting of all the muscles from your hip joints to your knees several times a day. However, if you have a hernia, a mild hernia or a weakness toward a groin hernia, be careful to note the exercises in the Daily Yoga Program that are to be avoided or used with care.

BALDNESS

Baldness, which occurs commonly in men, can result from heredity, from infections of the scalp, from too much or too little secretion from the pores in the scalp, and from deficient blood supply and general weakness.

Practicing yoga can relieve many of the conditions that contribute to baldness. It automatically promotes better circulation and contributes to better general or overall health, both of which are essential for healthy hair. Yoga also relieves tension and tension produces a tight scalp, which restricts the supply of blood to the hair and affects the secretion from the pores. The Daily Yoga Program leads to a healthier scalp and the retention of hair. Two specific exercises that will help are the Head Stand and Nose to Knee.

In addition, once a week before shampooing, massage coconut oil into the scalp with a brisk finger movement to stimulate circulation. This will add some needed nutrients to the hair while giving the scalp a good massage, which will help relax the scalp and stimulate the flow of blood to the head.

LARGE STOMACH

Many men, especially as they get older, develop a large or bulging upper abdomen. While it is more pronounced in men that are overweight, even a thin man can develop a large stomach. Most excess weight seems to accumulate first above the belt in most men. Whether it comes from drinking too much alcoholic beverages or eating too much food, the reasons for the bulge above the belt are a weakening of the muscles in the abdominal wall and the accumulation of fatty tissue both inside and outside the abdominal wall.

By concentrating more on the exercises involving the abdomen in the Daily Yoga Program, the large stomach can be brought under control. The Diaphragm Lift is very good for getting rid of the accumulated fat inside the abdomen, and Shooting Legs Out, the Spinal Twist, and Sit-Ups are particularly good for strengthening the abdominal wall muscles. In addition, a good habit for a man with a bulging stomach problem is to practice contracting the muscles from knees to waistline when standing and sitting.

ROUND SHOULDERS

Round shoulders or a thick upper back is very common in men, and usually comes from bad posture, being muscle bound, and the range of common male activities requiring them to bend forward. Most time spent at a desk involves leaning forward. Even while standing, it is easier to slump forward than to stand straight. As the back muscles are used less with advancing age, they tend to follow the shape the person provides most of the time, and this is usually a round upper back.

The problems that stem from round shoulders are many. The worst is a spine that is out of alignment. Lower back problems and upper back problems can come from round shoulders. Since all bones and muscles are directly or indirectly connected to the spine, an unhealthy spine can lead to unhealthy arms, legs, neck and many other parts of the body.

Round shoulders restrict the space that the lungs require for full or deep breathing. Thus, respiratory problems can result, in part, from round shoulders.

The Daily Yoga Program is designed to prevent and correct round shoulders. All exercises that require placing the hands above the head, including Back Against the Wall and Full Body Stretch, provide the opportunity to straighten the shoulders. The Full Locust, the Bow, and the Fish are specific exercises for the upper back.

In addition, Push-Ups provide several benefits that combine to prevent and correct round shoulders. They strengthen the arms, chest, shoulders and abdominal muscles, which stops the chest from sagging and the shoulders from getting round.

To begin the Push-Ups, lie on your stomach, palms next to your chest on the floor. With your fingers, point straight ahead and curl your toes on the floor. Keeping your body absolutely straight and stiff, push your body up by straightening your arms while you breathe in. Then, lower your chest to within one inch of the floor, keeping your body straight. Start with three Push-Ups, once a day, increasing to ten.

SHORT GLUTEUS MAXIMUS MUSCLES

This problem is the lack of flexibility in the muscles from the lower back to the feet, but mostly in the gluteus maximus muscles, or upper buttocks, and the hamstring. These muscles become so short in most men that they cannot bend over and touch the floor without bending their knees. Some cannot even reach their knees. This condition comes from years of inactivity in these muscles, mostly from sitting at a desk, a position which specifically permits the muscles to become shorter. To maintain full flexibility in the muscles of the lower back, the gluteus maximus and the hamstring must be stretched.

To stretch these muscles, concentrate on the forward bending exercises and postures such as the Triangle, Touch and Sit, and Reach Forward with your Daily Yoga Program. Gradually, these muscles will stretch, allowing you to have greater flexibility of movement, which among other things, will permit you to derive more benefit from all of the yoga exercises and postures that you do.

Won't it be great to get rid of these problems and be a fully healthy man again?

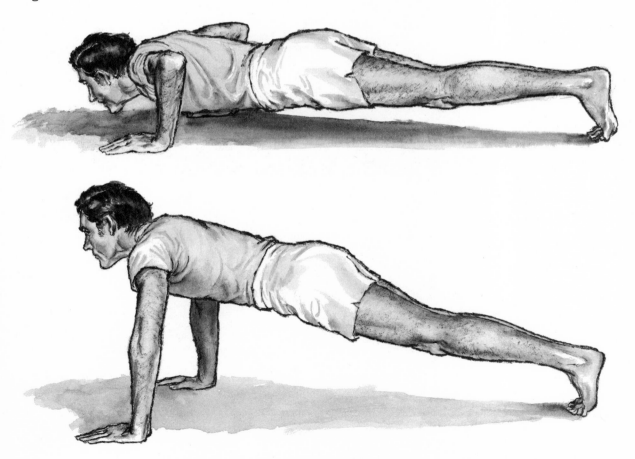

The Head Stand provides many of the same benefits as the Shoulder Stand. A difference is the Head Stand gives extra stimulation to the entire nervous system, particularly the brain.

To save the beautiful woman's neck from getting muscular and thick, I do not teach my women pupils this posture. Instead, I encourage them to do the Shoulder Stand.

For the Head Stand, your mat should be doubled to be two inches thick, and wide enough for your elbows to be on it. Always practice near a wall, so if you lose your balance you will have support.

* Kneel on the floor. Interlock your fingers. Bring your head and elbows to the floor. Place the top of your head on the floor so that the back of your head is supported by the palms of your hands when you begin to go up. Your elbows should be about twelve inches apart. Hold your hands tightly against your head. Your hands, head, elbows and forearms will be your sole support. Breathe freely and regularly throughout this exercise.

* Slowly, straighten your knees until you are balancing on your head, hands, forearms, elbows, and on the balls of your feet. Now, slow, slow, step by step, one foot at a time, walk toward your chest; be sure to keep your knees straight. Walk on the tips of your toes until your thighs are close to your chest. Do not change the position of your hands, head or arms. Keep your elbows down tight.

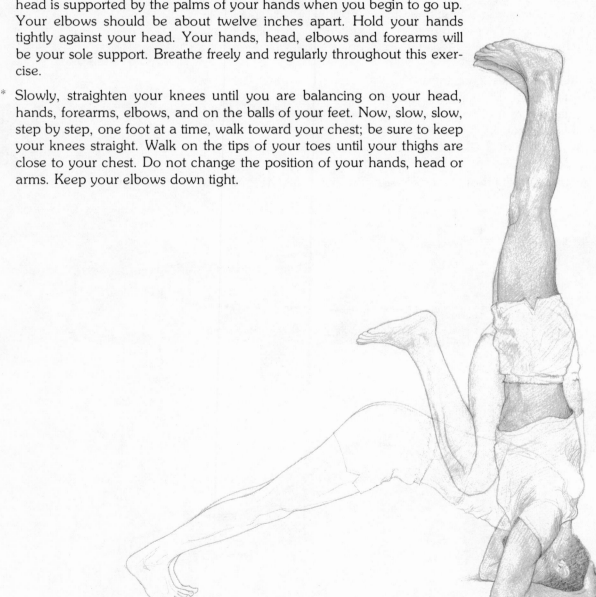

* Slowly, and with balance and control, lift your feet off of the floor. Do not jerk and don't push or kick to go up or you might fall over backward. When your time comes to go up, you will feel and get a natural push that comes from your balance and the distribution of your weight.

* Bend your knees and bring your legs up, with your thighs close to your chest, still holding your head and elbows in the same position. Remain there briefly, holding your balance until you have confidence; then slowly raise your legs up straight. Contract your buttocks and keep your legs together.

* To come down from the Head Stand, bend your knees and slowly bring your feet to the floor. You should never come down with straight knees or you might lose your balance.

* If you want to go up again, rest a few minutes before you do. While up, your balance is mainly on your elbows and forearms, rather than directly on your head. My advice is that you never stay more than five minutes in the Head Stand. For a month or so, start with half a minute and reach, if you wish, to no more than five minutes at a time.

BENEFITS

Strengthens and builds up neck muscles.
Good for the growth of your hair.
Rejuvenates the brain cells.
Stimulates the circulation of your whole body.
Increases vitality.
Reverses the influence of gravity on your internal organs.
Relieves pelvic congestion.

DO NOT DO

If you have neck problems.
If you have high blood pressure, low blood pressure, heart trouble, or weak eye capillaries.
If you are suffering from congestion of the ears.

K. *Multiple Sclerosis*

Nowhere does the self-discipline of yoga bring greater rewards than in helping the crippled to walk again, to use muscles thought to be long dead and to control previously uncontrolled internal organs.

The beneficiaries of this rebirth through yoga were all victims of multiple sclerosis, a disease of the central nervous system. It may block messages from the brain to the eyes, arms, legs, bladder, or anywhere in the body. When the doctor diagnoses this disease, the patient often says, "This is it!" I say, "This is not it! Don't ever give up. There is such a thing as help yourself and God helps you."

They came to my class in wheelchairs or leaning on canes or walkers. It was the first yoga class for victims of multiple sclerosis in the country. At first they thought I was mean, but then realized that I feel and care about them and had to be firm. Doctors marveled at the effects of yoga on my pupils.

A woman in a wheelchair whose pet phrase was "I can't," changed her thinking to "I will." She walked without help across the room. A girl who couldn't even sit up on her exercise mat without bracing her back, gradually managed to sit up without leaning, and then to stand and finally to walk the width of my studio with television cameras recording her smiling progress. A girl whose bladder was so uncontrolled that she had to get up several times nightly, now sleeps through the night. A girl whose neck trembled all the time, with the discipline of yoga, has learned muscle control and now she has her neck under control.

It was the magic combination of their own self-discipline and the self-confidence I was able to give them that made yoga their hope for a new life. Like the beautiful flowers that come back year after year to reward you for your care of their garden, yoga rewards the faithful with a heightened self-discipline that becomes part of their whole life.

After faithfully following my Daily Yoga Program, now it has become an important part of their everyday lives. By contracting their lower body muscles for their bladders, by breathing for their lungs and relaxation, and by stretching and contracting all of their muscles to sit up and walk, the bodies of my pupils with multiple sclerosis are waking up again.

6
Woman and Her Beauty Regime

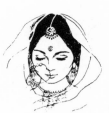

Now that yoga exercises and proper eating are changing the shape of your body, now that yoga breathing is feeding your bloodstream with an ever-fresh supply of oxygen, and yoga discipline is strengthening your mind and your will, your self-image is changing. You visualize yourself as younger, more vital, but what does your mirror say?

Look at those frown lines running between your eyes and creasing your forehead, the tension lines like parenthesis marks at the corners of your mouth, the bags under your eyes, the suggestion of a double chin. Your life before yoga created those premature signs of age. Your life with yoga can bring your face closer to your new image of yourself.

Nobody can erase all the signs of living, and you wouldn't want to because the experiences of a full and happy life can make a pleasant face beautiful. But you can go to work on the wrinkles created by tension, disagreements, dissatisfaction with yourself. If you realize that one sad expression can create one wrinkle, one tightening of the lips in anger can produce a new line, you can understand that regular facial exercises—what I call my "faces"—can get rid of some of the lines that add nothing to your looks but unwanted age.

The faces you make, while my skin-nourishing treatment covers you from forehead to neck, will give your skin a gentle massage without the stretching and pulling you would get from a hand massage.

The hair treatment will leave your hair glowing, looking more alive. My hand exercises will make your fingers supple and ache-free, while my foot exercises will put a spring back into your walk. Last but not least, my exercises and recommendations to tone and care for the breast will make a complete picture of a new you from head to toe.

My beauty regime should now make you look as good as you feel with your yoga way of life.

A. *Making Faces for Wrinkle-free Youthfulness*

When you feel good, you smile. And that's the most effective wrinkle remover of all. To prevent wrinkles before your time, do the following exercises according to instructions. Your goal is to tone your facial muscles, keep them elastic, and improve the circulation without stretching or harming the skin.

MOUTH OPEN FACE

Open your mouth wide, as if you were yawning, your eyes as wide as you can, and lift your eyebrows. Hold for half a minute. Then close your mouth and eyes tight and feel the muscles contracting. Do this twice.

This is for drooping cheeks and for circulation all over your face.

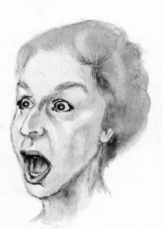 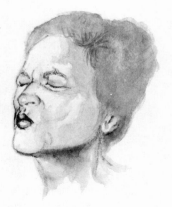

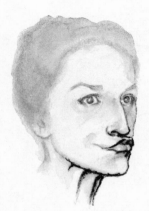

MONKEY FACE

Bring your upper lip up to touch your nose. Then bring your lower lip to meet your upper lip. Hold for half a minute and release.

This is for picking up hanging jowls and helps the chin line.

"O" FACE

Make an "O" with your mouth, pull your eyebrows up. With your eyes wide open, try to move your lower eyelids up and down without moving the upper lids. You will learn this by concentrating on the lower lids. Do for half a minute.

This is to get rid of the bags under your eyes.

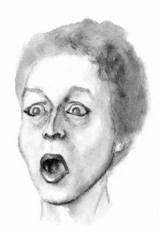

BLOW FACE

Close your lips, fill your cheeks with air as in a balloon, pushing the air upward and keeping it in. Hold your lips firm but not too tight, to avoid vertical lines above your upper lip. Hold for half a minute.
This is for your smiling lines and all the furrows.

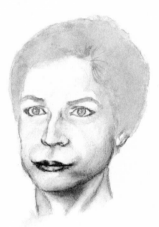

FISH FACE

Suck your cheeks in as if you were whistling and, while your mouth is in that position, move your jaws from side to side, at least three times each side.

This is very good for your neck muscles and your double chin.

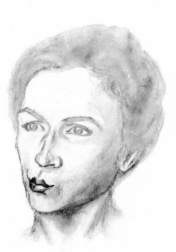

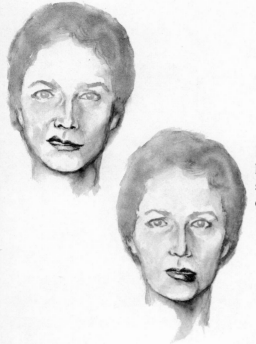

UGLY FACES

Hold your lips a little apart and very relaxed. Move the four corners of your lips, one at a time: pull up the right corner lightly, without any strain or stretch, as if you were sneering; then the left corner up; then the right corner down, and then the left corner down. Repeat this exercise twice.

This is for vertical lines above your upper lip.

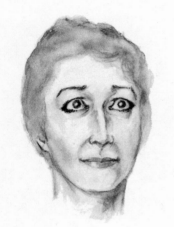

EYEBROWS UP AND DOWN

Your face relaxed, move your eyebrows up and down without moving any part of your face. Do this three times.

This is for the frown lines between your eyes.

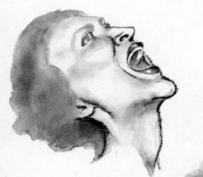

HEAD BACKWARD AND FORWARD

Drop your head back as far as you can, while leaving your mouth fully open. Come forward slowly, then push your chin forward toward your chest and keep the skin under your chin contracted, not folded. Do this three times.

This is for the double chin.

CROW'S FEET

Open your eyes fully, eyebrows up. Now, close your eyes slowly and while they are closed, raise your eyebrows up and down, concentrating on your upper lids and resisting opening your eyes. Do this three times.

This is for your crow's feet.

These facial exercises will help you to get rid of the stale and set expressions.

B. *Skin Care*

Give your skin an extra glow by keeping it clean and nourished. Learn to treat it lovingly. Whatever climate you live in, whether cold, hot, dry or humid, and whatever type of skin you have, whether normal, oily or dry, cleanliness is a must. Many people with dry skin think they should not clean it often. On the other hand, those with oily skin think they should wash it frequently. Dry, oily or normal, what all skin needs is tender cleaning, morning and evening.

Everything I advise for treating the skin comes from the kitchen. The advantages of these ingredients are that they are pure, nourishing and safe, and what is good internally is also good externally. These are the items from your kitchen for your skin care:

almonds	eggs
almond oil	honey
avocado	lemon
banana	milk
bread	oatmeal flour
chick-pea flour	wholewheat flour
corn flour	yogurt (plain)
cucumber	

EVERYDAY SKIN CARE TREATMENT

For dry skin, put a teaspoonful of plain yogurt in the palm of your hand and apply it to your face as if it were soap. For normal skin, mix in your palm half a teaspoonful of plain yogurt with half a teaspoonful of any of the four flours, making a paste, and apply it to your face. If your skin is oily, take a full teaspoonful of one of the flours in your hand, add a little water

SAVITRI'S WAY TO
PERFECT FITNESS
THROUGH HATHA
YOGA

and make a paste of it, to use as a soap. Whatever kind of skin you have, be gentle with it. Whatever mixture you use, wash it off with lukewarm water and then sprinkle your face with cold water. This is the best all-purpose way to clean your face. Now, pat your face dry with a towel. Your skin is clean.

If you have oily skin, you need nothing more after cleaning it. If you have normal or dry skin, apply a small amount of pure almond oil, without perfume. This is your regular, daily skin care.

Before I give you the Seven-Days-a-Month Facial Treatment, here are a few important hints for everyday care:

* Whenever your skin feels dry, take a soft cloth, dip it in rosewater, and pat it on your face and neck.

* Drink a lot of water to keep your face and skin young. It is also good for your body.

* Use a little lemon juice to remove blackheads. A touch with your fingertip daily is enough.

* Before you go to a party, refresh your skin by making a paste of one peeled cucumber and one tablespoonful of honey, mixing it in a blender. Apply this to your face and neck and leave it on no longer than five minutes. Wash off with plain water. The remaining paste can be stored in the refrigerator for a few days.

* Be sure to include your chin and neck in any face treatment. Your neck is an important part of your appearance.

REMEMBER THESE NEVERS:

* Never be harsh to your skin; no pulling, no stretching, no rough massaging. That will damage it.

* Never go to bed with makeup on. Your skin will not have a chance to breathe.

* Never wash your face with hot water. It takes away the natural moisture.

* Never use facial tissues for removing makeup. Use only some form of sterilized cotton.

* Never use a washcloth for washing your face. It is too rough for the delicate facial skin.

* Never use heavy creams. If you use any creams, I recommend oils, such as almond oil, salad oil, avocado oil, mustard oil or sesame oil. Apply with upward and outward movements, and keep away from your eyes.

* Never expose your face to too much sun or frost. Your skin will age.

* Never frown. It gives you wrinkles.

* Never use too much makeup. It clogs your pores.

The health of the body is reflected in the skin.

THE SEVEN-DAY-A-MONTH FACIAL TREATMENT

This treatment is for seven days each month. It should be done for seven consecutive days or if this is not convenient, it can be spaced throughout the month. It is for the face, but would be beneficial for the neck, arms and hands, too. Be careful to keep it out of the eyes. Clean your skin before applying these treatments.

It is important that the treatments be done in the following sequence.

FIRST DAY

1 teaspoon chick-pea flour (or corn flour)
1 teaspoon of egg white

Mix together and apply to skin. Leave on for forty minutes. After twenty minutes, when mixture begins to dry, start doing my facial exercises. Wash with warm water, then with cold water (no soap). Dry well.

SECOND DAY

Almond Oil

Apply almond oil to your face and neck. Then, with a pan of boiling water, cover your head with a towel and steam your face. Gently wipe off.

NOTE: Put five shelled almonds in one tablespoonful of milk to soak overnight for use on the Third Day.

THIRD DAY

5 shelled almonds soaked in milk

Skin the almonds that have been soaking in milk overnight, grind them, and mix them with the same milk. Put the paste on your face and leave it there for ten minutes. Then wash it off with warm water, then cold.

FOURTH DAY

Freshly cut tomato half

Rub your face lightly, all over, with the cut half of a tomato. After a few minutes, no more than five, wash with plain water.

FIFTH DAY

1 slice avocado
1 piece of banana

Mash the avocado and banana together and apply the mixture to your face. Leave it on for forty minutes. Do my facial exercises during that time. Wash off with warm, then cold water.

SIXTH DAY

1 teaspoon chick-pea flour (or corn flour)
Juice of ½ lemon

Mix to form a paste. Apply to face and leave on for forty minutes. Do facial exercises during this time. Wash off with warm, then cold water. Apply oil or light moisturizing cream.

SEVENTH DAY

½ slice bread (any plain bread)
1 tablespoonful of milk

Mash together with hands and apply to face. Leave on for five minutes. This has a moisturizing effect on the skin. Wash off with plain water.

Your skin will feel fresh like morning dew.

C. *About Hair*

Hairstyles and fashions come and go—long, short, curly, straight, but healthy and well-groomed hair always will be in fashion. Whatever we wear, however we are dressed, we never feel well dressed without clean and shining hair.

If your health is not good, your hair cannot be healthy either. If you do not feel good, your hair will show it. If you are to have healthy hair, you need good circulation to your scalp and a proper diet. Unless you have a medical problem such as a scalp disease, these few suggestions will help to make you happier about your hair:

* Your Daily Yoga Program will stimulate the circulation of your blood, which will provide more oxygen and nutrients to your hair.

* Washing and keeping your hair clean is very necessary. Washing once a week is sufficient; washing more often tends to take away the natural oil.

* Brush your hair every night before going to bed, using a real bristle brush, not a nylon one. This is necessary to stimulate the circulation in the scalp and allow the hair to breathe.

* When you brush, put your head down and brush the hair from the back toward the front. Then brush side to side. Do not brush the scalp.

* Give your hair an oil treatment once a week. Massage pure coconut oil (which is at room temperature) into your scalp. Massage briskly with your fingertips. Wiggle and circle your scalp. Press both thumbs into the base of your skull and move with a circular motion. Then, place all your fingers, including your thumbs, on your head, moving your forehead and scalp as you massage your head briskly. Do this one to two hours before shampooing. After shampooing, rinse your hair with one-half cup of

plain yogurt, and then rinse again with clear water. This entire treatment keeps the head cool and gives nourishment to the hair.

* Try to dry your hair naturally rather than with electric heating.

* Trim your hair at least once a month to keep it growing healthily.

* Massage your hair once a day by grasping handfuls of hair and pulling it up, around, and back and forth until the scalp tingles. This head self-massage can be done any time you find convenient.

This entire treatment will help prevent baldness and even has restored hair in many cases.
Aren't you pleased you gave lasting health to your unhealthy hair?

D. *Eye Exercises*

Your eyes are too important to overlook. They reveal the state of your health. They reflect your mood. They express your personality.

To return the sparkle to your eyes when you are tired and tense and to give them a treat, try these exercises:

* Sit in a comfortable position, with your spine erect. Take one or two deep breaths. Look straight ahead, your eyes sharply open. Do not blink for as long as you can. When your eyes start watering, close them gently. If they do not water at first, this means your eyes are tense. Close your eyes and then try again.

The following exercises will reduce the tension in your eyes. As you master them, your eyes will be able to water easily.
Now, work with your eyeballs only, without moving your head.

* Open your eyes sharp, again. Look up toward your eyebrows, then to your right side, then your left side, down toward your chin, and finally, straight ahead. Close your eyes briefly, open them wide again. This time, look down, left, up, right and back straight ahead. Close your eyes. Do this exercise two times.

* With eyes open, roll your eyes clockwise and then counterclockwise, in one continuous motion. Do two rounds, each side (like Eddie Cantor). Close your eyes. Open eyes wide and look side to side (right to left, left to right). Then look up to down, down to up. Do this exercise two times.

* Imagine a spot in the middle of your forehead, look up there; and one on the tip of your nose, look there. Go back to looking straight ahead, eyes wide open. Do this twice.

* Open eyes wide, try to feel that you are pushing your eyeballs out and in. Close your eyes. Do this twice.

* Finally, put the palms of your hands on your closed eyelids, with your eyeballs fitting comfortably in heels of your hands. With a light touch,

revolve your hands clockwise and then counterclockwise, without stretching the skin of your eyelids. Repeat two times. Open your eyes and enjoy the refreshing light.

All of these exercises strengthen the eye muscles, stop you from frowning and get rid of headaches caused by eye strain.

Don't do these exercises if you have any eye disease, and do not force them.

Smile with your eyes, not with your mouth only.

E. *For Supple Hands*

Hands were created for more than just performing the everyday tasks of life. A woman's hands can open the door to romance with a telling gesture, a gentle touch, an artfully careless flick of the wrist. Shapely fingers invite sparkling jewels from dinner rings to wedding rings. For the hands, my yoga exercises offer twin benefits. They will insure the shapeliness of your fingers and keep them supple. They also can free your hands from the arthritic aches that attack joints and the stiff fingers that destroy the hands' natural grace. Hands were made for loving, not hiding.

To make your hands more flexible and supple, do these exercises. Sit in the Lotus position if you can. Otherwise, sit straight in any comfortable position:

* Put the palms of your hands together in front of your chest (but not touching it) with your fingertips pointing up. Press the heels of your hands together hard. You must hold your elbows up at *all* times. Breathe in and hold; release when you have to breathe out. This exercise strengthens the pectoral muscles, thus firming the bust. Do this exercise three times.

* With elbows and hands in same position, press the fingers of your right hand hard against the fingers of your left, and bend only the fingers back as far as you can. Repeat with left fingers pressing against the right ones. The palms of your hands stay together at all times. Breathe normally while doing this exercise. Do three times each side.

* While elbows and hands stay in the same position, pull the fingers of each hand away from the other hand, with palms still together and without dropping your elbows. Take a deep breath, hold; release when you have to breathe out. Do this exercise three times.

* With elbows and hands in the same position, press your fingers together while separating your palms. Breathe in, hold; and release when you have to breathe out. Do this exercise three times.

* With elbows in the same position and hands at the same level, clasp your fingers. Take a deep breath and pull, but don't let go. Hold until you have to breathe out, then release. This exercise also strengthens the pectoral muscles. Do this exercise three times.

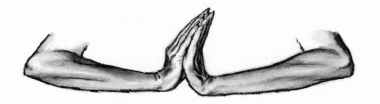

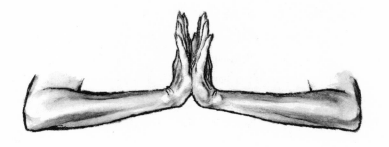

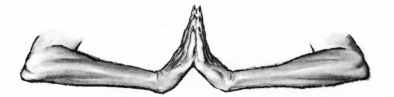

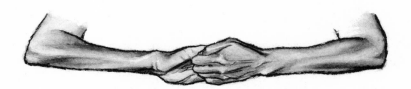

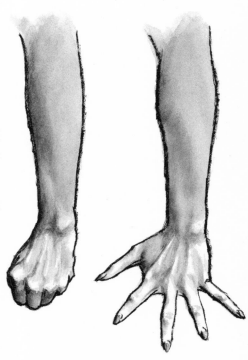

* Put your hands to your sides. With palms facing the floor, open all fingers sharply, then close to make a tight fist. Release, and drop your fingers down and shake hands loosely. Breathe normally. Do this exercise three times.

You will be surprised how your hands will be not only more flexible and supple, but more beautiful, too.

F. *For Feet and Ankles*

Our feet are our weight-bearing silent servants. Why should they suffer from lack of exercise and lose their strength, flexibility and good looks? You can prevent the accidents of muscle tears, pulls and strains by keeping your feet and ankles in condition. Healthy and well-balanced feet are the result of preserving the arches and maintaining the full range of movement in the joints, particularly the joints connecting the toes with the foot bones.

Proper foot care includes:

* Wearing comfortable shoes that fit properly.

* Walking and/or running with proper shoes.

* Avoiding high heels because they throw your balance off and your body forward. This unnatural posture leads to backache and tired feet.

* Not standing on one foot. This throws the body out of line, causing muscle imbalance in the back, and also brings back problems. While standing, especially for long periods of time such as in a receiving line or at a party, stand evenly on both feet and equally on your toes and heels. This keeps your foot, leg and back muscles in balance and prevents fatigue.

Do these feet and ankle exercises:

* Sit on the floor with both legs in front of you, feet six inches apart. Move your toes inward (touching the big toes if possible) then outward, then forward and then backward. Do not bend your knees. Do this six times, twice a day.

* Lie on your back with your legs straight up in the air, soles of your feet facing the ceiling. Move your toes up (toward the ceiling) then out or apart, while your heels are touching. Then move your heels apart while your toes are touching. Do this cycle six times, twice a day.

* Stand with the front half of your feet on a large book that is about two inches thick. Standing erect, try to lower your heels to touch the floor. Raise your heels to a level with your toes, then try to touch the floor with them again. Try touching the floor with your heels six times, twice a day.

* Standing flat on the floor, lift your toes off of the floor so you are standing on your heels only. Then lower your toes to the floor and stand on your toes only. Do this six times, twice a day.

One evening each week, before going to bed, soak your feet in warm water for ten minutes. Dry your feet and gently massage them with Vaseline petroleum jelly or oil. Put on an old pair of socks and sleep that way.

Your feet and ankles will silently thank you for this extra care.

G. *The Female Breast*

The female breast provides a continuous source of wonder for everyone—infants as well as people of all ages. Not only is it attractive, but it serves the useful purpose of providing nutrition for babies.

Contrary to what many people believe, the breasts are not composed of muscular tissue, but a combination of fibrous and fatty tissue, which determines their size and shape. The breasts are supported by the pectoral muscles. If these muscles are weak or lose their tone, the breasts will sag and lose their shape. A beautiful body does not permit sagging or pendulous breasts, which can result from lack of exercise, exercising without proper support, wearing improper-fitting brassieres, or a shortage of hormones usually due to aging.

To prevent such sagging, a woman needs to wear proper-fitting bras—especially when she's exercising; to develop correct posture; to maintain a proper position while feeding a baby, and to exercise the pectoral muscles regularly.

Size and shape are not the only considerations for a beautiful breast; suppleness and healthy clear skin are also important. Daily, the breasts

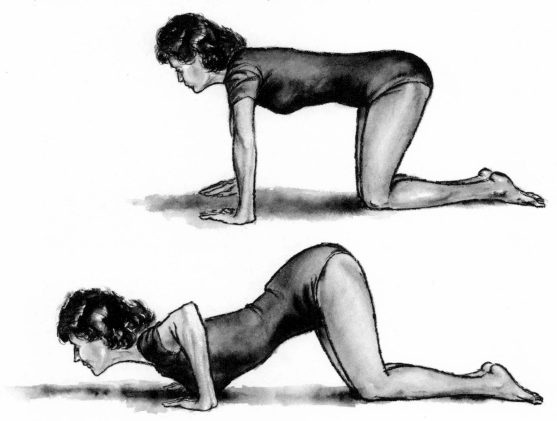

need a gentle fingertip massage and washing with a damp cloth. This serves the dual purpose of cleanliness and improving the circulation.

The following exercises strengthen and help tone the pectoral muscles. They may not prevent sagging of the breast entirely, but they will help maintain its youthful appearance.

Three exercises that should be a part of your Daily Yoga Program: the Full Body Stretch; Knee Touch to the Forehead, and the Grand Cobra will be beneficial. Two of the hand exercises which are described in this chapter, in the section "For Supple Hands," strengthen the pectoral muscles. One presses the palms together and the other clasps the fingers and pulls.

There is a third exercise specifically designed to strengthen the pectorals. It also exercises the shoulders and tones the underarm muscles. This is the push-up for women.

Start on your hands and knees. Place your palms on the floor at shoulder level with fingers turned inward and opposite fingertips about ten inches apart. While you are on your hands and knees, push your body and head forward as much as you can. Then, try to touch your chest to the floor, not your face. Hold for a second. Bring your body straight up, not back. Lower your body to touch your chest again, and straighten up again. Touch your chest three times at first, increasing to six times later.

7

Savitri's Recipes for Healthful Eating

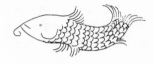

In Chapter 4, I discussed Proper Eating and Weight Control, regardless of what kind of food you eat. Over the years, however, my students and my friends have asked me to write down some of the dishes they have eaten in my home that they enjoyed.

The recipes in this section, therefore, fulfill most requirements for a healthful eating regimen. They do emphasize my own personal preference for vegetables and fish because these foods are usually more fresh and much more healthful, pound for pound, than most other things you can eat.

In addition, doctors tell me that the real secret to weight reduction is to reduce intake and calories.

To help you achieve this, these recipes are measured for small servings and call for foods that are low in calories. They were developed from Indian dishes that are lightly spiced for those who are not accustomed to highly seasoned food, and were created with emphasis on nutritional values.

The recipes are for two people. It is easier to increase from two to four or six than it is to reduce from six to two without spoiling the dish.

The ingredients in these recipes were selected with the idea that they are available everywhere. As I mentioned in Chapter 4, eat more frequently, but each time in small quantity. Four small meals a day are better for your health, your figure, and your energy supply than are three large ones. With this in mind, my recipes have been measured for smaller quantities.

You are now ready to plan and prepare your meals. For planning purposes, the recipes are all easy to prepare and especially designed for busy housewives and working people with little time to spare, but a genuine desire to avoid useless foods. Even the people who are not fond of cooking will have fun making these dishes.

Since you will be eating smaller quantities at one sitting, you must eat well-balanced meals and good, nutritious food. Meals are nutritious if prepared properly and with fresh supplies whenever they are available. To get the most benefit from what you cook, baking and broiling are far better than frying or boiling, which takes away the very nutrients, vitamins, and minerals you do not want to lose. And overcooked food loses most of its value.

To save the vitamins and minerals, the recipes have been prepared using high protein liquids in place of water wherever possible. I use yogurt or milk.

We already know how important proper food is for our health. When you try these recipes, you will find them tasty as well as healthful.

I emphasize cooking foods that can be prepared in advance and then warmed later. None of the foods in these recipes have to be eaten the moment they are cooked.

You will even enjoy cooking for yourself—cook for two and freeze the leftovers for another meal.

The recipes are colorful as well as easy and quick. They have less quantity and more quality, presented in an attractive way. They are creative— many you may never have tried before. All of them have been measured, timed, and sampled.

And they are delicious.

BREAD (*Chapati*)

¾ cup fine wholewheat flour (stone ground)
¼ cup water
1 teaspoon oil (for hands)

Set aside a quarter cup of flour to use in rolling.

Place a half cup flour in a bowl and slowly add water, stirring until it forms a dough that can be kneaded. Not all the water may be needed, but the dough must be soft and easy to roll. Knead the dough for ten minutes and roll it into a ball. Cover it with a damp cloth and leave it for at least a half hour. It will keep this way for as long as three hours and can be refrigerated, wrapped in plastic, for twenty-four hours.

When it is ready to cook, put a heavy cast-iron griddle over medium heat. Oil hands and knead the dough while the griddle heats. Divide dough into four balls.

Using flour set aside, flour both the rolling surface and rolling pin. Oil hands again. Take one ball, roll it in the hands, and flatten it. Dip into the dry flour. Roll it out evenly and gently into a round piece six inches across, or longer and thinner if preferred. Keep the surface thinly floured. To keep the dough from sticking, it may be dipped into the flour once or twice, but only enough flour should be used to help it roll easily; too much will dry it out.

When the griddle is smoking hot, put the bread on it for about a half minute, or until air bubbles appear. With tongs, turn it over and cook the other side about a half minute, or until it shows light brown spots. Turn it again, leaving it one or two seconds on each side, until it puffs up.

If cooking over gas, after the bread is lightly browned, lay it on another burner over medium flame until it puffs up. Turn with tongs and cook the other side one to two seconds.

Two pieces of bread should be kept for later. They will keep in foil in refrigerator up to three days. To prepare, place the bread, still in the foil, in a 350° oven for fifteen minutes. This recipe makes four chapatis, two for immediate use (one per person), two for later.

CHICKEN CURRY (*Murg Kari*) *

½ *frying chicken*
1 *medium onion*
2 *tablespoons vegetable oil*
2 *bay leaves*
2 *cloves*
small amount water
1 *tablespoon ground coriander*
1 *tablespoon ground cumin*
1 *teaspoon curry powder*
1 *teaspoon red chili powder*
½ *teaspoon ground ginger*
¼ *teaspoon ground cardamom*
½ *teaspoon ground turmeric*
½ *teaspoon garlic powder*
¾ *teaspoon salt*
1 *cup plain low fat yogurt*
2 *tomatoes*
1 *tablespoon unsweetened shredded coconut*

Chop chicken into two-inch pieces, bone and all. Remove and discard skin.

Chop onion fine and sauté in oil with cloves and bay leaves.

Use enough water to make a paste of the dry spices and add to the onion. Cook over medium heat until the oil separates from the spices or they no longer have a sharp aroma.

Beat yogurt. Peel tomatoes. Add yogurt, tomatoes, chicken, and then coconut to spice mixture. Bring to a boil and cook then over low heat for forty-five minutes, stirring once or twice.

If more gravy is needed, add more yogurt.

* Lamb curry can be prepared the same way.

BAKED CHICKEN PATTIES (*Murg Tikkya*)

1 whole breast of frying chicken
1 tablespoon fresh ginger (or 1 teaspoon ground
ginger)
½ medium onion
1 fresh hot green chili pepper
1 teaspoon soy sauce
1 egg
1 tablespoon wheat germ flour, cornmeal flour, or
crumbled cornflakes

Garnish: 2 tablespoons fresh lemon juice
freshly ground pepper
salt, if desired
sprigs of parsley

Skin chicken, rinse, and remove bones. Split chicken meat in half. With back of knife, pound chicken until each half is broad and flat.

Grate ginger, chop onion fine, slice chili pepper fine. Blend all ingredients except chicken, egg and flour into a smooth paste, using blender or hand beater. Cover both sides of chicken with the mixture and leave it covered in refrigerator at least one hour, or overnight if possible.

Beat egg lightly. Spread flour on flat surface. Dip chicken pieces first into beaten egg, then coat lightly on both sides with flour.

Cook in preheated 400° oven for fifteen minutes on each side or until golden brown. To make it crisper, cook a little longer.

If desired, garnish before serving.

CHICKEN AND SPINACH (*Murg Palak*)

2 legs of frying chicken (thighs and drumsticks)
2 tablespoons vegetable oil
2 bay leaves
2 cloves
1 teaspoon fresh ginger (or ½ teaspoon ground)
1 cup fresh spinach
1 hot green chili pepper (more if desired)
¼ teaspoon ground cardamom
⅛ teaspoon salt

Cut chicken into small pieces, bone and all. Remove and discard skin.

Put oil, bay leaves, and cloves into heavy cooking pot and sauté chicken in it until light brown.

Grate ginger; chop spinach and chili pepper. In a blender, blend spinach, ginger, cardamom, chili pepper, and salt into a smooth paste. If no blender is available, chop the ingredients very fine. Add mixture to the chicken. Bring to a boil and simmer twenty-five minutes.

This recipe can be used with any leafy vegetable, such as kale, mustard greens, collard greens, etc.

CHICKEN WITH YOGURT (*Murg Dahi*)

1 whole breast of frying chicken
1 tablespoon fresh ginger (or 1 teaspoon ground)
½ cup skimmed milk yogurt
¼ teaspoon red chili powder
¼ teaspoon ground cumin
1 bay leaf
⅛ teaspoon curry powder
1 tablespoon vegetable oil or margarine

Skin chicken, rinse and remove bones. Cut chicken into small pieces, about one inch.

Grate ginger. Mix spices, yogurt, and oil thoroughly. Place chicken in the mixture and marinate two hours (or overnight).

Put marinated chicken on baking tray lined with foil. Broil seven minutes, turn and cook the other side seven minutes, until golden brown. Adjust broiling level to avoid browning too quickly.

CHICKEN WITH SOY SAUCE (*Murg Chatni*)

1 whole breast of frying chicken
¼ cup soy sauce
½ teaspoon sugar
1 tablespoon white wine
2 tablespoons corn oil
¼ teaspoon salt
5 drops Tabasco sauce
1 teaspoon cornstarch
2 tablespoons water

Skin chicken. Rinse and remove bone. Cut into one inch pieces.

Make a marinade of the soy sauce, sugar and white wine. Put chicken in it and marinade at least one hour or overnight.

Put oil and salt into a heavy skillet. Use medium heat and when oil is hot, add chicken and whatever marinade is left and sauté until brown. Add Tabasco sauce.

Dissolve the cornstarch in cold water. Pour over chicken, mix well, and simmer over low heat for twelve minutes.

CARROT DESSERT (*Gajar Helva*)

4 medium carrots
1½ cups skimmed milk
2 tablespoons brown sugar
1 tablespoon unsalted butter (or margarine)
4 cardamom pods
1 tablespoon chopped almonds
1 teaspoon white raisins

Peel and grate carrots. Cook in the milk over medium heat for about a half hour, or until most of the liquid is absorbed. Stir and mash with fork.

Add sugar and cook five minutes. Add butter, crushed cardamom pods, chopped almonds and raisins.

Reduce the heat. Cook until butter floats on the top of the mixture.

Stir and place the carrots in two serving bowls. Serve hot or cold.

SEMOLINA PUDDING (*Suka Halva*)

1 tablespoon unsalted butter
¼ cup semolina (Cream of Wheat)
½ cup milk
⅛ teaspoon saffron
¼ cup sugar
1 teaspoon white seedless raisins
1 tablespoon slivered almonds
¼ teaspoon crushed cardamom seed

Heat butter in a skillet. Add semolina and cook over medium heat— stirring constantly to prevent burning—until golden brown.

Add milk slowly and carefully, then saffron, and cook over low heat for five minutes, or until milk is absorbed. Stir frequently.

Add sugar, raisins, almonds and cardamom seed and stir well. Simmer for ten minutes and serve hot.

JEWEL DRESSINGS

The jewel dressings take their names from favorite jewels of India—coral, amber, pearl and jade. They add color to your table and joy to the taste. These dressings can be served over any kind of fresh fruit or vegetables, not just salad greens.

CORAL DRESSING (Pink)

1 medium fresh beet (or 1 tablespoon beet root
    extract)
1 cup low fat plain yogurt
⅛ teaspoon Tabasco sauce
1 tablespoon honey
1 tablespoon pimento

Boil the beet until tender when tested with a fork. Remove from water, peel, and chop.

Put chopped beet in blender and blend to a paste, or mash well with a fork.

Add yogurt, Tabasco sauce and honey to beet mixture. Blend well or mix thoroughly with hand beater.

When serving, top with chopped pimento.

Any leftover dressing will keep well for a week if refrigerated and tightly sealed.

AMBER DRESSING (Gold)

2 garlic cloves
1 egg
½ cup olive oil
¼ cup white wine vinegar
1 teaspoon honey
½ teaspoon dry mustard
¼ teaspoon fresh ground black pepper

Peel garlic and rub against the inside of the serving bowl. Discard garlic. Hard-boil egg and chop it fine.

In same serving bowl, mix with a fork the oil, vinegar, honey, mustard, chopped egg, and pepper.

This dressing can be mixed at the time you're preparing the salad, or mixed in advance and refrigerated for as long as a week, tightly sealed.

PEARL DRESSING (White)

1 cup low fat plain yogurt
2 garlic cloves
⅛ teaspoon white pepper
1 teaspoon roasted sesame seed
1 teaspoon salt
1 tablespoon large curd cottage cheese

Put yogurt in blender. Add garlic (skinned and chopped), pepper, sesame seed, and salt. Blend thoroughly in blender, or mix well with hand beater.

When ready to serve, add cottage cheese and stir carefully, to mix well but not enough to break the large curds. The dressing can be made in advance and refrigerated for as long as a week, if tightly sealed.

JADE DRESSING (Green)

½ avocado
2 whole limes
2 tablespoons fresh lime juice
1 teaspoon fresh parsley
¾ cup skimmed milk
¼ teaspoon salt
¼ teaspoon ground white pepper
¼ teaspoon grated lime peel
¼ teaspoon crushed dry mint leaves

Peel avocado half and chop. Wash limes, grate the skin, and squeeze two tablespoons of juice. Chop parsley.

Put avocado and lime juice in blender and blend until smooth, or mash well with fork.

Add chopped parsley, skimmed milk, salt, and white pepper. Blend well or mix well with hand mixer.

When serving, sprinkle lime peel and mint leaves on top. Any leftover dressing can be kept for one week if sealed tightly and refrigerated.

FRUIT OMELET (*Phel Chila*)

1 tablespoon fresh peach
1 tablespoon fresh strawberries or other berries
1 tablespoon pitted dates
1 tablespoon white seedless raisins
3 eggs
1 tablespoon milk
2 tablespoons vegetable oil

Peel peach and chop. Wash and chop other fruit fine. Mix well.
Beat eggs until foamy. Add milk and mix well.
Heat oil in eight- or ten-inch omelet pan or skillet until it sizzles. Pour in eggs and cook over medium heat until slightly puffy.
Place fruit along center of eggs and fold edges of eggs over it. Turn quickly with large pancake turner and cook one minute.

VEGETABLE SCRAMBLED EGGS (*Sabzi Anda*)

1 tablespoon onion
1 tablespoon tomato
3 eggs
2 tablespoons skimmed milk
1 teaspoon sweet butter
¼ teaspoon brewer's yeast
¼ teaspoon wheat germ
¼ teaspoon soya powder
⅛ teaspoon salt
⅛ teaspoon fresh ground back pepper

Chop onion and tomato fine. In saucepan, beat eggs until foamy.
Mix all ingredients except salt and pepper. Add mixture to eggs.
Cook on medium heat three to five minutes, stirring constantly, until they begin to form soft creamy curds.
Remove from heat. Add salt and pepper.

SPLIT LENTIL (*Moong Dahl*)

½ cup split lentil (yellow or green)
3 cups water
¾ teaspoon salt
⅛ teaspoon ground turmeric
¼ teaspoon red chili powder (or 1 fresh hot green
    chili pepper)
1½ tablespoons vegetable oil
1 medium onion
½ teaspoon cumin seed
2 whole cardamom

Put lentil in a sieve or colander and rinse under cold running water until water runs clear. After rinsing, put lentil into a heavy cooking pan with two cups of water. Soak for at least one hour, or overnight.

Return lentil to colander and rinse again. Put one cup fresh water into the heavy cooking pan, add lentil, salt, turmeric and red chili powder (or chili pepper). Stir, and bring to a boil over high heat, then lower heat, cover and simmer for half an hour, or until lentil is soft.

While the lentil is cooking, put the oil in a small skillet, slice the onion and sauté it until light brown. Add the cumin seed and cardamom and cook five minutes, or until dark brown (but not burned).

When lentil is ready, stir gently and then place in serving bowls. Ladle the entire contents of the skillet over top of it and serve.

MEAT BALLS (*Kheema Kofta*)

1 teaspoon onion
1 heaping teaspoon fresh ginger (or ½ teaspoon
    ground ginger)
½ pound ground lean lamb or beef
1 egg
¼ teaspoon rosemary
⅛ teaspoon salt

Chop onion very fine. Grate ginger.

Mix meat with all ingredients and knead well together. With moist hands, form into twelve one-and-a-half-inch balls. Place on greased baking sheet and bake in preheated 300° oven, five minutes on each side.

If well-done meatballs are desired, cook longer.

SKEWERED MEAT (*Sheekh Gosht*)

½ pound boned lamb or beef
2 cloves garlic
1 teaspoon fresh ginger (or ½ teaspoon ground
    ginger)
¼ teaspoon mustard seeds
½ teaspoon poppy seeds
¼ teaspoon ground turmeric
½ teaspoon ground coriander
⅛ teaspoon cayenne pepper (optional)
2 cloves
2 bay leaves
⅛ teaspoon salt
¼ cup red wine or yogurt

Cut meat into one-and-a-half-inch pieces.

Crush garlic, grate ginger, crack mustard seeds. Combine spices with wine or yogurt for marinade. Put meat into marinade for at least two hours.

Thread the meat on skewers.

Place skewers under broiler or over charcoal. Turn and baste frequently with the marinade. Continue turning and basting until meat is brown.

LAMB SHANKS (*Mamna Bhuna*)*

2 lamb shanks
2 garlic cloves
1 tablespoon fresh ginger (or 1 teaspoon ground
        ginger)
½ cup yogurt
1 teaspoon ground cumin
1 tablespoon ground coriander
½ teaspoon red chili powder
¼ teaspoon black pepper
¼ teaspoon ground cloves
½ teaspoon ground turmeric
½ teaspoon salt
1 medium onion
2 tablespoons vegetable oil
1 large tomato
1 tablespoon slivered almonds

Chop each lamb shank into four pieces, leaving the meat on the bone. Remove skin and fat.

Chop garlic; grate ginger. Beat yogurt and add spices. Marinate lamb pieces in the mixture at least one hour at room temperature, or in refrigerator not more than twelve hours.

Chop onion and in a heavy pan, sauté it in the oil. Cut tomato into six to eight pieces, add to onion, and cook five minutes. Add lamb and marinade. Cover pan, bring to a boil and simmer fifty minutes. Uncover pan no more than once, or the steam and flavor will be lost.

Add almonds. Cook ten minutes more.

GROUND MEAT (*Sukha Keema*)

1 large tomato
2 tablespoons corn oil
½ teaspoon ground sweet basil leaves
½ pound ground lean lamb or beef
¾ teaspoon salt
½ teaspoon black pepper

Remove the skin and chop the tomato. Heat the oil in a small cooking pan over medium heat. Add the tomato and basil and sauté until the oil separates from the tomato—about fifteen minutes.

Add the meat and salt. Mix well and cook ten minutes over medium heat, or until meat changes color. Stir frequently.

Add freshly ground black pepper and simmer for five minutes.

---

* This is two meals for two persons. Half may be refrigerated or frozen. It will keep four or five days in refrigerator.

LIVER AND WINE (*Kalaga Wine*)

½ pound liver (beef, calves or lamb)
4 tablespoons white flour
1 teaspoon salt
½ teaspoon ground black pepper
4 tablespoons butter (or margarine)
2 garlic cloves
1 teaspoon lemon juice
2 tablespoons dry white wine

Wash and clean membrane from liver. Pat dry. Cut the liver into two-and-a-half by one-half inch strips.

In a plastic bag, put the flour, salt and pepper. Place liver in the bag, shake until it is well coated. Remove the liver, after shaking off excess flour, and put aside.

In a medium-sized skillet, melt the butter and add the garlic, chopped. Sauté lightly.

Add the liver and continue sautéing, turning it frequently to keep it from sticking, until it is lightly browned.

Add the lemon juice and wine, cover and cook over medium heat for five minutes. Serve hot.

ONION AND TOMATO MIX (*Piaz Tamatar Kachumbar*)

1 teaspoon dry roasted peanuts
1 medium onion
1 medium tomato
½ teaspoon salt
⅛ teaspoon red pepper
1 tablespoon fresh lemon juice (or lime juice)

Chop or grind peanuts. Chop onion. Peel tomato and chop it into one-half-inch cubes. Mix onion and tomato in a serving bowl.

Add salt, pepper, and lemon juice, and stir.

Cover and refrigerate for one half hour.

Sprinkle with peanuts and serve.

One tablespoon per person per serving is sufficient.

LEMON PICKLE (*Nimbu Achar*)

12 lemons
1 tablespoon salt

Wash and dry six of the lemons. Cut each into four pieces. Put the cut lemons into a one pint, sterilized jar, and add the salt. Cover it tightly and shake well.

Expose the covered jar to the sun every day for at least one hour for two weeks. Shake occasionally.

After two weeks, extract the juice of the remaining six lemons, or more if needed, and cover the lemons in the jar with the juice.

Refrigerate and leave in jar for at least two more weeks before eating. This pickle can be kept for several months.

This is a good accompaniment with meat dishes, and one-quarter piece of lemon per person is enough to serve at mealtime.

MINT CHUTNEY (*Podina Chutney*)

½ cup fresh chopped or dry mint leaves
1 hot green chili pepper
½ cup grated unsweetened coconut
1 teaspoon fresh chopped ginger (or ½ teaspoon
    ground ginger)
½ teaspoon salt
½ teaspoon ground cumin seed
½ teaspoon sugar
2 tablespoons lemon juice

Blend all ingredients in blender. Add a few tablespoons of water, if needed, to make a smooth paste. Bottle and refrigerate.

One tablespoon per person per serving is sufficient.

PLAIN BOILED RICE (*Chawal*)

½ cup any long-grained rice (or Indian basmati rice)
1 ¼ cups water
2 tablespoons oil
½ teaspoon salt

Put rice into the thick-bottomed pan in which it is to be cooked. Wash rice well in cold water, rinsing it four or five times, until the starch is washed away and the water runs clear.

Soak rice one hour in water, covered. Drain.

Add one and a quarter cups water, oil, and salt, and mix well. Cook over medium heat until all water is absorbed. Stir thoroughly once or twice while cooking.

Set heat at low simmer, cover pot, and simmer twenty minutes.

RICE PULAO (*Chawal Pulao*)

Any addition to rice makes it a *pulao,* of which there are many varieties. Almost all are flavored with saffron, then another ingredient.

½ cup any long-grained rice (or Indian basmati rice)
½ teaspoon saffron
1 teaspoon water

Mix saffron and water.
Rice with carrots: 1 small carrot, scraped and grated
Rice with peas: ¼ cup peas
Rice with onions: 1 medium onion, minced

Rice with raisins: 1 tablespoon white seedless raisins
Rice with chicken: ¼ cup cooked chopped chicken
Rice with meat: ¼ cup cooked chopped meat
Rice with seafood: ¼ cup cooked chopped fish (any kind) or shrimp

Wash and cook rice as directed for plain rice. Before simmering, stir in saffron, then carrots, or peas, or onions, or raisins, or chicken, or meat, or seafood, mixing well. Cover and simmer over low heat for twenty minutes.

TANDOORI SHRIMP (*Tandoori Jhinga*)

½ teaspoon fresh ginger (or ¼ teaspoon ground)
4 garlic cloves
1 teaspoon fresh lemon juice
½ cup yogurt
1 teaspoon ground coriander
1 teaspoon ground cumin
⅛ teaspoon ground red pepper
⅛ teaspoon ground cloves
⅛ teaspoon paprika
⅛ teaspoon salt
1 tablespoon vegetable oil
½ pound fresh or frozen shelled shrimp or prawns

Grate ginger. Combine all ingredients except shrimp and mix well in blender or with hand beater.

Put mixture in a baking dish, add shrimp, and marinate two to three hours.

In oven preheated to 375°, bake shrimp twenty minutes, stirring once or twice.

GREEN PEPPERS STUFFED WITH CRABMEAT (*Simla Mirch Kakra*)

½ pound fresh crabmeat
1 large onion
¼ teaspoon chili powder
¼ teaspoon ground turmeric
⅛ teaspoon sweet basil
⅛ teaspoon salt
½ teaspoon fresh lemon juice
2 green peppers
1 medium onion
1 tablespoon vegetable oil
1 tablespoon white wine

Chop crabmeat fine. Mince large onion.

Mix crabmeat, minced onion, chili powder, turmeric, basil, salt and lemon juice. Clean green peppers and stuff them with the mixture. Set aside.

Slice medium onion. In a large skillet, heat oil to medium temperature and sauté sliced onion until brown. Remove onion from pan and place on top of stuffed pepper. Place peppers in the same skillet and add white wine. Cover and simmer fifteen minutes or until peppers are tender.

FISH WITH TOMATOES (Machi Tamatar)

½ pound filet of sole or flounder
4 garlic cloves
1 green chili pepper
2 tablespoons olive oil
⅛ teaspoon ground turmeric
2 whole dry hot red peppers (optional)
2 bay leaves
⅛ teaspoon salt
2 large tomatoes

Cut fish into serving pieces.

Chop garlic fine; slit green chili pepper lengthwise.

Heat oil in a heavy pan, add garlic, green chili pepper and spices, and sauté one minute.

Peel and quarter tomatoes. Add tomatoes and fish to spices. Cover tightly and bring to a boil. Lower fire and simmer about twenty minutes, or until fish is tender when tested with a fork.

POACHED FISH WITH GRAPES (Dumm Machi Angoor)

½ pound any fine-grained white fish filet
¼ cup dry white wine
⅛ teaspoon salt
⅛ teaspoon ground white pepper
¼ teaspoon sweet basil
¼ pound white seedless grapes (or large white
    grapes)

Wash fish well under cold running water. Pat dry.

Put wine and seasoning into shallow pan and bring to a boil over low heat. Add fish and simmer gently ten minutes. Add grapes and simmer five minutes longer.

White seedless grapes may be used whole. Larger grapes should be split lengthwise and seeded.

MUSTARD FISH (Rai Machi)

2 medium white fish filets
½ lemon
1 teaspoon dry mustard
⅛ teaspoon salt
½ onion

Wash fish under cold running water. Pat dry. Juice lemon half.

Make paste of mustard, salt and lemon juice. Spread over fish. Chop onion fine and sprinkle over fish.

Bake on foil-covered cookie sheet in preheated 400° oven for fifteen minutes. *Do not turn.*

FISH STUFFED WITH SPINACH (*Machi Bhara Palak*)

1 pound whole white fish (any kind)
1 tablespoon vegetable oil
1 cup fresh spinach
1 teaspoon fresh ginger (or ½ teaspoon ground)
1 teaspoon dried mint flakes
⅛ teaspoon ground cumin
1 fresh green chili pepper
⅛ teaspoon salt

Clean and bone fish and wash it under cold running water. Pat dry. Rub fish well with oil, inside and out.

Chop spinach and grate ginger. Place all ingredients, except fish, in blender (or use hand mixer) and blend well.

Slice fish lengthwise and spread mixture evenly between the two pieces.

Wrap fish carefully in aluminum foil and place on baking sheet. Cook for thirty-five minutes in preheated 350° oven.

FISH FLAT KABOBS (*Machi Tikkya*)

¾ pound fish filets (any kind that is not oily)
¼ cup milk
2 eggs
1 small onion
1 teaspoon fresh ginger (or ½ teaspoon ground)
½ tablespoon rice, corn or chick-pea flour
5 whole black peppercorns
⅛ teaspoon red pepper
½ teaspoon ground coriander
⅛ teaspoon salt
1 tablespoon fresh parsley

Clean fish under cold running water. Steam fish over water or simmer in one-quarter cup milk for ten minutes until fish flakes with a fork. Mash fish.

Separate eggs. Chop onion fine; grate ginger.

Combine fish, egg yolks, flour and spices. Mix well.

Divide into small balls, about one-and-one-half inches in diameter, then shape into small patties.

Beat egg whites until stiff and brush over both sides of each pattie. Place on lightly oiled foil-covered cookie sheet and place in lower part of broiler. Cook five minutes. Turn and cook five minutes more until golden brown. Before serving, sprinkle with chopped parsley.

To cook in oven, preheat to 350° and bake seven minutes each side.

CHILLED CUCUMBER SOUP (*Thanda Khira Rasa*)

1 medium cucumber
½ clove garlic
2 cups skimmed milk
½ teaspoon caraway seeds
½ teaspoon ground white pepper
⅛ teaspoon salt
2 walnut halves

Peel cucumber and slice into rounds. Mince garlic. Simmer milk, cucumber and seasonings for five minutes. Chill before serving. Garnish each bowl with a walnut half. This will keep in a refrigerator two days but no longer.

MODIFIED MULLIGATAWNY SOUP (*Mulligatawny Rasa*)

⅓ pound chicken (with bones)
3 cups water
½ teaspoon salt
2 tablespoons vegetable oil
1 small onion
¼ teaspoon ground ginger
¼ teaspoon turmeric
⅛ teaspoon red chili powder
½ teaspoon ground cumin
1 tablespoon corn or chick-pea flour
1 tablespoon cooked rice

Bring water to boil. Put in chicken and salt. Reduce heat to low and cook until chicken is tender. Take chicken out and let cool, reserving the stock. Skin chicken and remove meat from bones. Cut into one-eighth-inch cubes and set aside.

Heat oil in the pan to be used for making the soup. Chop onion and sauté it lightly. Add spices and sauté one minute, stirring constantly. Add flour and sauté one minute more.

Strain chicken stock into soup pot. Add chicken. Bring to a boil, then reduce heat to medium-low, and simmer one half hour.

This soup is served in a bowl over one tablespoon of boiled rice and should be very hot.

SPICED TEA (*Masala Chai*)

1 cup milk
1 cup water
2 teaspoons sugar or honey
3 whole cardamom pods
½ teaspoon crushed fresh ginger
½-inch stick cinnamon, broken up
2 teaspoons tea (not in a teabag)

Combine all ingredients except tea and bring to a boil. Add tea, cover, and turn off heat. Let it stand five minutes. Strain and serve immediately.

SPINACH WITH MIXED VEGETABLES (*Palak Belavat Sabzi*)

1 pound or 2 cups fresh spinach
1 medium onion
2 tablespoons oil
1 small potato
1 tomato
1 cup mixed green vegetables such as zucchini, green
*   beans, and peas (may be leftovers)*
1 teaspoon mango powder (or 1 lemon)
½ teaspoon celery seed
½ teaspoon cayenne
⅛ teaspoon salt

Wash spinach and remove stems. Chop and then puree in blender to a smooth paste.

Chop onion and sauté in oil until transparent. Chop potato and tomato. Add to onion with other vegetables and spices. Sauté about five minutes and then simmer twenty minutes.

Mix in spinach paste and heat.

If mango powder is not available, serve with lemon quarters.

STUFFED OKRA (*Bhara Bhindi*)

½ pound okra (8 pods)
1 tablespoon ground coriander
1 teaspoon ground cumin
½ teaspoon fennel seed
¼ teaspoon ground turmeric
⅛ teaspoon red chili powder
1 teaspoon parsley flakes
1 tablespoon fresh lemon juice
⅛ teaspoon salt
2 tablespoons oil

Clean okra with damp cloth or wash and dry quickly. Remove stem ends. Slit pods on one side and open slightly.

Mix all spices with salt and lemon juice. Fill each okra pod with the mixture.

In well-oiled or Teflon skillet, heat oil, add okra, cover pan tightly, and cook ten minutes over medium heat. Turn okra pods, cover again, and cook ten minutes on other side. To brown, remove cover and cook ten to fifteen minutes longer.

CAULIFLOWER WITH MUSTARD SEEDS (*Phoolgobhi Rai*)

1 small head cauliflower (about 1 pound)
⅛ teaspoon salt
2 tablespoons oil
1 teaspoon mustard seeds
½ teaspoon ground white pepper

Trim stem and leaves from cauliflower. Break the head into flowerets one to one-and-a-half inches long, using a knife to cut into the heavy stem. Wash and dry well on paper towels. Sprinkle pieces with salt.

Over medium heat, warm oil in heavy skillet, then sauté mustard seeds. As seeds begin to pop, add cauliflower and sauté until it has a golden tinge. Cover skillet and cook ten minutes more, when flowerets should be tender with crispy edges.

Sprinkle with white pepper.

ZUCCHINI CASSEROLE (*Tori Dumm*)

4 small to medium zucchini, or yellow squash
1 tablespoon oil
3 ounces low fat cottage cheese
¼ teaspoon garlic or onion salt
¼ teaspoon basil
1 egg
1 or 2 slices bacon

Clean zucchini and slice them about one-quarter-inch thick. Pat dry.

Spread oil on bottom of one-quart casserole. Put in one layer of zucchini and one layer of cottage cheese. Sprinkle with seasoning. Add another layer of zucchini and another of cottage cheese, and sprinkle with remaining seasoning.

Hard-boil egg and crumble it. Cook bacon crisp and crumble it.

Top casserole with crumbled egg and bacon.

Bake in preheated oven at 350° for fifteen minutes, or until zucchini is tender.

COLD CHOPPED EGGPLANT (*Bharta Baigan*)

2 medium eggplants
4 spring onions (without tough green ends) or 2 small
  yellow onions
1 fresh hot green chili pepper
3 tablespoons fresh mint (or 2 tablespoons dried mint)
½ teaspoon ground cumin
¼ teaspoon freshly ground black pepper
⅛ teaspoon salt
1 tablespoon fresh lemon juice

Wash eggplants and place in shallow baking dish. Bake in 350° oven thirty to thirty-five minutes until soft when tested with a fork.

Remove eggplants and peel under cold running water, making sure all the skin is removed. Mince pulp or chop finely.

Chop onion, pepper, and fresh mint fine. Combine with spices and lemon juice and add to chopped eggplant. Chill in refrigerator before serving.

This will keep three to four days in refrigerator.

BAKED EGGPLANT (*Bhuna Baigan*)

1 large eggplant
1 medium onion
2 tablespoons sesame oil (or any vegetable oil)
1 bay leaf
¼ teaspoon red chili powder
1 teaspoon mustard seeds
1 tablespoon dried unsweetened shredded coconut
1 or 2 medium tomatoes
⅛ teaspoon salt

Wash eggplant and place in shallow baking dish. Bake in 350° oven thirty to thirty-five minutes until it feels soft when tested with a fork.

Remove and peel under cold running water, making sure all the skin is removed. Chop fine and set aside or refrigerate.

Chop onion fine and sauté in oil about five minutes until translucent. Add bay leaf, chili powder, mustard seeds, and coconut. Cook five minutes.

Peel and chop tomatoes, and add with salt to onion mixture. Cook about five minutes.

Add eggplant, mix well, and heat over medium fire. Serve hot.

CARROTS WITH GINGER (*Gajar Adarak*)

4 medium carrots
1 tablespoon fresh ginger (or ½ teaspoon ground
*   ginger)*
1 ½ tablespoons oil
⅛ teaspoon salt
1 tablespoon honey

Scrape carrots and cut into slices one-quarter-inch thick. Grate ginger.

In a saucepan, sauté grated ginger in oil over medium heat for five minutes. Stir in carrot slices and salt, and sauté ten minutes. Add honey, stirring well, and sauté five minutes more. Cover pan and cook an additional five minutes.

Ground ginger may be used if fresh ginger is not available, but fresh ginger gives an entirely different and more interesting taste to the carrots.

FRESH MIXED VEGETABLE PATTIES (*Melavat Sabzi Tikkya*)

½ cup potatoes
½ cup fresh beets
½ cup zucchini
½ cup fresh green beans
½ cup fresh peas
½ cup eggplant
1 egg
1 small onion
⅛ teaspoon marjoram
1 teaspoon cracker crumbs
1 chili pepper (optional)
1 tablespoon oil

Peel and dice potatoes and beets. Wash and chop vegetables, except onion, into small pieces. In steam basket, over water, steam all vegetables until soft. Drain well to remove excess moisture and mash with potato masher.

Separate egg. Beat yolk lightly; beat white until stiff.

In a mixing bowl, put the mashed vegetables, the onion—finely chopped—marjoram, beaten egg yolk, cracker crumbs and chopped chili pepper, if desired. Mix well.

Shape into four patties and coat with beaten egg white.

Pour half of the oil onto a flat baking sheet, arrange patties on it, and, in a 350° oven, bake or broil them five to seven minutes until golden brown. Brush remaining oil over top of patties after turning, and bake or broil until golden brown.

SKEWERED VEGETABLES (*Sheekh Sabzi*)

1 green pepper
2 large mushrooms
1 small zucchini
4 cherry tomatoes
4 small white onions
2 tablespoons vegetable oil (or olive oil)
1 teaspoon fresh lemon juice
1 teaspoon garlic salt

Wash and prepare the vegetables. Cut pepper in chunks, cut mushrooms in half, and slice zucchini in one-inch pieces. Alternate vegetables on skewer.

Mix oil, lemon juice, and garlic salt. Brush vegetables with the mixture.

Place skewers under broiler or over charcoal. Turn and baste frequently with remaining mixture. Cook about ten minutes, or until tender.

TURNIP AND APPLE (*Shalgam Sav*)

1 large turnip
1 large tart apple
3 tablespoons vegetable oil
¼ teaspoon salt
¼ teaspoon freshly ground black pepper
¼ teaspoon ground cardamom
¼ teaspoon lemon juice

Peel turnip. Peel and core apple; cut it in half and quarter each half. Cut turnip in two and cut each half into one-quarter-inch slices.

Sauté turnip in oil for ten minutes over medium heat. Add apple slices and sauté ten minutes.

Add salt, pepper, and cardamom. Mix well. Cover and simmer five minutes.

Before serving, sprinkle with lemon juice.

SPICED CABBAGE (*Masala Bundhgobi*)

1 small head cabbage
1 medium onion
1 medium tomato
1 teaspoon fresh ginger (or ½ teaspoon ground
    ginger)
½ lemon
1 tablespoon safflower oil
1 teaspoon salt
¼ teaspoon ground turmeric

Trim outer leaves from cabbage. Wash and quarter it, remove stem and core. Shred or chop cabbage fine.

Chop onion fine. Peel and chop tomato. Grate ginger. Juice lemon.

In heavy frying pan over medium heat, sauté onion in oil until golden brown. Add cabbage, tomato, salt, turmeric, and ginger. Mix and cover.

Cook twenty minutes over medium heat. Remove cover, increase heat, and cook quickly until all liquid is absorbed.

Before serving, sprinkle with lemon juice.

PEAS WITH POWDERED MILK (*Martar Dudh*)

1 large tomato
2 tablespoons powdered skim milk
½ cup water
2 tablespoons vegetable oil
½ teaspoon ground cumin
½ teaspoon ground ginger
½ teaspoon ground coriander
¼ teaspoon ground cardamom
¼ teaspoon ground turmeric
¼ teaspoon red chili powder
1 ½ cups fresh peas
1 teaspoon salt

Peel and chop tomato. Dissolve powdered milk in water.

Put oil into heavy skillet over medium heat. Add spices and stir for two minutes. Add peas and cook five minutes. Add tomato and salt and cook five minutes.

Add milk to mixture and bring to a boil. Cover and cook on low heat for ten minutes.

STRING BEANS WITH MUSHROOMS (*Same Guchi*)

½ pound string beans
2 large or 4 small mushrooms
¼ cup water
⅓ teaspoon salt
1 tablespoon butter
½ tablespoon slivered almonds
¼ teaspoon paprika
⅛ teaspoon tarragon

Clean beans and cut into one-inch pieces. Slice mushrooms.
Simmer beans in salted water until water is absorbed.
In small frying pan, melt butter and sauté mushrooms and almonds. Pour over beans and mix well.
Sprinkle paprika and tarragon over top.

POTATO AND ONION CASSEROLE (*Alu Pyaz Dumm*)

2 medium potatoes
1 medium onion
1 ½ tablespoons butter or margarine
½ cup skimmed milk
1 teaspoon salt
½ teaspoon freshly ground white pepper
2 eggs
¼ cup cheddar cheese
1 tablespoon fresh chives
1 tablespoon wheat germ

Scrub potatoes and boil in jackets until half done—approximately fifteen minutes. Remove from water, peel and slice fine. Peel onion and slice fine.
Lightly butter a casserole dish and put the milk in it. Add one layer of potatoes, dot with butter and sprinkle with salt and pepper; one layer of onions, and one layer of potatoes. Dot with butter.
Beat the eggs well and pour over the ingredients. Sprinkle with remaining salt and pepper, then the cheese, shredded; chopped chives and wheat germ.
Cover and put in a preheated 325° oven and bake for twenty minutes. Uncover, and cook ten minutes more, or until golden brown.

SAUTÉED ZUCCHINI (*Bhuni Tori*)

2 medium zucchini (or yellow squash)
2 tablespoons corn oil
½ teaspoon instant minced onion
½ teaspoon garlic salt

Clean zucchini and slice it fine.
Put oil into heavy skillet over medium heat. When it is hot, add all ingredients and sauté for fifteen minutes.

CUCUMBER YOGURT (*Khira Raita*)

8 ounces plain yogurt
⅛ teaspoon ground ginger
¼ teaspoon sugar
⅛ teaspoon salt
½ small cucumber
15 white seedless raisins
¼ teaspoon parsley flakes
⅛ teaspoon freshly ground black pepper
⅛ teaspoon paprika

Beat yogurt with ginger, sugar, and salt. Peel and grate cucumber. Squeeze out most of the liquid. Combine yogurt, cucumber, and raisins, mixing well. Mix parsley, pepper, and paprika and sprinkle over top. Serve cold.

This will keep up to four days in refrigerator.

For variations, instead of cucumber and raisins, combine:

1. ¼ cup grapes, cut in two and seeded and
   ½ banana, sliced thin, or
2. 1 small potato, peeled, boiled, and diced and
   ½ avocado, peeled and sliced, or
3. ½ green pepper, grated and
   1 small tomato, chopped

8
One Thing More

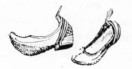

To my students generally, I am a very private person. I am their teacher; to them an institution rather than a woman. I yell at them when they let themselves go. I usually end up laughing with them as they laugh at my mispronounced and made-up words like "jelly-pulley," which I use to illustrate what I mean by hanging flesh.

For those in desperate need of understanding, however, I sometimes reveal myself. I let them know that I, too, have gone through disappointments and losses like theirs. My own experience with yoga has given me the strength and the ability to help others.

SELF-UNDERSTANDING

In the course of this book, I have stressed that one of the treasures yoga offers is self-understanding. It is only when a person understands himself—both his mind and his body—that he can deal with life's realities and with whatever life demands of him. The lesson of this book, the lesson of my own life, and the lesson I try to teach all of my students is that yoga—faithfully and regularly practiced—can and does make coping with life easier.

Because yoga has carried me through happy childhood delights and some challenges, as well as adult frustrations, problems and difficulties, I feel I can help others go through similar trials. My students come to me unbelieving, brought by concerned friends who know how much yoga has meant in their own lives.

Almost all problems my students bring to me can happen to every human being, including me. Thus, I can say to them that I, too, have suffered as they are suffering; that I, too, never thought I would make it, but here I am—teaching, helping others, drawing strength from the very yoga I am offering them.

People who join my class join for lots of different reasons. Some of them have problems; most of them do not. The majority of my students come to renew themselves physically. They come to learn to breathe properly, to lose the weight that slows them down, and to learn to live with themselves even with aches and pains. Some simply come to enjoy an exercise session with friends and to gain more self-discipline. Most of my students are healthy and wish to stay healthy. That's what yoga is all about.

COPING WITH STRESS

People also join my classes because they are under stress or are trying to cope with a special problem. They are all placed in classes with the other students—from beginners to the advanced. At first, improvement for the emotionally bothered centers on exercises designed to relieve the tension that they are living with. Their tensions can be seen in stiff shoulders or aching backs, lost appetite or compulsive eating—all the areas of tension I have described in this book. I soon feel they want to talk and need to talk. And I listen.

I listen well because at a very young age, I learned how to deal with life's disappointments. I was the fifth of six children and I was proud of my family. I had all the normal experiences with happiness and disappointments that are usual in a large family. But my disappointments began when I was a child. I wanted to be a dancer, and my family was not in favor of it. They did everything to discourage me, but yoga gave me the strength to take it, to keep on dancing, because it was so important to me.

Sometimes, today, when I talk about discipline in my classes, my pupils say, "That is easy to say—but hard to do." I tell them I know it is hard, but we have to try and try again. One of my pupils, a skier, was tense before an upcoming race. Another, a tennis player, was nervous about a tournament. A swimmer was uptight about a meet. A dancer was shaking before a stage performance. A singer was choking before a concert. A runner was out of breath before running. What is my yoga telling them? "So what if you are nervous—do yoga and be better the next time."

Among the many who have brought their frustrations to me was a woman very upset with what had happened to her marriage. She called me one evening to say she could not deal with it anymore. She said she had the pills ready to put an end to her misery.

We talked for a while. I suggested she might want to start pulling herself together with a full hour of yoga. She said she was too upset to exercise. I said to her, "Then why are you calling me?" She agreed to do the exercises and to stay in touch with me.

After doing yoga, she called me. I advised her to take a warm bath and to eat a good, nourishing meal to counteract the acid in her stomach from tension and too many cups of coffee. Following several more calls, her final call was to let me know that she was ready for sleep. She felt better. I felt better, too.

The next day, she called to tell me she had slept well and felt really rested for the first time in weeks. Later on, she came in to say, "Thank you for saving my life." And all I told her to do was practice some yoga.

MY CHILDHOOD

My childhood experiences have helped through my adult life. I was eleven years old when I lost my mother. Shortly before her death, the two of us took a trip together. On that trip she said to me, "I have polished you as a diamond. If you are ever thrown in the trash, you will always shine." We were very close. It was hard for me to believe that I would have to live without my mother.

That very loss of mine made it possible for me to help a wealthy and well-known woman who had had a truly ideal marriage. She went to pieces when her husband died suddenly. She was plump and happy in her married life. After her tragedy, she stopped coming to her yoga class. Her friends started saying to her, "Go back to Savitri." At first, she resisted. "What will yoga do for me?" she would ask. A friend finally brought her back to class. When I looked at her, she started to cry. I told her, "You are welcome to cry, but before you do, why don't you finish your class? Then we can talk and then you can cry."

After the class was over, we talked. I said to her, "You will never feel the same again but you have to go on. Since today's yoga class made you feel better, why don't you come to class every day for a while?" For six months she took yoga daily. She lost weight. She found herself a good job. Now, I see nothing on her face but smiles. Yoga had made her understand that loss is loss, but we have to adjust ourselves and go on.

While growing up, another experience taught me a lesson in adjustment. I got married at 13 and had to become a grownup overnight while I was still a child. I had to leave my father's home where we had a staff of servants. I left behind my dancing and my yoga as well, and moved into my husband's home. There, as the eldest son's wife, I was expected to take charge of everything.

HAPPY DUTY

My life pattern totally changed. Yet, I was determined that neither my family nor his would ever know the extent of the emotional changes I was going through. My yoga discipline taught me to accept his family as my family. In India, although they say a daughter-in-law is never liked, his family grew to love me. With the help of yoga, I learned to adjust myself to live their kind of life and to do things that were pleasing to them. I thought that was my duty and God expected me to do this duty.

The difficulties of that long-ago life experience made it possible recently for me to help a teenager who told me she could not stand the sight of her family. She was the daughter of a high government official and so miserable that she wanted to get away from home and stay away. After a few yoga lessons, she asked if she could talk to me alone. She said there was something about me that made her feel I would understand.

I told her how lucky she was to have a well-to-do family, a good school to go to, everything that so many others lacked. I asked her what she was missing. "I'm missing love, affection and understanding," she replied.

"A lot of teenagers feel that way," I told her, "but have you ever thought of trying to understand your family?"

I suggested that she stop listening to her friends who were against her going back to school. She might start listening to her own better judgment and to her parents. I said that if she would go back to school and show her parents that she could study, then they would be proud of her and she would find out how much they really loved her.

As she progressed in yoga, she would say, "I feel different, I feel better. I like what you are giving me."

Before she took yoga, she confessed she could not concentrate on any one thing for as long as five minutes. Now, she can read for hours. She is doing well in school, working part-time, loving her parents, and making them proud of her, as I was sure she would.

Yoga carried me through another major change in my life-style when my husband was transferred to Washington. I had to leave both my family and my professional life as a dancer and yoga teacher behind. I faced the challenges of being a diplomat's wife in a different world with an unfamiliar way of living. Additionally, I no longer had servants to help me with the entertaining that was required.

To continue my dancing and to teach yoga was another problem. As a diplomat's wife, I had to get special permission from the government of India. I got the permission to perform and to teach because I was bringing the art of India to America.

I started teaching yoga with one pupil in my home, and gradually, by word of mouth, my classes grew to such an extent that I had to move to a large studio. At the same time I was teaching yoga, I was lecturing and performing all over the United States.

ACCEPTING CHANGE

Before coming to Washington, D.C., American women in India who were my yoga pupils and were my dancing students told me about their difficulties in adusting to the Indian way of life while their husbands were assigned to missions there. At the time, I would tell them to get to know the people, understand their way of life, and learn the good things about them.

Now, in America, I had to practice what I had taught there. With my own experience, it was easy to help other wives of diplomats who had similar problems.

Several of my students from the diplomatic corps in Washington have told me they miss the food of their homeland, their relatives and friends, the slower tempo. They were used to the way they had lived at home. Often they found the changes to be too much. They would become so upset they could not sleep, could not adjust.

One ambassador's wife told me she had migraine headaches ever since her husband was posted to Washington more than a year earlier. I showed her how yoga would give her the ability to accept changes in her life and help her to relax. And it did. She has had no more headaches since she has started yoga.

Another crisis came in my life when I lost my younger son. I never thought I could live through that. We were still fairly new to Washington, far from home and family, and had not yet made close friends when tragedy struck.

I really thought that was the end of my life. When I was in shock, I wished many times that I could follow my son. I thought I had lost love for my God and the strength to tell myself that life must go on. But yoga gave me the ability to live with sorrow and to slowly fill a big hole in my life. That's why I feel that yoga does give people the strength to adjust their lives, to find peace and serenity, and to understand themselves. Because of my experience, I believe I have helped three mothers who lost children. Today, they, too, are adjusting each with a big gap in her life.

Not long ago, a depressed young man went to the top of a building in Washington and jumped, but did not die. A friend went to visit him in the hospital and told him, "I want you to go to Savitri and take yoga. She will help you to want to live again." After taking yoga for a while, his attitude changed. Once he asked, "You have gone through a lot in your life, haven't you?"

"Yes," I said, "but I did not ever try to take my life." Sometimes in class I would say to him, "Aren't you feeling better now? Aren't you glad you finished law school? Think how many people you will be able to help." He agreed.

SUBSTITUTE MOTHER

I take all my pupils as my children. They call me all hours of the day and night with physical as well as emotional problems. They call to say, "My wife has nonstop hiccups," or, "My husband has a stiff neck," or, "I have such a back pain I can't move," or, "I sleep three hours and can't go back to sleep," or, "I'm grinding my teeth." One had dizziness, another diarrhea. They complain of "just feeling lousy, no energy at all." These are mostly problems for doctors, but when a doctor examines them and finds nothing wrong, he tells them they are just tense. Then I get the call. Yoga does help everyone deal with all the big and little stress situations we face daily.

Every day I get the products of tension; problems they want yoga to solve. After a student has been with me for a few months, I don't hear as many complaints. Instead, I hear them telling each other how good they feel.

SAFE HARBOR

As I kept hearing the same complaints over and over, day after day, year after year, I began to realize that if my brand of yoga could help relieve all these problems for my pupils, perhaps my message should go further. My pupils kept urging me to put my teaching on paper, particularly since many of them were in Washington only for a short tour of duty. When they left Washington and me, they wanted to take me with them in book form. Many of them said they came sad and depressed, but left cheerful and happy.

People do come out of depression through the yoga experience. It is my aim to give them health and an understanding of themselves to make them comfortable with themselves. I like to think I steer my students through a sea of emotions into a harbor of peace.

Index of Recipes

For information about yoga classes, cassettes and related literature and activities,
write to Savitri's Studio, P.O. Box 5671, Washington, D.C. 20016

DIVERSITY BY DESIGN

"Some people have accused us of aspiring too high ... But we believe that ideals are like stars, you may not succeed in touching them with your hands, but like navigators at sea, you may be guided by them."

Ernest E. Howard

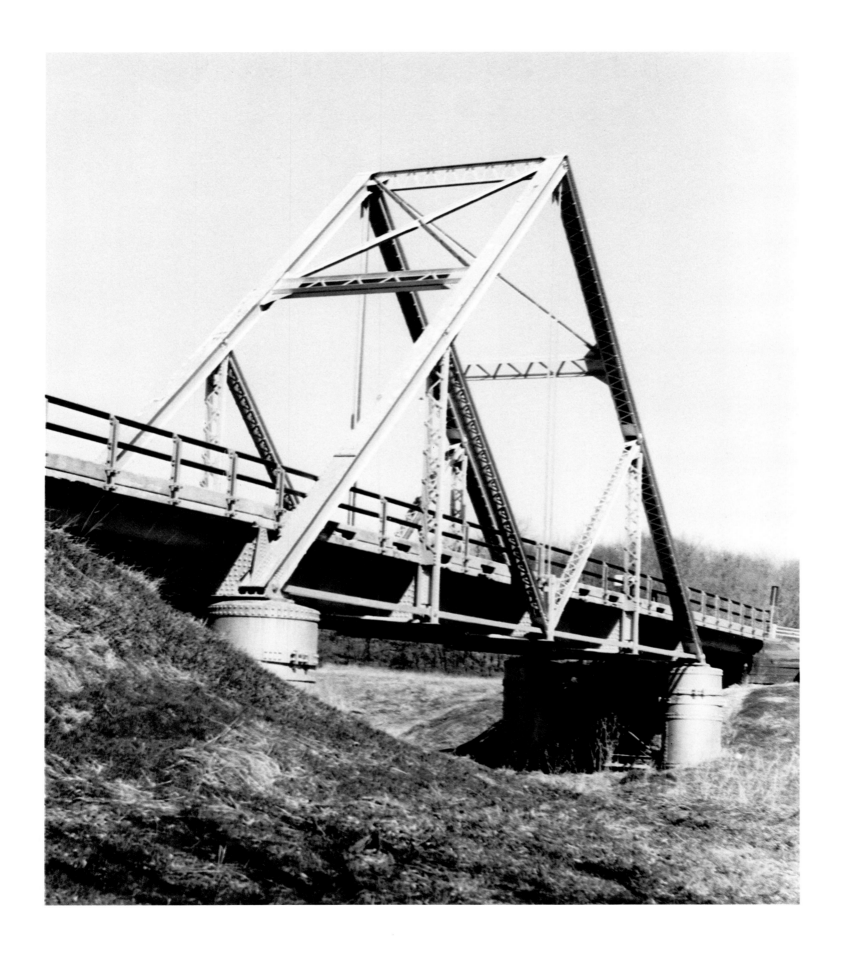

DIVERSITY BY DESIGN

Celebrating 75 Years of
Howard Needles Tammen & Bergendoff
1914-1989

Researched and Written
by
Kathi Ann Brown

Published by
Howard Needles Tammen & Bergendoff

(facing page) The A-Truss Bridge was an early design of John Alexander Low Waddell, a pioneer in structural engineering consulting. The design was ideal for use by the railroads in the late 1800s, and more than 100 A-truss bridges were eventually built.

FIRST EDITION
Copyright 1989 by Howard Needles Tammen & Bergendoff
L.C. 89-50600   ISBN 0-932845-34-7

Printed in the United States of America
The Lowell Press, Kansas City, Missouri

PHOTO CREDITS

H. Armstrong Roberts: pages ii, iv, 23, 26

UPI/Bettmann Newsphotos: pages iv, 6, 18, 28, 30, 39, 41,45, 47, 57, 63,
66, 73, 74

Missouri Valley Special Collections,
Kansas City, Missouri Public Library: pages 1, 6, 8, 9

Local History Section-Wichita Public Library: pages 7, 123

The Texas Collection-Baylor University: page 41

Kansas State Historical Society: page 42

CONTENTS

FOREWORD

I n January 1959, HNTB engineer Walter Keller wrote to retired partner Henry C. Tammen with a request. Would Tammen consider writing a short history of Howard Needles Tammen & Bergendoff for publication in the firm's in-house magazine? Henry Tammen had retired in 1950, after 42 years with HNTB and its predecessor firms. He had been a partner in the firm for more than two decades.

"It surprises me," explained Keller, "how eager our people are to know more about the beginnings of the firm and [those] who brought it all about. The subject comes up every time anyone sees photos of older bridges. As a matter of fact, lunch-time conversations, especially with newer [employees], often turn to speculation on the men who started the partnership. I don't think such questions are prompted by mere curiosity. To my way of thinking they show a large amount of respect for and some awe of [people] who have achieved as much as you. In any case, the interest is real and alive."

Henry Tammen never submitted the article that Walter Keller urged him to write. He died two years after receiving Keller's request. A few years later, Henry's daughter Margaret found among her father's personal papers a handwritten draft of a firm history which Henry had started shortly before his death in 1961. He had filled a dozen sheets with notes and anecdotes about the early days of his career. A chapter outline attached to the draft hints that Henry had planned to turn his reminiscences into a book someday. Unfortunately for us, death claimed him before he could fulfill his intentions.

The history of HNTB which follows is an attempt to pick up where Henry Tammen left off 30 years ago. Our hope and our wish have been to capture and preserve in this book some part of the unique, long legacy that the founders of HNTB have bequeathed to us and to future generations of HNTB employees.

Time has been both friend and foe in this effort. During the 75 years since the founding of Harrington, Howard & Ash in 1914, much has happened. The firm has been blessed with its share of successes and triumphs, as well as tested on occasion by adversity and personal trials. Those times, both good and bad, have made HNTB what it is today — and will help shape what it will be tomorrow. We are fortunate as an organization to possess a richly textured past that offers so many valuable lessons for the future.

We, the current partners of HNTB, are proud to offer this publication — *Diversity by Design: Celebrating 75 Years of Howard Needles Tammen & Bergendoff, 1914-1989* — as our generation's contribution to the preservation of the firm's history. At the time that Henry Tammen was at work on his memoirs, many of us were among those who, according to Walter Keller, wanted "to know more about the beginnings of the firm and those who brought it all about." We hope and trust that 30 years later interest in the firm's early partners and projects is still "real and alive." It is to HNTB's founders and to its employees — past, present, and future — that this diamond anniversary history is dedicated. ■

1989 Partnership

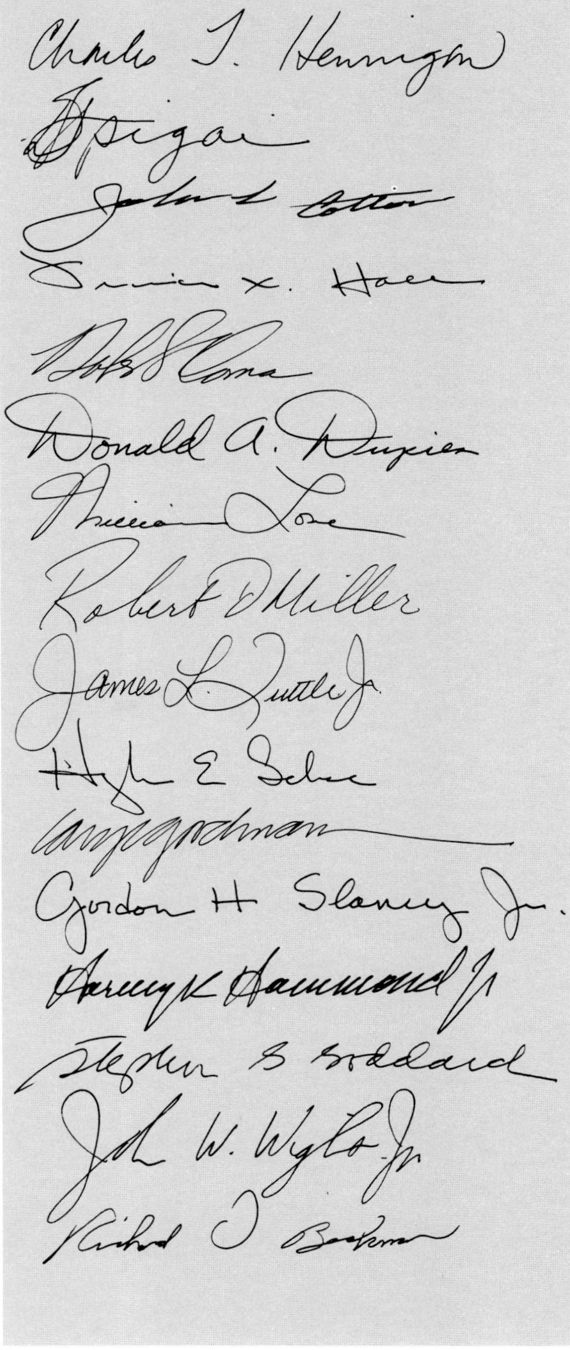

[handwritten signatures:]

Charles T. Hennigan

T. Pigai

John L. Cotton

Irwin X. Hall

Rolf S. Como

Donald A. Dupier

Theresa Lowe

Robert D. Miller

James L. Tuttle Jr.

Hugh E. Schur

Larry Goodman

Gordon H. Slaney Jr.

Harvey K. Hammond Jr.

Stephen B. Goddard

John W. Wyly Jr.

Richard J. Beckman

i

INTRODUCTION

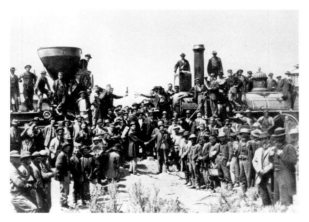

Grants of free land from the federal government and the promise of great wealth created intense competition in the second half of the 19th century among hundreds of American railroad companies looking to strike it rich during the country's rapid expansion. Independent consulting engineers made successful careers of designing bridges for rail routes across the rivers and canyons of the West. (above) Completion of the first transcontinental railroad on May 10, 1869, at Provo, Utah, inspired an entire generation of American railroaders to head West. For many, the dream went bust during the 1893 Depression, when hundreds of railways were bankrupted. In spite of the nation's financial chaos, Waddell's business thrived.

In 1914, John Lyle Harrington, Ernest Emmanuel Howard, and Louis Russell Ash joined together to form the civil engineering partnership Harrington, Howard & Ash in Kansas City, Missouri. Since the founding of Harrington, Howard & Ash, the surname Howard has been carried forward in the firm's name without interruption for 75 years. Today, the "H" of HNTB stands as a symbol of permanence and of continuity with the past.

HNTB can trace its roots back as far as 1886, when maverick bridge engineer Dr. John Alexander Low Waddell opened a consulting practice in Kansas City. Waddell quickly distinguished himself in the design of railroad bridges, a specialty which for a half century supplied a steady stream of work for the successive partnerships which evolved from Waddell's original firm. By the time that the third successive partnership — Harrington, Howard & Ash — opened its doors in 1914, the firm's design boards were overflowing with work on bridges in every corner of the United States and abroad.

Harrington, Howard & Ash could easily have remained a small but successful Kansas City firm, glorying in the heyday of American railroading, content to fade into relative obscurity with the passing of the railroad era. Destiny, and the firm's partners, however, had other plans. Between 1914 and 1989, Harrington, Howard & Ash slowly transformed itself into one of the nation's premier engineering and architectural firms: HNTB, Architects, Engineers & Planners. Today, HNTB boasts a far-flung network of 31 local design offices in 25 states across the country. Sixteen partners share responsibility for the firm's projects and internal operations. The partners are supported by an experienced staff of 40 associates and more than 2,200 technical and administrative employees. Together, HNTB's team of professionals handle more than $168 million of design work for clients annually.

The growth of HNTB over the years has come hand-in-hand with an increased diversification of the firm's services to clients. Building on a solid reputation in bridge design, HNTB soon branched out into other pursuits. The firm's expertise in roadway design has been well-established since the beginning of the modern turnpike and interstate highway eras following World War II. Airport planning and design has been a major activity at HNTB for more than 25 years. More recently, the firm has developed expertise in environmental engineering. Participation in rapid transit projects and in construction supervision also keeps HNTB staff busy.

The most dramatic evolution in HNTB's services has been the addition of architecture to the firm's portfolio. Many engineering firms have tried — and failed — to integrate architecture into their practices. HNTB, however, has enjoyed tremendous success in that arena. Since the merger of the Kansas City architectural firm of Kivett & Myers with HNTB in 1975, architecture has become an increasingly important component of HNTB's business. Today, architecture contributes as much as one-fourth of the firm's fees each year.

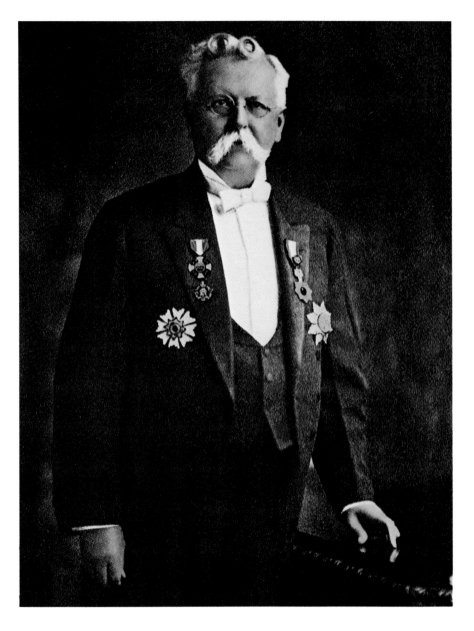

John Alexander Low Waddell
(1854-1938)

After several years in academe in the United States and abroad, Waddell opened an engineering consulting practice in Kansas City in 1892. Independent engineers like Waddell were a new breed of American entrepreneur who came of age during the country's most intense period of industrialization. Young engineers Ernest Howard and Henry Tammen learned about the intricacies of bridges and business partnerships while working in the shadow of the brilliant Waddell.

iii

Although three-quarters of a century has passed since the first days of Harrington, Howard & Ash, the legacy of the past is everywhere evident at HNTB. Especially prized by the firm are the many long-standing client relationships which have developed through the years. HNTB frequently has been invited to design an upgrade or replacement for a bridge or roadway which was originally designed by the firm for a client 30, 40, or 50 years ago. In other cases, the firm has provided services to a client on an

(right and below) The firm's earliest years were set against a backdrop of major advances in transportation, aviation, and communication.

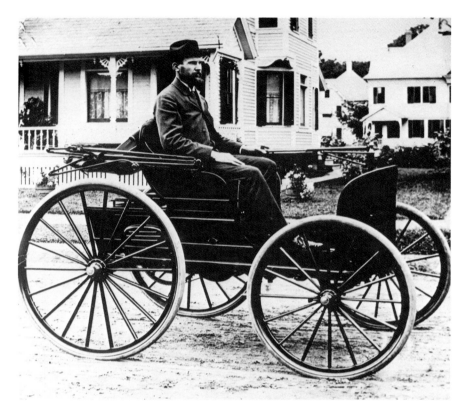

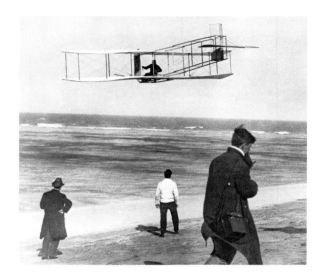

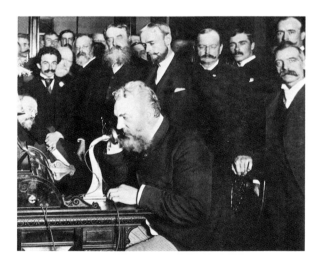

ongoing basis for so many years that the work has occupied two or more generations of HNTB engineers.

Less easy to quantify than long-term clients — but equally vital to HNTB's success and longevity — are the core values of integrity and quality which have been passed down from generation to generation. The firm's long tradition of exceptionally high ethical and technical standards continues to be a point of great pride to partners and employees, especially as HNTB continues to grow and thrive in an increasingly competitive business environment. A satisfied client, a fee honestly earned, and a job well done remain as important today as they were 75 years ago.

Like most histories, the history of HNTB is actually several tales woven together. One tale recounts the story of the people who founded and guided the firm from its early days to the present. Another tale highlights the projects which earned the firm its cherished reputation and rank among its peers. And a third tale places those people and projects in the larger framework of the country's political and economic development. Taken together, these three threads tell the story of HNTB. That story is found in these pages. ■

PART ONE

Pioneering Bridge Design

"A growing country, coupled with technological advances in transportation, could only mean a prosperous future for far-sighted engineers who possessed the necessary know-how and determination to take advantage of the opportunities."

CHAPTER ONE
The Beginning (1886-1914)

B undled up to stave off the chilly winds of New York Harbor, Ernest Howard and his elderly companion boarded the Staten Island Ferry. To fellow passengers that wintry day in 1936, the pair appeared to be an aging, but hale father and his middle-aged son on an afternoon outing in the midst of the nation's worst depression. But neither man was particularly interested in the city's waterfront sights. The two, in fact, spent most of the cruise deep in conversation, discussing what fascinated them both perhaps more than anything else: bridge engineering.

To anyone acquainted with either of the two men, the choice of topic that day would have come as no surprise. Born a generation apart, the pair nonetheless shared an intense interest in every aspect of the civil engineering profession, most especially of bridge design. An afternoon of collegial talk about their favorite topic could only have been pleasure to them both. What might have surprised anyone who knew both men, however, was the identity of Ernest Howard's companion. The 82-year old man sharing the rail at Howard's side was none other than his former employer, Dr. John Alexander Low Waddell.

Two decades earlier, Howard and Waddell had parted professional ways. Waddell, often considered the father of twentieth-century bridge design in America, had been Howard's boss during the younger engineer's formative professional years. That relationship had ended abruptly in 1914, when Waddell withdrew from his partnership with John Lyle Harrington, and Howard remained with Harrington to form Harrington, Howard & Ash. Standing on the deck of the ferry 22 years later, the pair might have discovered that their common interests and experiences outweighed any differences. Both men were native Canadians; both were devoted to their profession, delighted in world travel, and shared a scholarly bent. Both, too, had savored the rewards and frustrations of senior partnership in successful engineering firms. Standing as equal colleagues at the rail as the boat chugged along on its route across the Harbor, the formidable Waddell and his former protégé could well have wondered how things might have turned out if other choices, other decisions, had been made.

A Maverick

John Alexander Low Waddell was born in Port Hope, Ontario, in 1854, the oldest of nine children of Robert Needham Waddell of Ireland and Angeline Esther Jones of New York. Sickly as a youth, Waddell received his basic education at the hands of private tutors. In 1872, he enrolled at the Trinity College School in his hometown. A subsequent five-month stint at a business college in Toronto led the restless Waddell to cross the border into his mother's native country to attend Rensselaer Polytechnic Institute in Troy, New York, one of the first professional engineering schools in the United States. Waddell graduated from RPI in 1875, only six years after the first transcontinental railway in North America had been opened with a golden spike at Provo, Utah.

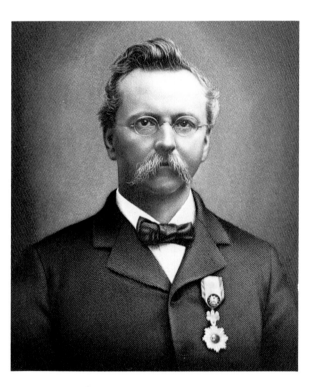

(above) A young J.A.L. Waddell's movable bridge designs allowed bridges to be built at sites where ordinary fixed spans that would interfere with river traffic were not feasible.

(facing page) Waddell gained experience designing bridges across the country and around the world, such as the Willamette River Bridge, Salem, Oregon.

1

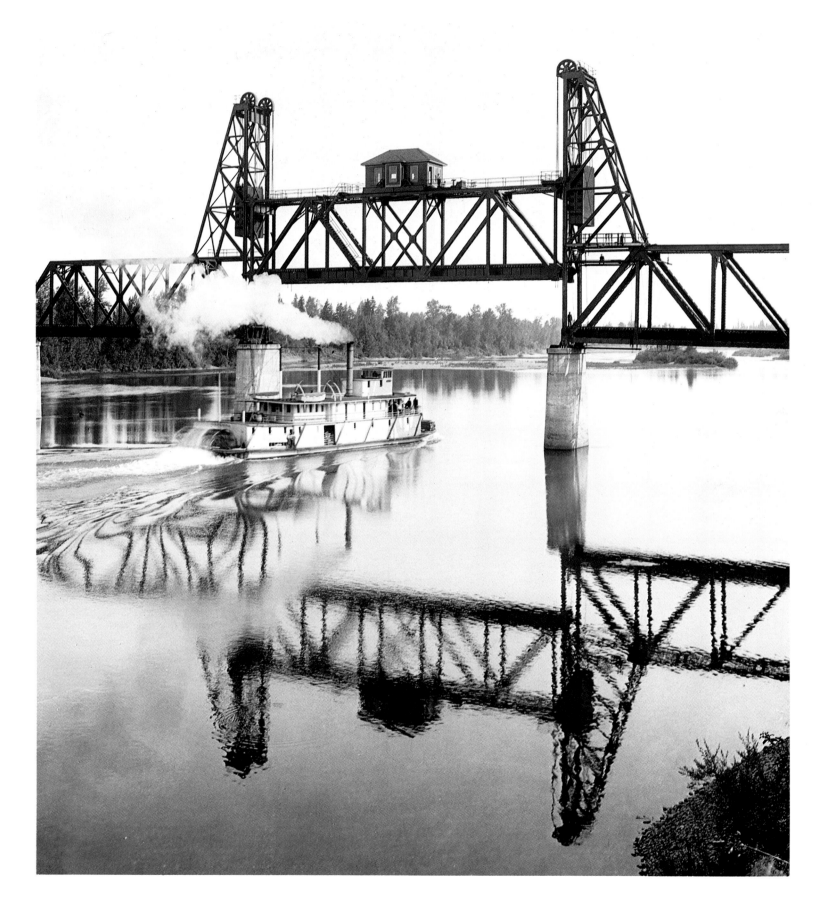

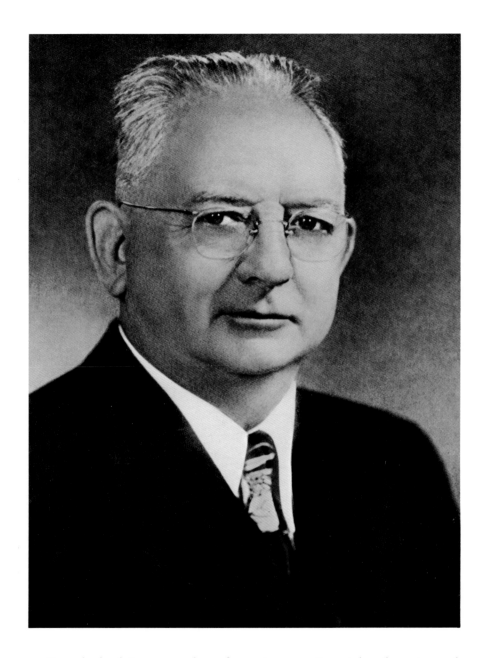

Ernest E. Howard
(1880-1953)

*Ernest Howard joined Waddell &
Hedrick in 1901, where he learned the
art of bridge design from J.A.L. Waddell,
and later, John Lyle Harrington. Known
and respected both as an engineer and
a scholar, Howard guided the firm that
bears his name through two world wars
and the Great Depression.*

3

Canada had its own plans for a transcontinental rail route and
Waddell wanted to be part of the project. He returned to his native
country and spent the next three years as a government draftsman
in connection with the location and construction of the Canadian
Pacific Railway. But Waddell also had a scholarly itch that his
assignments on the CPR couldn't satisfy. He was soon back at RPI,
this time as a faculty member. That didn't last long either.
Obviously torn between his academic interests and the challenges
of real-life engineering problems, Waddell left RPI to spend a year
as the chief engineer of Raymond & Campbell, a bridge design firm
in Council Bluffs, Iowa.

Waddell was soon off again, this time to the Orient. The offer of
a professorship in the Civil Engineering Department of the Imperial
University of Tokyo proved to be too tempting to pass up. While
abroad, he published his first book: *The Designing of Ordinary
Iron Highway Bridges (1882)*. But, after four years in Tokyo,

Waddell decided to return to the States and settle down. In 1886, he moved to Kansas City, Missouri, and the following year hung out his shingle — as an official agent of the Phoenix Bridge Company of Phoenixville, Pennsylvania, and as a private engineering consultant.

Waddell's decision to return to the United States was timely. Developments around the nation pointed to a bright future for professional engineers. The League of American Wheelmen, forerunner of the American Road Builders Association, had been founded in 1880 by avid bicyclists. The group was busy promoting its "better roads movement," a campaign which would eventually lead to federal action to create the nation's network of highways. In 1883 John Augustus Roebling's Brooklyn Bridge was opened by President Chester Arthur to great fanfare. The next year brought the unveiling of architect William LeBaron Jenney's Home Insurance Company Building, Chicago's first skyscraper. And the four decades bracketing the turn of the century witnessed the mind-boggling boom-and-bust cycles of American railroad building.

With his experience on the Canadian Pacific Railway and his bridge design work for Raymond & Campbell and the Phoenix Bridge Company, Waddell was in an excellent position to make the most of the frenzied competition among American railroad companies. Bridges on the new rail routes became Waddell's specialty. By 1892, Waddell was confident enough of a steady market for his services to resign from Phoenix to devote himself full-time to his own consulting practice.

South Halsted Street Bridge

Just as Waddell was launching his new business, the Depression of 1893 hit the country. In the course of a few months, 74 railroads fell into receivership, 600 banks closed and 15,000 commercial houses collapsed across the nation. Waddell was not among those to lose his shirt in the financial chaos. In fact, he was hard at work on a project which ultimately became his best-known work: the South Halsted Street vertical lift bridge in Chicago, Illinois.

Although European designs of movable short-span bridges had come earlier, Waddell's bridge over the South Chicago River was his own invention and the first large-scale, high-clearance lift span of its type in the United States. The bridge's center span of 130 feet could be lifted to a height of 155 feet, to let ships pass, by means of wire ropes passing over sheaves (pulleys), 12 feet in diameter, on top of two towers on the river banks. The weight of the span was balanced by counterweights of cast iron. Intentional or not, Waddell's selection of Chicago as the location to showcase his new invention was well-timed; that year the city hosted thousands of visitors to the World's Columbian Exposition.

Waddell & Hedrick

When Waddell tendered his resignation as agent of the Phoenix Bridge Company, he decided that it was time to take on an assistant. He hired Ira G. Hedrick. Hedrick worked as Waddell's right-hand-man until 1899 when Waddell made him a partner and created Waddell & Hedrick.

Among the first to join Waddell & Hedrick's growing staff was Ernest Emmanuel Howard in 1901. Howard was born on February 29, 1880, in Toronto, Canada to a London-born Presbyterian minister and his wife. His mother's ill health, however, sent the

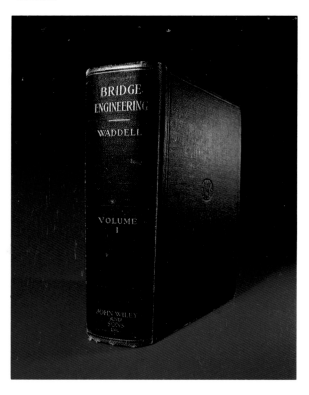

(below) Like his protégé Ernest Howard, J.A.L. Waddell was a brilliant engineer, scholar, and writer. His textbook, "The Designing of Ordinary Iron Highway Bridges" (1882), is considered a classic.

4

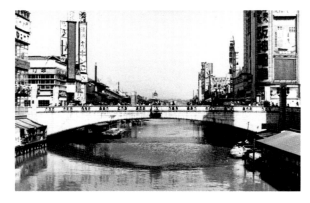

(above) While a professor at the University of Tokyo, Waddell established an international reputation as both teacher and designer. The Ebisu Bridge in Japan is a Waddell design.

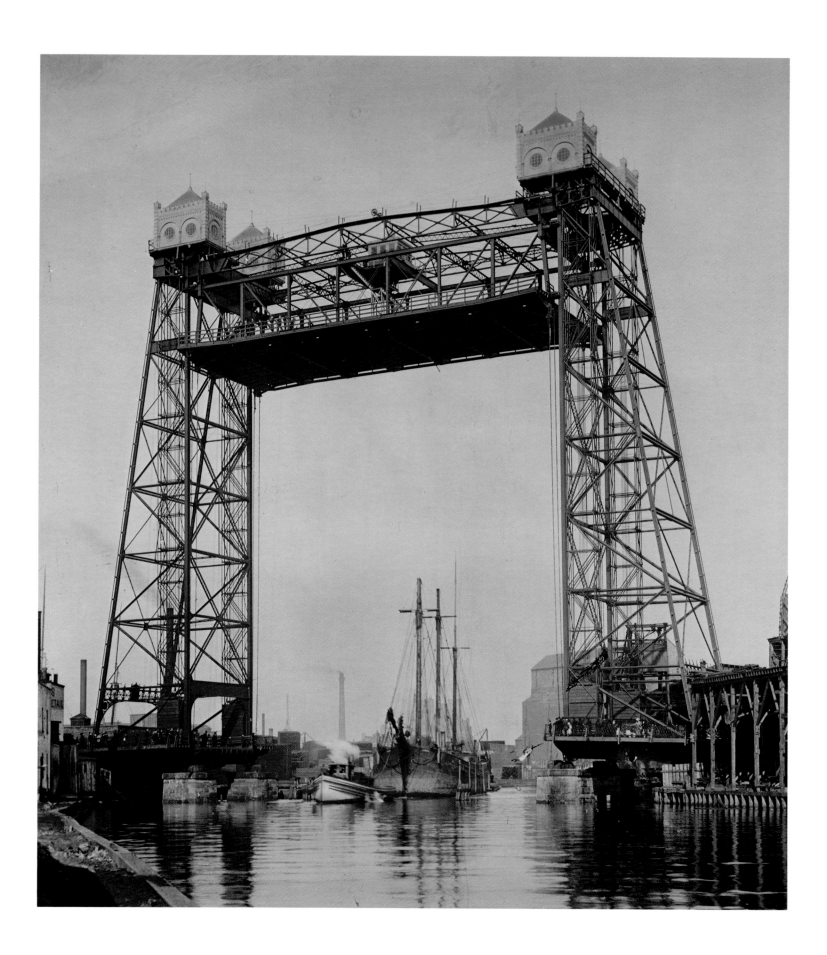

family south to Jacksboro, Texas, in 1893, "out in cattle country 40 miles from a railroad." Far from his genteel roots, Howard "lost [his] English accent the hard way."

Howard's boyhood curiosity about how the world worked blossomed early. Later in his life he reminisced about those early days. When he had gone swimming with the boys he "spent most of the time building water wheels in the creek. [He] hung around the carpenter shop, the blacksmith shop or anywhere that men were working with tools." The interest was so strong that Howard enrolled at the 1,000-student University of Texas, graduating in 1900 with both a B.S. and a degree in civil engineering.

After a short stint on some irrigation works for rice lands in lower Louisiana, Howard returned to the university as an instructor. Like Waddell — who would soon employ him — Howard loved the academic life as well as the adventure of the railroad. Fate soon wrested from the new engineer's hands any need to choose between the two paths. Howard's boss, University of Texas Dean Thomas U. Taylor, took the liberty not only of recommending Howard for a slot on Waddell's staff in Kansas City, but of wiring the young man's acceptance before Howard had even had a chance to think over the offer.

Ernest Howard dutifully arrived on the doorstep of Waddell & Hedrick in June 1901 and settled into work at the grand salary of $30 per month. His first few years with the firm were a whirlwind. After a bit of office work, he took the assignment of assistant engineer on the construction of the Red River bridge at Alexandria, Louisiana, until its completion in 1902. He returned to the office for a year and then the firm sent him to Mexico as assistant engineer on the extensive bridge work of the Veracruz and Pacific Railway. He became resident engineer in charge in September 1903. His work there was completed in 1904. Next he took charge of the construction of the James Street Bridge and the reconstruction of the Ohio Street Bridge, both over the Kaw River in Kansas City. From March 1905 until its completion, he was in charge of the construction of the $3 million Sixth Street-Intercity Viaduct in Kansas City.

Howard was not the only engineer to join Waddell & Hedrick's growing staff in 1901. Twenty-eight year old Louis Russell Ash also left an academic career to enter the Waddell & Hedrick fold. Born in Kentucky in 1873, Ash was graduated from the University of Arkansas with a B.C.E. degree in 1893, the same year that Waddell was designing his South Halsted Street bridge. The next year he took a B.E.E. degree and accepted a position as professor of mathematics at Coe College in Cedar Rapids, Iowa. There he stayed until 1901 when the lure of private practice proved to be too enticing to ignore. His new job with Waddell & Hedrick, however, did not stymie his academic pursuits. In 1902 he took a C.E. degree from his alma mater, and in following years he pursued post-graduate work at the University of Chicago.

Howard and Ash joined the world of private engineering consultants during a fascinating period in the country's development. The spring of 1901 had witnessed a monumental collision of banking interests which nearly destroyed the Great Northern and North Pacific railroad lines, as well as the country's entire banking structure, until a settlement was forced on the rival parties. The railroad companies faced other problems as well: the United Mine Workers mounted a massive strike against railroad owners of the nation's mines which ended only when President Theodore Roosevelt threatened to send in federal troops.

Of more professional interest perhaps to Howard and Ash were

(facing page) The mechanical design of the South Halsted Street lift bridge in Chicago (1893) was innovative and helped establish Waddell's firm as a leader in the design of movable bridges.

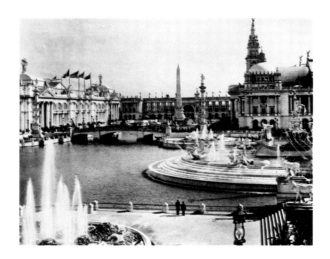

(above) Visitors to the World's Columbian Exposition in Chicago in 1893 would have been able to see Waddell's unique movable bridge at South Halsted Street. The exposition drew thousands to wonder at the latest marvels of American scientific invention.

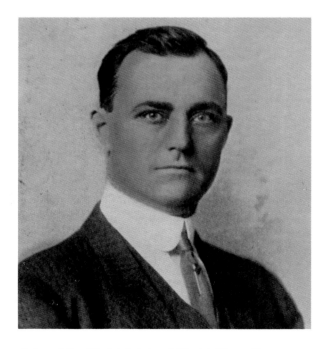

(above) Ira Hedrick joined Waddell's staff as an assistant and became his partner in 1899. Both talented and ambitious engineers, Waddell and Hedrick were soon at loggerheads. Hedrick withdrew from the partnership in 1906.

6

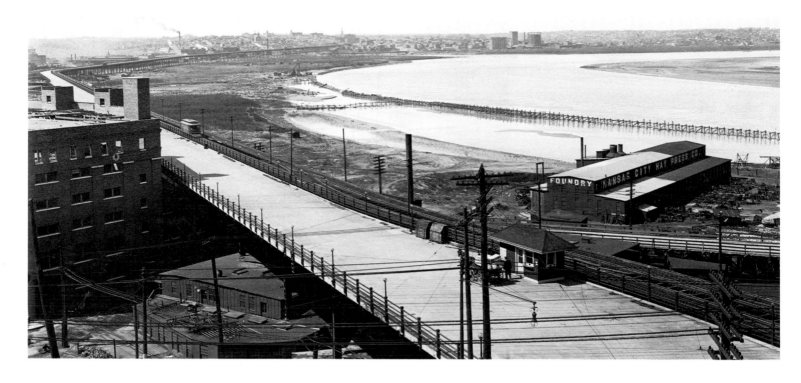

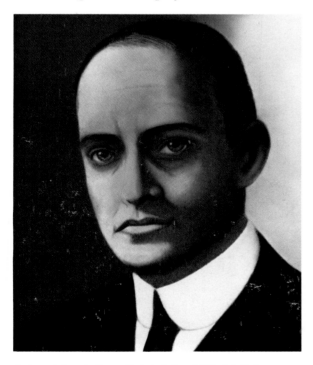

(top) Kansas City's 8,400-foot Intercity Viaduct accommodated automobiles and street cars when it opened in 1906. Ernest Howard was the resident engineer on the project.

(above) Louis Russell Ash joined Waddell & Hedrick in 1901, the same year Ernest Howard joined the firm. After leaving with Ira Hedrick in 1907, Ash returned to become a partner in Harrington, Howard & Ash in 1914.

developments in the transportation field. The establishment of the American Road Makers (formerly part of the League of American Wheelmen) and the American Automobile Association in 1902 ushered in the age of the automobile, an invention which Ernest Howard would live to see revolutionize his firm's practice. In 1903, Henry Ford founded his car company with start-up capital of $100,000. That same year, Dr. H. Nelson Jackson, a prominent surgeon from Burlington, Vermont, completed the first transcontinental car trip in 52 days, driving along railroad rights-of-way and dirt paths in a 20 HP Winton touring car. And, the Wright Brothers launched the first successful airplane flight at Kitty Hawk, North Carolina on December 17, 1903.

These developments heralded a future filled with engineering challenges. A growing country, coupled with technological advances in transportation, could only mean a prosperous future for far-sighted engineers who possessed the necessary know-how and determination to take advantage of the opportunities.

For even the most talented and ambitious engineers, however, the path into the future would be mined with its own troubles. By 1906, the "dignified and bemedalled" Waddell and the "brilliant and spirited" Hedrick were at loggerheads. Men of strong personalities, the pair did not see eye to eye on a number of issues. At the end of the year Hedrick withdrew.

Waddell & Harrington

Before Ira Hedrick had emptied his desk drawers at Waddell & Hedrick's headquarters, Waddell found another partner. Thirty-nine year-old John Lyle Harrington had worked for Waddell for two summers during his undergraduate days at the University of Kansas in the 1890s. In 1907 he returned to Kansas City to join his former employer in creating the new partnership of Waddell & Harrington.

A native Kansan, Harrington had grown up in the rich farmland of Johnson County, near DeSoto. In spite of limited formal

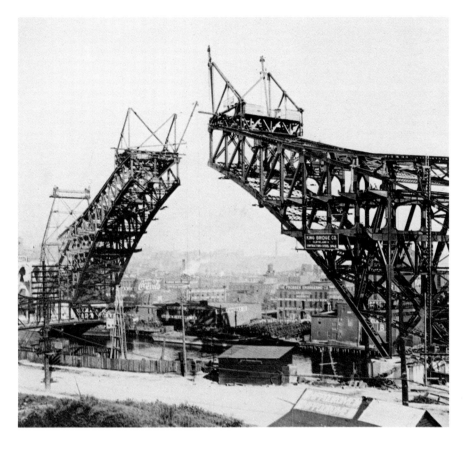

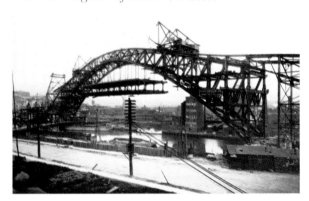

(left and below) The Detroit-Superior Bridge in Cleveland, Ohio, was one of the firm's earliest projects. Today the bridge is listed on the National Register of Historic Places.

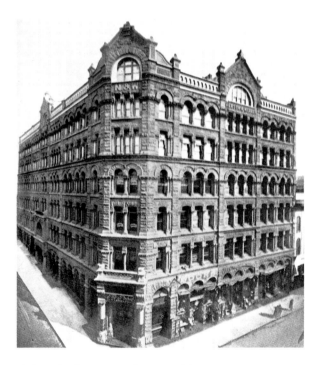

(above) The New Nelson Building in Kansas City housed the first offices of Waddell & Harrington.

schooling, he was admitted at age 22 to the University of Kansas by examination, working his way through college to earn simultaneous B.S., A.B. and C.E. degrees in 1895. Harrington during the next dozen years took a succession of jobs with bridge, steel, railroad, and construction firms in various parts of the country. He stayed only long enough at each to absorb the experience he felt useful. While working in Montreal as chief engineer and manager of the Locomotive and Machine Co., Harrington received both a B.S. and M.S. from McGill University.

Harrington's sudden reappearance in Kansas City to become a partner in a firm by which he had been employed for only two summers might seem unusual. In fact, since his college days, Harrington had kept in close touch with Waddell. The young engineer compiled and edited a volume of 22 of Waddell's articles on engineering in 1905 while working in Montreal, a full two years before becoming Waddell's partner.

In Harrington, Waddell perhaps felt that he had found a devoted protégé. With Ira Hedrick on the way out the door and his own travel and research activities increasing each year, Waddell needed someone he could depend on to handle the day-to-day operations of the firm. The "imperial, political, and polished" Harrington seemed to fit the bill.

Henry Casper Tammen, who joined the firm in 1908, regarded Harrington "as the driving force of the firm, getting most of the business done by the firm, and seeing that it was carried through." His boss was a "charming, cultured gentleman, of striking appearance, a super salesman, an able structural and mechanical engineer [who] kept closely in touch with everything that was going on in the office."

(below) John Lyle Harrington replaced Ira Hedrick as Waddell's partner in 1907. Energetic and restless, Harrington had worked for Waddell during summers as an undergraduate at the University of Kansas in the 1890s. His training as a mechanical engineer was critical to perfecting and popularizing Waddell's movable bridge designs. When Waddell and Harrington parted in 1914, the latter invited employees Ernest Howard and Louis Russell Ash to become his new partners.

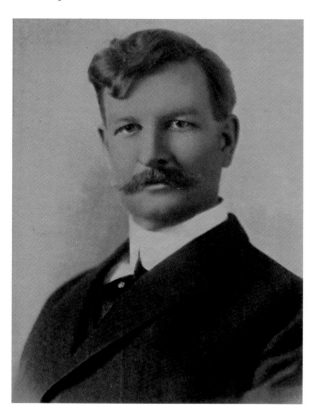

(above right) While most of the bridges designed by Waddell and Harrington were steel, the firm also designed concrete bridges. One of the most spectacular is the beautiful Arroyo-Seco Viaduct in Pasadena, California.

(facing page) This high-rise ribbed-spandrel arch bridge, completed in 1908, is still in use

Tammen was 24 years old when he walked through the doors of Waddell & Harrington in the New Nelson Building in Kansas City. "The word 'new' was a misnomer," recollected Tammen years later, "in that the building was old, dirty, dingy and was located in the most unprepossessing neighborhood." Tammen had come to Kansas City from two years as a rodman and draftsman on the Western Pacific Railroad. Born in Yankton, South Dakota, on November 15, 1884, Tammen had studied at the University of California, finishing his studies in 1906.

Despite his first, unfavorable glimpse of his new employer's

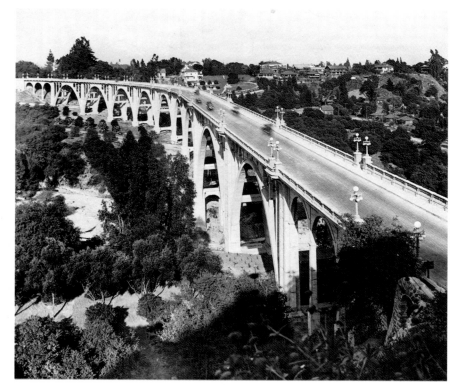

location, Tammen was quite impressed by the men with whom he worked and the projects to which he was assigned:

> *"... the firm was wide awake, with exceptionally competent partners and assistant engineers, able supervisors and a group of ambitious young men in the drafting room, all trying to get ahead. When I arrived, the drafting room staff was small, about 15. Work was plentiful and varied, with plenty of opportunity to learn and to advance — an ideal situation."*

Harrington proved to be no easy taskmaster. Tammen noted that he had the boss to "thank for many, many evenings of studying and hard work necessary to accomplish the tasks he thrust upon me. I owe[d] him a great deal."

Waddell was less accessible to the new engineer from South Dakota; he devoted most of his time to roaming the United States and Canada developing work, so it was a few years before Tammen came to know him.

Tammen's entry into the firm brought him immediately into contact with a man who first became his boss, then later his

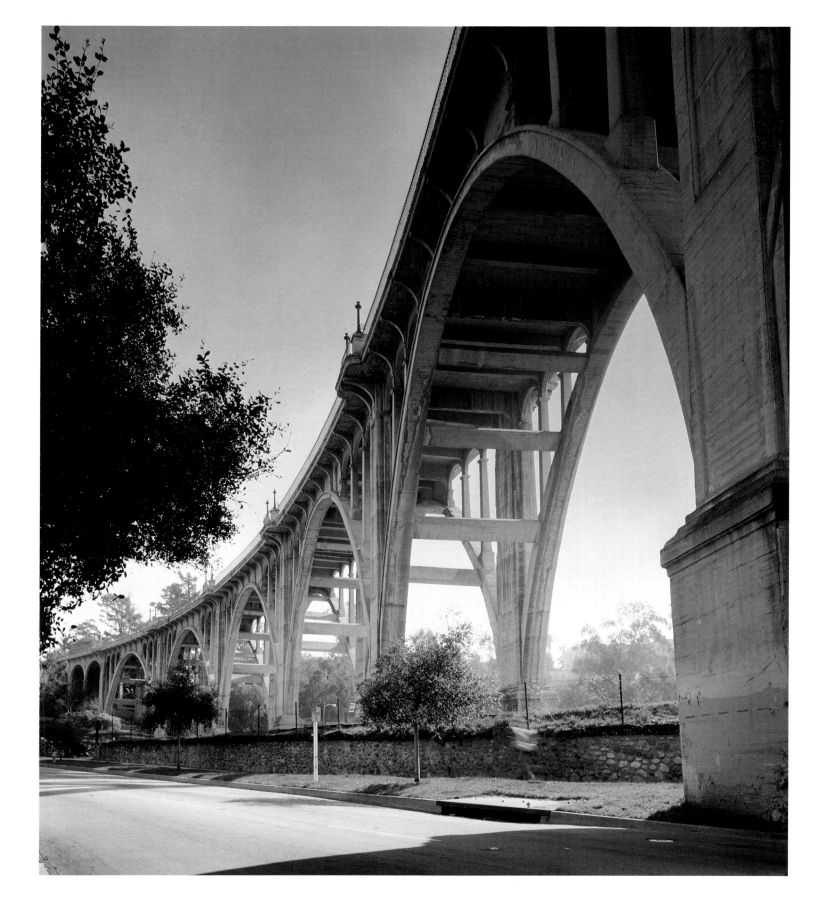

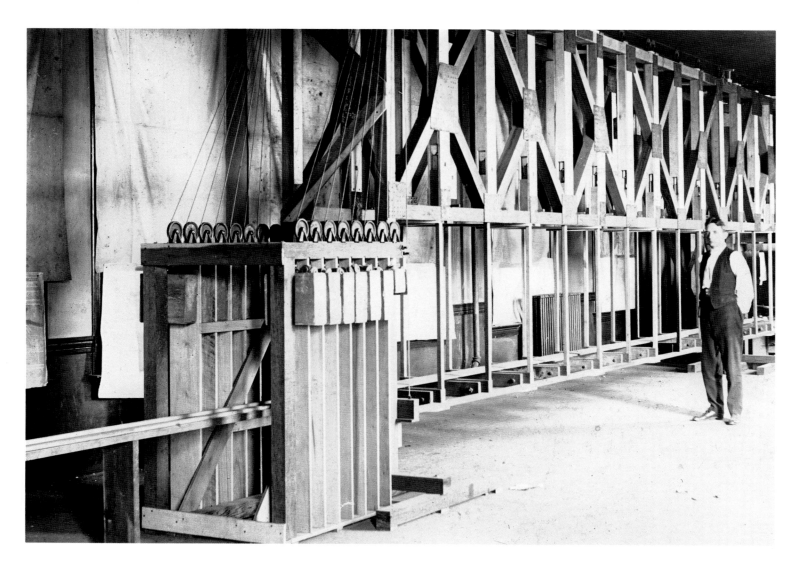

(top) When Henry Tammen joined Waddell & Harrington in 1908, Ernest Howard, not yet 30 years old, was hard at work on a 29-foot long demonstration model of the Armour-Swift-Burlington (ASB) Bridge. The design included a lower deck supported by hangers that "telescoped" into the upper truss. Howard's successful model persuaded a skeptical client to accept the innovative design.

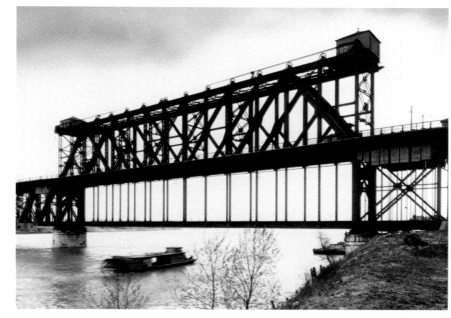

(right) Howard and Tammen mastered the intricacies of movable bridge design under John Lyle Harrington's watchful eye. The ASB Bridge, spanning the Missouri River at Kansas City, was their first project together. Completed in 1912, the bridge carried automobile traffic on an upper deck and railroad traffic on a lower deck that could be raised to allow passage of riverboats.

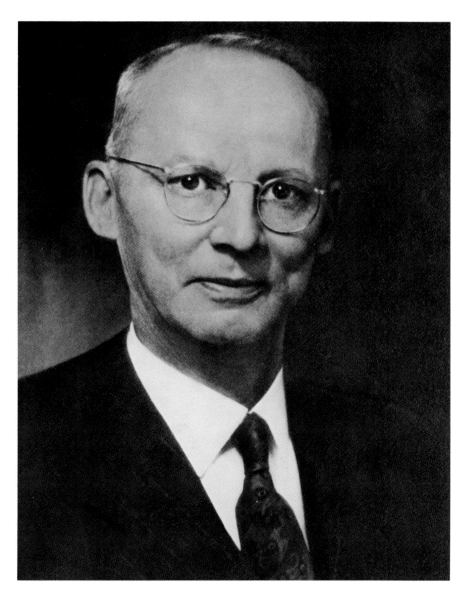

Henry C. Tammen
(1884-1961)

Henry Tammen joined Waddell &
Harrington in 1908 and worked under
the demanding John Lyle Harrington.
One of Tammen's first projects was the
mechanical design of the Armour-Swift-
Burlington Bridge in Kansas City,
Missouri. Tammen worked side by side
with future partner Ernest Howard to
perfect the bridge's unusual design.
Tammen's meticulous technical
standards and renowned engineering
abilities won him a place in the
partnership and in the firm's name in
1928.

12

partner: Ernest Howard. Howard had elected to stay with Waddell when Hedrick departed in 1907. In the reorganization of the firm which followed, Howard had become principal assistant engineer. When Tammen joined Waddell & Harrington in 1908, Howard was hard at work on a 29-foot long working model of the proposed Armour-Swift-Burlington (ASB) bridge over the Missouri River at Kansas City. Tammen was assigned to work with Howard. The new employee was quick to spot Howard's strengths:

> *"I was always impressed by his incisive thinking in the*
> *solution of a difficult problem and above all by his*
> *calmness 'under fire.' He held to the thought that there*
> *was no problem so difficult and no mishap so serious*
> *that an acceptable solution could not be found by calm,*
> *thorough investigation and analysis."*

Howard's "calm, thorough" efforts on the ASB bridge model paid off; his demonstration of the model's lifting deck won the support of the client, and the bridge was completed in 1912 under Howard's direction.

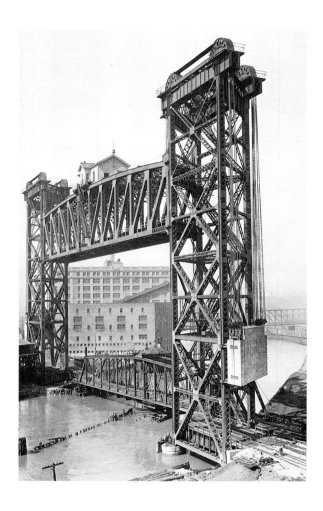

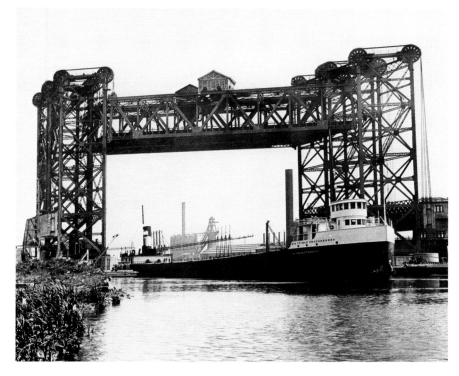

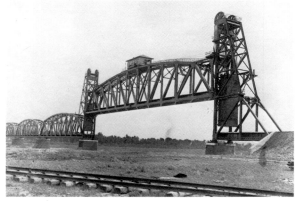

(this page) Harrington's mechanical design concepts were refined and brought to life by Howard and Tammen. The firm developed many innovations in lift mechanisms that were put to use in a variety of bridges. (top left) Pennsylvania Railroad Bridge over the Chicago River, Chicago, Illinois. (top right) Pennsylvania Railroad Bridge over the Calumet River, Chicago, Illinois. (above) Missouri River Bridge, Snowden, Montana, for the Great Northern Railroad.

Clouds on the Horizon

The Armour-Swift-Burlington Bridge was only one of more than two dozen bridges using vertical lift elements that Waddell & Harrington designed between 1907 and 1914. The Waddell & Harrington bridges were the first of their kind since the construction of the original South Halsted Street Bridge in Chicago more than a decade earlier. Although Waddell had won acclaim for his innovation, the lift mechanism of the South Halsted Street structure needed a better design. Not until 1909 was another built in the United States: the Pond Creille Bridge at Sand Point, Idaho, designed by Waddell & Harrington.

Several biographical sources suggest that Harrington brought the vital mechanical engineering skill needed to develop Waddell's invention into a rational, well-integrated design. Harrington put both Henry Tammen and Ernest Howard to work on experiments to refine Waddell's original efforts. The assignment proved to be challenging and rewarding. Both future HNTB partners laid the foundations of their professional careers in the feverish perfection of vertical lift mechanisms.

Refinement of the new bridge type sowed seeds of discontent between Harrington and Waddell. The firm was flooded with orders to design vertical lift bridges. Harrington, naturally perhaps, basked in the glow of his success. Waddell — not known for his humility — did not revel in the firm's popularity. As a consequence, the firm's achievement was offset by an "undisclosed controversy" between the two principals which "because of Harrington's inflexibility and Waddell's vanity left a legacy of bad feeling on both sides," according to Harrington's biography. By the end of 1914, Waddell & Harrington had been dissolved. From then on, Waddell and his protégé Ernest Howard would take different paths through the engineering world — until their paths crossed again on an afternoon ferry ride in 1936. ■

CHAPTER TWO

A New Firm: Harrington, Howard & Ash (1914-1920)

The firm of Waddell & Harrington was destined to last only seven years. During those seven years — from 1907 until 1914 — a great deal had happened. The "perfected" vertical lift bridge in which the firm specialized was in great demand. To handle the work, the firm in 1910 had taken over the entire top floor of the Orear-Leslie Building at 1012 Baltimore Avenue in Kansas City, Missouri. The firm opened another office, too. Harry G. Hunter was sent to Vancouver, British Columbia, to set up a small office in connection with work for the Canadian Northern Pacific Railway. Business was booming for the small Kansas City firm.

Ernest E. Howard

Important changes in staff had also taken place during the Waddell & Harrington years. In September of the same year in which the firm moved to the Baltimore Avenue address, Ernest Howard was named associate engineer. Just 30 years old, Howard had impressed his superiors with the same attributes which Henry Tammen had noticed during his assignment with Howard on the ASB Bridge working model.

Being named associate engineer of a growing firm was surely an honor for the young Howard. He had come a long way since his boyhood days of building water wheels in the local creek. Yet, as much as bridge design absorbed his attention and considerable talents, Howard was also intensely interested in subjects beyond bridge engineering. The activities which would give rise to his reputation as the "firm's scholar" — a reputation which still resonates 36 years after his death — were already well-loved in his young adulthood. His interests in archaeology, the Bible, theatre, travel, and education took up what free time he had when he was not working on a bridge design.

Howard's mind was always at work on projects even when he relaxed with friends. In 1911, as a young man canoeing with companions on the Blue River near Kansas City, he prepared a large map of the Blue, which he envisioned as a potential boat course of beauty "comparable to the Thames in England." Industrial development put an end to Howard's dreams, but with friends he built a weekend cottage on the river banks, which they named "Shack-en-Bleu."

The final days of Waddell & Harrington had also witnessed the return of former Waddell & Hedrick employee, Louis Russell Ash. In 1907, when J.A.L. Waddell and Ira Hedrick went their respective ways, Ash had decided that his immediate future lay with Hedrick. He stayed with Hedrick for only three years, however, before taking a position as head of bridge design for Kansas City. As city engineer, Ash probably came into frequent contact with his old colleagues at Waddell & Harrington. Howard's ASB Bridge was built while Ash was employed by the city. In 1913 Ash was offered the position of principal assistant engineer with Waddell &

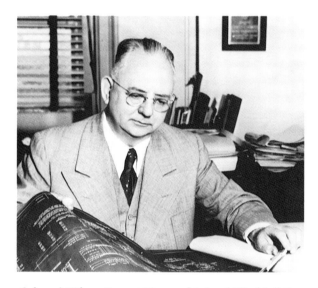

(above) When Ernest Howard joined Waddell & Hedrick in 1901 he earned $30 a month. His earliest duties included drafting, inspection, and supervision of construction of bridges as far away as Mexico. He quickly gained his superiors' confidence and at age 34 became John Lyle Harrington's partner when the latter split with Waddell in 1914.

14

Harrington, and took over the general direction of all office engineering. His return to the firm might have been inspired by the offer of a partnership share in the new firm which would shortly rise from the ashes of Waddell & Harrington.

Harrington, Howard & Ash

The tensions between John Lyle Harrington and his former mentor, Waddell, came to a head in 1913. Henry Tammen, who was offered the top spot of chief designer with both of the firms which resulted from the impending split, charitably characterized the breakup as a simple case in which two principals "agreed to disagree ... and the partnership was dissolved." Now-deceased HNTB partner Ellis Paul, who joined Harrington's reorganized firm in 1922, offered a second-hand, but perhaps more human analysis of the dynamic forces at work. Paul suggested that the split was the result of

> *"... two brilliant and self-centered individuals with different ideas on the development of their firm and ... the division of the 'spoils.' Although John Lyle Harrington, the younger, was interested in the lift bridge, his chief interest was in the development of new business and the expansion of the firm. His interest in the 'spoils,' then and later, was not what it could buy for him, but in the power and prestige he would have."*

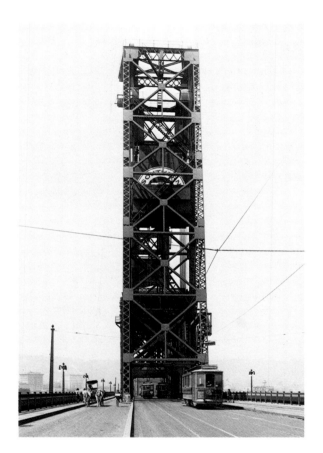

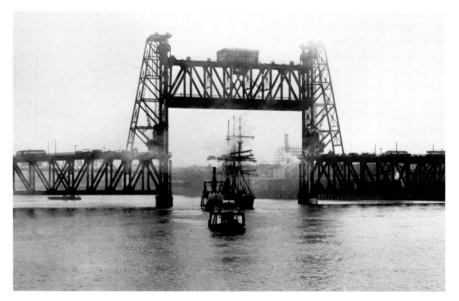

(above and right) Harrington, Howard & Ash's first job (#A1) was the Willamette River Bridge at Portland, Oregon (1914). Also known as the Harriman Bridge, and more recently as the "Steel Bridge," the structure featured the same ingenious lifting mechanism used on the ASB Bridge. The hangers on the lower deck could be drawn up into the superstructure of the overhead span. When necessary, both decks could be lifted. Ernest Howard designed the machinery.

(facing page) The "Steel Bridge" over the Willamette River at Portland is still in use and carries a light rail line.

Whatever the specific cause of the breakup — Harrington's "inflexibility" or Waddell's "vanity" — the two larger-than-life personalities parted by the close of 1913. Henry Tammen, who elected to stay as chief designer with Harrington, recalled that except "for Mr. Hardesty and Mr. Fox, who departed for new quarters with Dr. Waddell, everything continued as before."

But things were not quite the same. Although the new firm took over virtually all of the work in which Waddell & Harrington had been engaged, Harrington seemed to be determined to minimize his connection with his former partner. To symbolize a fresh start, a new job numbering system, beginning with #A1 (the Willamette

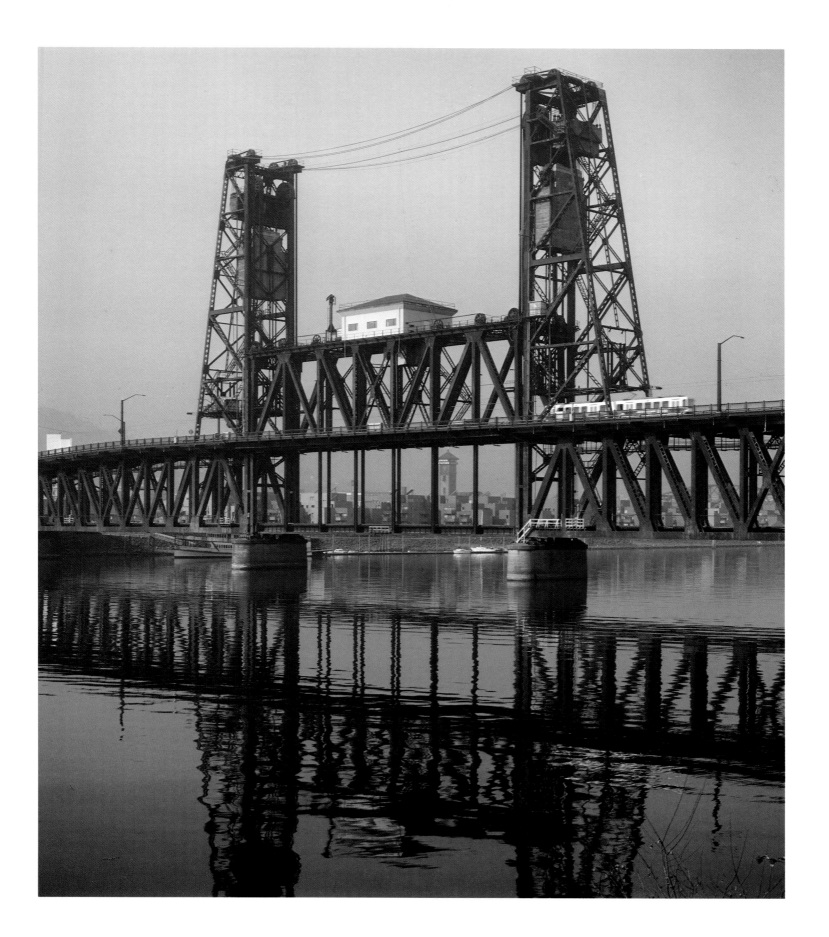

(right) In the 1920s, the Welland Canal bridges helped to see Harrington, Howard & Ash and its successor firm, Ash-Howard-Needles & Tammen, through the very earliest days of the Great Depression. The firm's connections to Canada date back to Waddell, a native of Port Hope, Ontario. Future partner Ellis Paul scrambled to learn enough mechanical engineering to devise an innovative design for the lift mechanisms on several spans.

(below) Experiments were conducted on the flexible cables for bridges in the series.

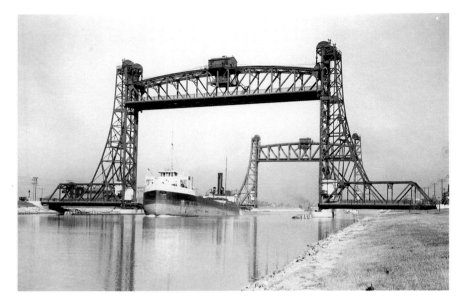

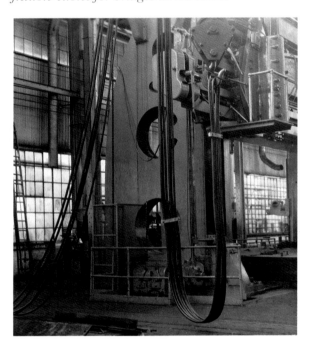

17

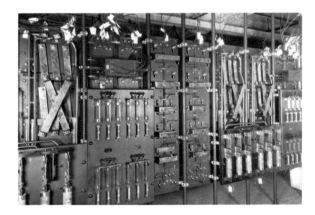

(above) The movable portions of the Welland Canal bridges required the design of switching controls to manage the speed and power of the lifting mechanisms. Henry Tammen was chief designer of the bridge series.

River Bridge at Portland, Oregon), was instituted.

Harrington also decided to exchange his role as junior partner for one more senior: he offered the much younger Ernest Howard and Louis Ash each a piece of the partnership. For the first time, the name Howard — the "H" of HNTB — appeared in the name of the firm. On January 1, 1914, the new firm of Harrington, Howard & Ash quietly opened its doors.

At first, the new combination of personalities in the partnership appeared to be a good mix. Each man handled different aspects of the business, according to Ellis Paul:

> "Harrington was a business getter and also a specialist in the mechanics of movable bridges. Howard took a major part of his time in developing plans and in preparing specs. Ash was very much a technical engineer."

Another employee summed up the division of labor quite simply: "Harrington got new work, Howard wrote all the specs, Ash reviewed plans."

A dozen or more years the senior of his two partners, Harrington was in a natural position to assume the dominant role. With business booming, however, he needed all of the help that his partners and his staff could give him. In addition to carrying on most of the projects of Waddell & Harrington days, the firm found itself in high demand for movable bridge designs across the continent and overseas. An informal tally by Henry Tammen lists more than 45 vertical lift bridges, 13 bascule bridges and six rolling bascule bridges designed by Harrington, Howard & Ash between 1914 and 1928.

U. S. railroad companies consistently topped the list of clients, but various bridge projects also took the firm to such faraway spots as Japan, Russia, and China. The Canadian government hired the firm in the early 1920s to design an extraordinary series of 18 movable bridges across the Welland Canal, a massive project for which Henry Tammen was primarily responsible as chief designer of the firm.

Ellis Paul worked for Tammen on the Welland Canal bridges shortly after being hired by the firm and quickly learned that Tammen held high expectations for his subordinates:

> *"The Canadian government had sent us a letter and told us that we were a bunch of copycat engineers. [That] in the design of these rolling bascules, we had followed [someone else's methods]. Tammen walked in with this letter, threw it on my desk — now I had NEVER seen a piece of mechanical engineering or design in my life — he threw it on my desk, and he said, 'Here, you solve what we're supposed to do.' About two hours later Tammen came back and said 'What've you got?' I said, 'I ain't got nothing.' I spent the noon hour talking to Jake Fast, our mechanical engineer, and I took the calculations home that night, fooled around with them, and that's how I got started on mechanical engineering. Mr. Tammen expected you to know what to do right when he wanted it 'did.'"*

Henry Tammen's high technical standards were rivaled only by those of his superiors, Howard and Ash. Howard, in fact, had already acquired a habit for which he would become well-known to at least two generations of engineers: marking up the painstakingly neat and clean drawings of his drafting staff with a black pencil. Ellis Paul recalled:

> *"Ash and Howard were the ones that paid most attention to what the design was. Howard would write 90% of the specs — he was very, very particular about them. In fact, both Howard and Ash would come out to the drafting room and look at your drawing, and Howard had a great habit of having a great big, very soft pencil, and he'd look at something — 'That's no good' — and he'd mess up your drawing ... they would pay all kinds of attention to what you turned out."*

Paying "all kinds of attention" to details paid off. From the opening volley of World War I until the end of the 1920s, a steady flow of business allowed Harrington, Howard & Ash to expand steadily. So encouraging did the future appear that eight years after its founding, the firm took the unprecedented step of opening another permanent office. In 1922, Harrington, Howard & Ash hung out its shingle in New York City.

New York City

The idea of establishing the firm in another location besides Kansas City was not an entirely new one. A small office had been run by Harry Hunter in Vancouver at the height of the firm's work for the Canadian Northern Pacific Railway during Waddell & Harrington days. But that office had been set up to accommodate one client and one project. No offices had been established with business development as the main goal. The New York City office was going to be different. Highway toll bridges were becoming an increasingly important segment of Harrington, Howard & Ash's practice. Not only was the East Coast a potential market for toll bridges, but such privately-financed projects required the confidence and backing of bankers. An office in the nation's main financial district could be an important adjunct to the firm's business.

The lion's share of credit for the initial concept of a New York City office probably belongs to John Lyle Harrington. Harrington was unabashedly ambitious to see the firm grow. Also, according to Ellis Paul, who moved to the New York City office a few years after it opened, "the old man knew all the bankers, and he made

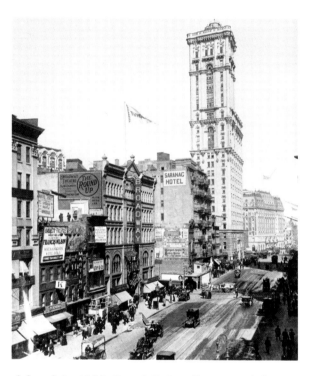

18

(above) In 1922, Enoch R. Needles opened the firm's first permanent office besides Kansas City. The office at 55 Liberty Street in the heart of New York City's financial district proved to be critical to the firm's survival during the Great Depression.

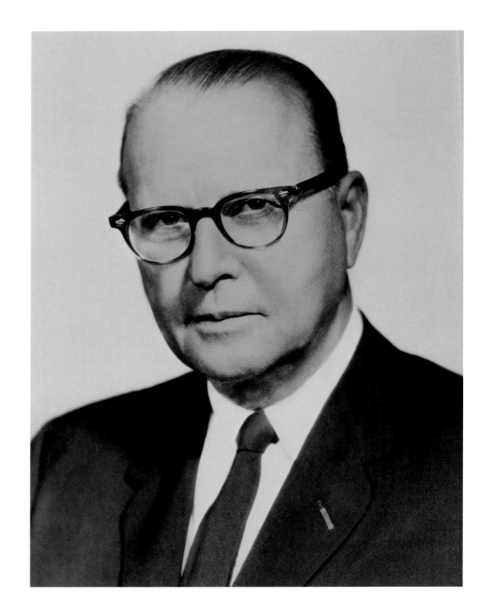

Enoch R. Needles
(1888-1972)

Enoch R. Needles started as a temporary employee of Harrington, Howard & Ash in 1917 but quickly became a valued worker and was sent to projects all across the country in his early years. His ability to cultivate friendships made him the top candidate to open the New York office in 1922. Six years later he was made a partner. His talent for building strong relationships proved invaluable in establishing the young firm with eastern financial markets as toll projects became more and more important to the firm's growth.

19

the first contacts." A biography of Harrington written after his death describes him as a man who "had few intimates." Any personal reserve on Harrington's side didn't seem to stand in his way when it came to knocking on the right doors and making professional acquaintances. Ellis Paul recalled:

> *"He was a good politician, a good presenter, a good business getter ... He was in the [Kansas City] office very, very little — you very seldom saw him — he didn't pay attention to the work that you did, like Howard and Ash did."*

Enoch R. Needles

By the autumn of 1922, the decision was made to send young Enoch Ray Needles to New York City to establish the firm's East Coast outpost. It was a decision which would soon boost Needles into the partnership and ultimately revolutionize the firm's entire practice.

Enoch Needles had been with Harrington, Howard & Ash only five years before accepting the New York City assignment. Born on October 29, 1888, in Brookfield, Missouri, to a farming family, Needles moved to Kansas City at the age of 12. While studying at the local classical high school, Needles discovered his interest in engineering:

> *"One of our mathematics professors … gave us some elementary field work in surveying and I remember distinctly the great pleasure of seeing the measured angles and sides of a polygon correspond rather closely with the calculated dimensions. About the same time, I read* The Winning of Barbara Worth, *the romance of a civil engineer in the west. I found myself rather pleased in thinking about highlaced boots, blueprints, the open air, and men working at building things."*

Family finances did not permit the young Needles to go to college immediately after high school. Instead, he signed up with the Kansas City Park Department for three years, working with a group assigned to survey the city's park and boulevard system. In 1909, Needles entered the freshman class at the Missouri School of Mines & Metallurgy, now the University of Missouri-Rolla. He continued working for the park department during summers. Although his mother had hoped that he would choose the ministry or medicine as a career, Needles remained enchanted by the dream of being a civil engineer. In 1914, less than a month before the outbreak of World War I in Europe, Needles was graduated with both B.S. and C.E. degrees.

Short stints with the Kansas City Southern Railroad (KCSR) and the Kansas City Terminal Railway (KCTR) gave Needles experience in field and mine surveying, mine drafting, and railroad evaluation work. A transfer to the bridge department of the KCTR added bridge design work to his professional portfolio. He also did his share of travelling during this period: "I guess the worst assignment was Louisiana," reminisced Needles four decades later. "I caught malaria and had to have shots every two weeks for a long time. The malaria bothered me on and off for several years."

In July 1917, Needles took a "temporary job" with Harrington, Howard & Ash. Such temporary hirings were typical of a period in which private consulting firms were formed and dissolved practically overnight. Several engineers might come together for a single project and break up immediately upon its completion. Or a cataclysmic national event like a war or financial panic might be the death knell for a small firm. In spite of the entry of the United States into the Great War in Europe in the spring of 1917, Harrington, Howard & Ash apparently had no intention of folding. Needles' initial three-month trial employment came and went without a pink slip.

His early assignments for Harrington, Howard & Ash kept the 30-year old Needles on the road. During his first year he was sent to Texarkana to work on the Red River Bridge at Bonham, Texas. After a short tour of duty in the Kansas City office, he headed southeast to Jacksonville, Florida, in 1918, to act as resident engineer on the St. John's River Bridge. The bridge was the first highway bridge to replace a ferry across the river at that location.

Needles returned to Kansas City in late 1921, but was off again in April of the following year. This time he headed for Delaware:

> *"My first job in Delaware was to make surveys and take borings for the design of a series of highway bridges over the Chesapeake and Delaware Canal. I recall that I*

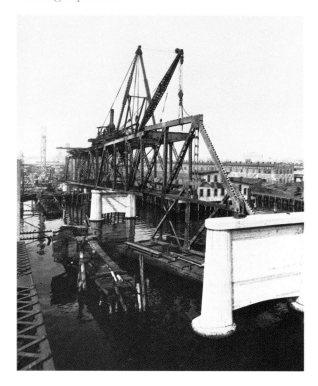

20

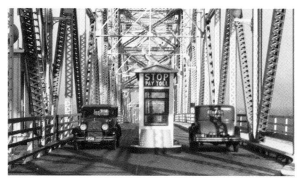

(above) Through its work on toll bridges in the early years of the century, the firm developed special expertise in revenue bond projects. Income and valuation reports became an important part of the services the firm provided to clients. This experience would prove providential when the modern turnpike era was launched in the late 1940s.

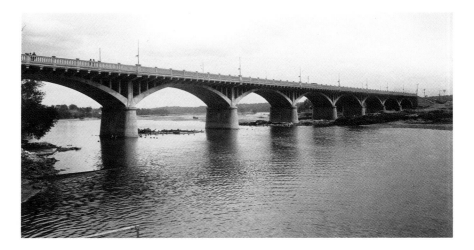

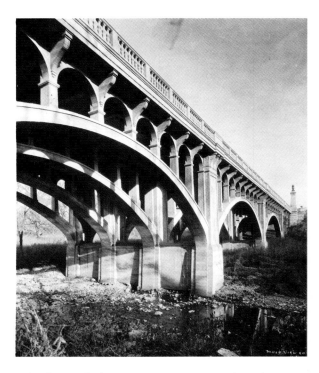

The firm's dedication to rigorous engineering standards in its bridges was matched by a strong commitment to the aesthetics of design. Over the years the firm earned a reputation for technical excellence and graceful structures. The Colorado River Bridge, Austin, Texas, (top) and the bridge over Brush Creek at Benton Boulevard in Kansas City (above) are fine early examples of ornate cast concrete bridge design.

drove a second-hand Model T Ford. We were to design six bridges which were to cost about $1 million. The U. S. Government had just purchased this historic canal from the private owners who had operated it for about 100 years."

The C&D Canal bridge project for the Corps of Engineers evolved into a long-term client relationship for the firm, one of many such relationships through the years. But Needles' primary mission in 1922 was to set up the new office. He secured "one room and a little entryway" on the eighth floor of 55 Liberty Street and went to work. The first days were anything but easy. Although the firm was already associated with toll bridges and already known to Wall Street — mostly through Harrington's contacts — Needles faced rough times ahead. Now-retired HNTB partner Josef Sorkin, who joined the firm in 1939, recalled stories of Needles' early days in New York City:

"During the first few years there was really nothing … there were no active jobs available. He utilized all that time in developing contacts, looking forward to the time when something would develop … He was very capable, outgoing … Needles had a quality of cultivating friendships and acquaintances in the right circles."

Like Harrington, the young engineer from Missouri had a knack for making professional contacts. Forty years after the opening of the New York City office Needles reminisced:

"I made it my business to attend the meetings of the Metropolitan Section of our Society [ASCE], and there I was privileged to form many wonderful friendships which have grown richer through the years."

His purchase of a farm in Delaware within a few years of settling in the East also brought Needles into neighborly contact with a man who would play a vital role in the future of the country's highway system, Francis duPont, Director of the Bureau of Public Roads during the opening days of the interstate construction era.

Needles' ability to cultivate "friendships and acquaintances in the right circles" soon became vital to the survival of the New York City office and of the firm. Less than a half dozen years after Needles moved to NYC, the firm faced two major crises: the withdrawal of John Lyle Harrington from the partnership, and the dark days of the Great Depression. ■

PART TWO

Surviving Adversity

"The loss of [Louis] Ash was a tragedy which was felt by the entire firm. But other events were soon to have an even greater impact on Ash-Howard-Needles & Tammen."

CHAPTER THREE

The 1920s and The Great Depression (1920-1940)

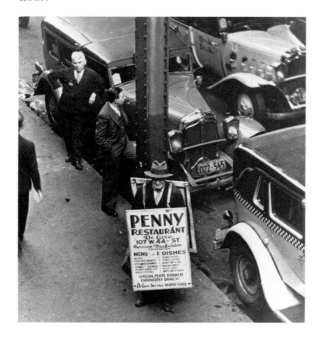

(below) The Crash of '29 and the subsequent Depression sharply curtailed the construction of new bridges. The firm was forced to lay off staff and depended upon a small number of bridge inspection assignments to keep the wolf from the door.

As Enoch Needles settled into his new assignment in New York City, Harrington, Howard & Ash basked in its recent successes. In 1921, Ernest Howard had won the prestigious Thomas Fitch Rowland Prize of the American Society of Civil Engineers for a scholarly paper on vertical lift bridges. "Old man" Harrington had served during 1923 as president of the American Society of Mechanical Engineers. Louis Ash had earlier taken a two-year leave of absence to serve as city manager of Wichita. And the two dozen engineers of the Kansas City office were awash with design work, stretching from the Don River in Russia to the state of Florida, where the legendary real estate mania of the 1920s had prompted a building boom.

The summer of 1922 — the same year in which Enoch Needles headed east in his second-hand Model T Ford — brought to the staff the addition of three men who eventually became HNTB partners.

James Powers Exum, a new graduate of Ernest Howard's alma mater, the University of Texas, was a native Texan who moved north to join Harrington, Howard & Ash straight out of school, as a draftsman and bridge detailer. He left the firm for a year during 1924 to work in the bridge division of the Texas Highway Department, but returned in 1925 to help design the Welland Canal bridges. Although the Great Depression would soon send him back to Texas for more than a dozen years, Exum later rejoined the firm and stayed until his retirement. Exum's exuberant Texas charm and his passion for golf were notable among his characteristics.

Ellis E. Paul also joined the firm in 1922, immediately after his graduation from the University of Kansas with a B.S.C.E. degree. A native of Kansas City, Paul also worked on the Canadian Welland Canal bridges, an experience which included his harried introduction to mechanical engineering at Henry Tammen's behest. Ellis Paul, according to more than one HNTB colleague, "had a bark that led you to feel that he was a very gruff, harsh, critical person ... but that was all exterior ... he also had a very, very warm heart, and a sense of humor." Like Exum, Paul spent most of his career with the firm working in the New York City office.

Yet a third future partner joined the firm in the summer of 1922. Ruben Nathaniel Bergendoff was born in Newman Grove, Nebraska, on January 4, 1899, to a Lutheran minister and his wife. The couple had emigrated six years earlier from the province of Smaaland, Sweden.

Bergendoff's natural talent for mathematics was fostered by his father, who "was a remarkable man" in his son's eyes:

> *"I remember a childhood of bobsledding, ice skating and a serious approach to the business of getting an education ... My father was very fond of mathematics and he was ambitious to see us get ahead in school. Father taught me mathematics as if it were a game. He did everything he could to give us an education, and*

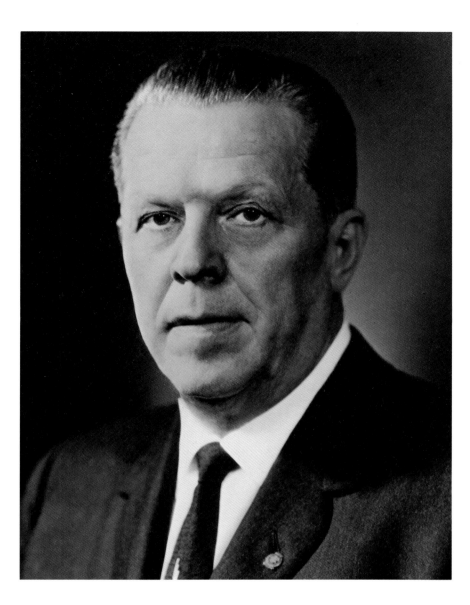

R. N. Bergendoff
(1899-1976)

Restless to work on bridges after a short stint with the North Carolina State Highway Department, R. N. Bergendoff joined Harrington, Howard & Ash in 1922, where he quickly advanced to the post of chief designer. The Great Depression, however, soon found him selling insurance and working for the state of Montana while waiting for the firm to find enough bridge work to hire him back. When he became a partner in 1940, Bergendoff brought with him a farsighted business approach and a strong sense of team play that proved to be critical during HNTB's most rapid period of growth in the 1950s and 1960s.

said he didn't care what we did, as long it was honest and we did it well."

Bergendoff graduated from South Philadelphia High School and entered Augustana College, a Lutheran school in Rock Island, Illinois, where he stayed for one year before transferring back to Philadelphia. A short stint in the military in the closing days of World War I took a year away from his studies. While working toward his degree at the University of Pennsylvania, Bergendoff took classes straight through his lunch hour and worked two or three hours a night at a bank. He was graduated in 1921.

Bergendoff's first job out of college was a short tour of duty with the North Carolina State Highway Department as a draftsman. At that time, North Carolina was one of only a handful of states to have its own highway department. Although Congress had passed the first federal-level highway legislation — the Federal Road Aid Act of 1916 — five years earlier, very little had yet been done to implement its call for "an integrated, nationwide system of interstate highways."

After two months of searching for a job, the young Pennsylvania

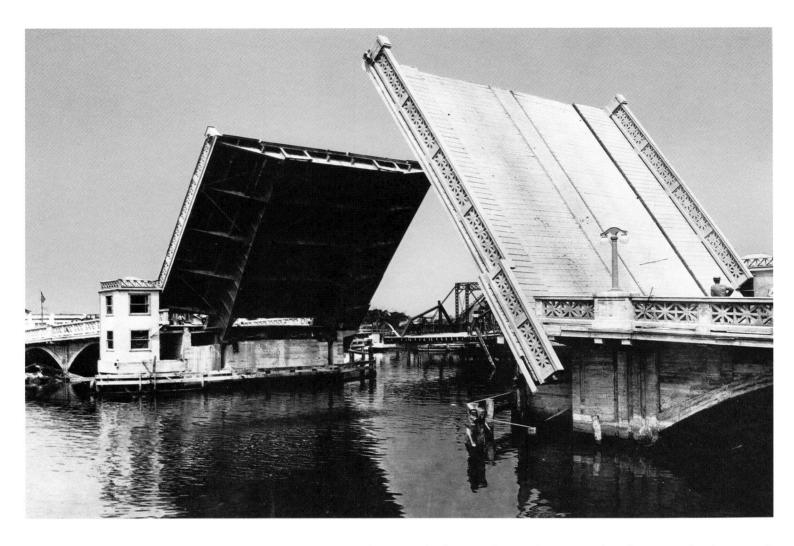

(above) To fulfill his dream of becoming a bridge engineer, R.N. Bergendoff "pestered" Harrington, Howard & Ash for a job. His first project for the firm was a series of small movable bridges in Miami, Florida.

graduate took the North Carolina post, but his eyes, he later said, "were on a job with a bridge-building firm." Bergendoff wrote letters to Harrington, Howard & Ash and to Waddell & Son, John Alexander Low Waddell's later firm in New York City, "pestering" them for a position. On June 1, 1922, he "landed the job with the Kansas City firm" at a salary of $135 a month.

His dreams answered, Bergendoff packed up and headed for Kansas City. In an anecdote which became one his favorites, Bergendoff recalled that John Lyle Harrington had only discouraging words for him soon after his arrival:

> *"Bergie, why do you want to get into this business? All of the big bridges have been built. The railroads have all they need. There just won't be any more big bridges."*

Bergendoff was unmoved. His first assignment was on one of several small movable bridges designed by the firm in the 1920s for the city of Miami, Florida. Florida at the time was in the midst of unprecedented real estate speculation, a financial frenzy in which thousands of people soon lost their shirts. The Florida real estate boom-and-bust was just a small taste of the gloomy panic which would hit the entire nation in 1929. In the meantime, bridges needed to be built where development in the state had taken place. Harrington, Howard & Ash was delighted to fill the bill.

End of a Partnership

As orders for bridge designs poured into the firm in the mid-1920s, seeds of discontent were germinating in the office at 1012 Baltimore Avenue in Kansas City. Harrington and his two younger partners were not getting along. Temperaments were partly to blame. Frank E. Washburn, who was acquainted with the trio, observed that the "imperial, political and polished Harrington was a far cry from the quiet, studious, modest Howard and Ash." The combination was wearing thin. By 1927, the differences in style had begun to tell.

Problems came to a head in early 1928. At least some of the staff was taken by surprise. More than four decades later, R.N. Bergendoff humorously recalled getting the news of the breakup:

> *"After [six] years with the firm, several of us thought we were so good that we ought to have better recognition. So we got up a petition, nicely typed. We got down [to the office] early one morning, laid it on each of the partners' desks. [The petition] said how valuable we were and how we ought to have more recognition from the firm. We never got an answer. Two months later, we were told the firm was splitting up. Harrington, Howard and Ash had lasted 14 years."*

However unaware the staff might have been of discord among their employers, Harrington decidedly did not consider either Howard or Ash "quiet, studious, modest." In a dramatic letter addressed to Enoch Needles, dated February 6, 1928, from Port Huron, Michigan, Harrington paints a quite different picture of his two partners. The strict factual accuracy of Harrington's comments to Needles is open to speculation; the emotional tone of the letter renders its objectivity suspect. The insight that the letter provides into its author's mind, however, is invaluable to understanding the human forces at work at a critical juncture in the firm's history:

> *Dear Mr. Needles —*
>
> *Mr. Ash had another flare up the day after bids were received on the Vicksburg job and announced that he wanted to pull out. He really wanted to segregate that job and do it himself, but that would violate the contract, and Mr. Howard objected.*
>
> *The great difficulty with the firm's work results chiefly from my continuous absence and consequent pressure upon me during my short periods at home, for that has left the management of the office to Messrs. Howard and Ash ... the divided authority has been ruinous. Hence, when Mr. Ash announced that he wished to withdraw, I consented for I will never urge anyone to stay with me. Mr. Howard then announced that he, too, wished to go alone, but on our way to Chicago Wednesday evening he dropped the fact that he and Mr. Ash plan to go together.*
>
> *Further talk made it clear that Mr. Howard and Mr. Ash want to be carried along in financial matters and share in the proceeds, although neither has shown any ability to share in the work. They are still unwilling to reorganize the office or to share in the outside work and travel, lethargically see no way to better the present, for me, intolerable conditions, hence have agreed upon details of separation, that is to carry out present contracts as a firm, to divide certain prospective business and the*

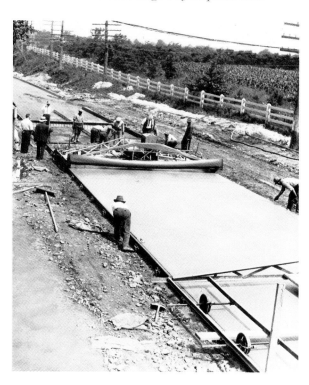

(below) Before Congress approved major funding to build an interstate highway system in 1956, a few states established their own road programs. R.N. Bergendoff's first job after graduating from college in 1921 was with the North Carolina State Highway Department.

26

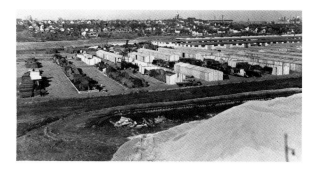

(above) Although the Great Depression ruined many firms, Ash-Howard-Needles & Tammen survived to receive some of the first public works projects funded by the Emergency Reconstruction Finance Corporation and Public Works Administration programs under the Roosevelt administration. The projects saved the firm from having to close its doors permanently.

returns therefrom, if any, in a definite manner, to deal each for himself with all other prospective business.

But Saturday morning Mr. Ash indicated that he really did not want to make the break and Mr. Howard made a like intimation. It seems to me they are seeking to force me to carry on in accordance with their views of financial matters, leaving other matters of organization as they are. That I can never do, if my doctor is any prophet.

So matters stand and will stand till I am next at home. When the matter took the open position, I felt like a boy just let loose from school, for the excessive pressure upon me, the necessity for constant travel, then for doing so much detail work when I come in that I never finish it before I must go again, the awfulness of a very badly managed office, the waste due to lack of planning and managment, have become a nightmare to me. Life has not been worth living for many years.

Please consider the whole matter confidential till it is cleared, one way or the other. So far I can see no hope of satisfactorily maintaining the present organization. I have held that you younger men must be made partners. I shall take reasonable time to work out my own plans. Travel delays doing so, but I hope to get matters in course by the end of the month.

Sincerely yours,

John Lyle Harrington

As the senior member of the partnership, Harrington might well have felt that his voice should dominate all questions of firm management and policy. Self-cast in the role of the firm's "business-getter," he might have resented any attempts by Howard and Ash to run things their way in the office. The note of world-weariness in Harrington's letter suggests that he felt a need to be in control of every aspect of the operation, even if it meant "excessive pressure" upon him. Reading between the lines, Howard and Ash — mature middle-aged men — might understandably have chafed under Harrington's "imperial" eye. And Harrington's obvious disdain for their management abilities would have provided ample grounds for dissension.

No written record remains of the thoughts of Howard and Ash on the split with Harrington. Failures of two bridges under Harrington's direction, however, undoubtedly heightened the growing discord among the three. A biography of Harrington notes that in September 1927, the timber falsework of a bridge under construction at Louisiana, Missouri, collapsed, and one man lost his life. A newly completed bridge over the Colorado River at Blythe, California, failed in June 1928 when a flood damaged the piers upon which the bridge rested.

Every firm occasionally experiences a design failure; a certain amount of risk is inherent in every type of engineering endeavor. Two incidents in less than nine months, however, would naturally have been quite upsetting. For Howard and Ash, the failures might only have exacerbated their discontent with Harrington. As younger partners who presumably would inherit eventual control of the firm from him, both probably were concerned about the long-term effect of Harrington's ambitions for the firm. Their

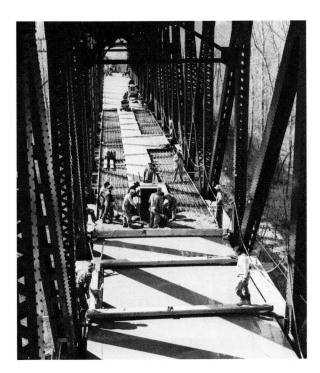

27

(above) One of the largest bridges designed by the firm in the days just before the Great Depression was located in Henry Tammen's hometown, Yankton, South Dakota. The soft banks along the river at Yankton provided more than one engineering headache. During construction of the bridge, one of the towers began to lean. Ash and Howard put their heads together to devise a solution to stabilize the offending column. The experience came in handy a few years later on the Vicksburg Bridge during summer floods on the Mississippi River.

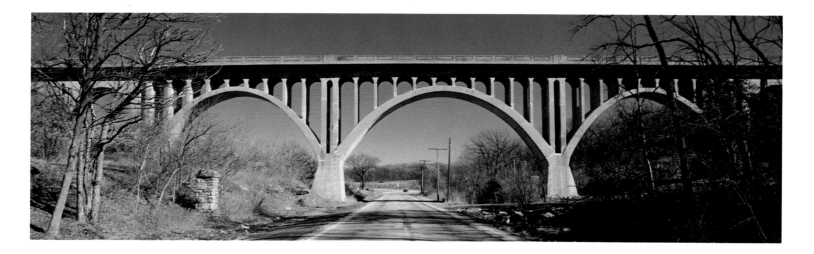

worries might have been well-founded. Harrington's biography notes that he found "himself in debt as a result of some land speculations" in the real estate craze of the 1920s and "may have been tempted to spread himself too thin in the highway bridge construction boom of the later 1920s." By 1927, Harrington was involved in the design and construction of no fewer than 30 bridges simultaneously. The two bridge failures might have prompted the more cautious Howard and Ash to question the wisdom of such frenzied activity, while Harrington might have seen the growth of the firm as vital to personal financial recovery.

A split became inevitable. A month after the second bridge failure, Harrington had moved out of the offices in the Orear-Leslie Building, taking with him Frank Cortelyou, principal assistant engineer, and several other staff members.

Ash-Howard-Needles & Tammen

One Harrington, Howard & Ash employee who might have been expected to depart for new quarters with Harrington did not. Enoch Needles, the recipient of Harrington's unhappy letter, stayed behind with Howard and Ash. Why Harrington had selected the young Needles as his confidant is impossible to know for certain six decades after the fact. It is also impossible to know how much sympathy Needles might have felt for his senior employer's troubles. Within 12 months of receiving Harrington's letter Needles accepted an equal partnership in the reorganized firm of Ash-Howard-Needles & Tammen. For better or worse, Harrington's wish that "you younger men must be made partners" had come true.

One of the first orders of business was to carry out the "agreed upon details of separation." Negotiations for the division of current and prospective work had to take place. The principals elected to send representatives to sort out the projects and make selections. Ellis Paul was chosen to represent AHN&T. He reminisced with some amusement 50 years later about bearing responsibility for the choices he made:

> "Howard appointed me. Ash said the only job he wanted to be sure to get in the firm was [the] Vicksburg [Bridge], and as I recall, we had the first choice, and I took Vicksburg. I asked old man Howard if he had any particular bridge he wanted — he said, 'No, use your own judgment.' From then on, every time he wanted a

(top) The railroads were still important clients to the young firm in the 1920s and 1930s. Ash-Howard-Needles & Tammen designed 25 single track bridges for the Kansas City Southern Railway, completed 1928-1930. The glory days of American railroading were, however, coming to an end. The firm's long tradition of railway bridge design began to give way in the late 1920s and early 1930s to the new challenges of designing toll bridges for the increasingly popular automobile.

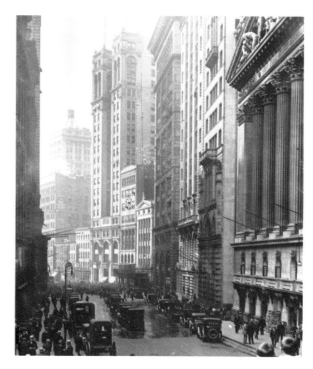

(above) The firm's long-standing ties to Wall Street and its solid reputation in revenue bond projects helped to win backing in the community for the toll bridges which Ash-Howard-Needles & Tammen helped to secure for its clients from the ERFC and PWA.

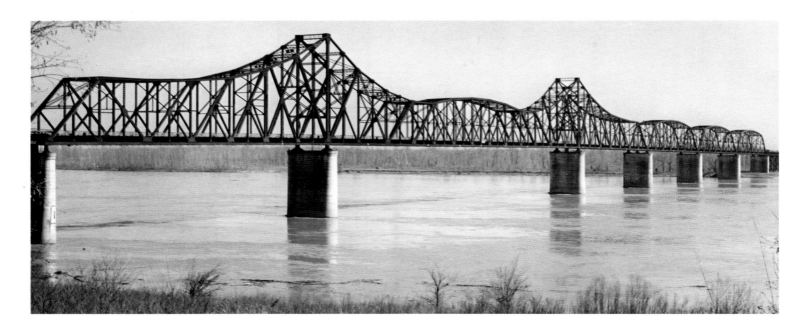

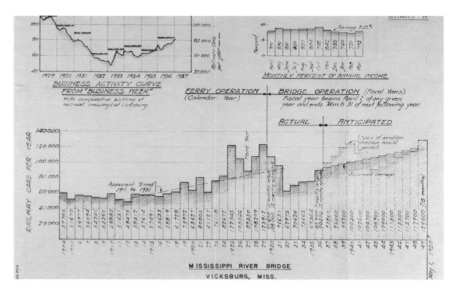

(top) The Vicksburg Bridge over the Mississippi River was a project of partner Louis Ash and he gave personal attention to a problem that developed on pier #4 during construction of the bridge in 1929. Ash felt obligated to make the final inspection of the troubled pier and descended ladders into the caisson under 45 pounds of air pressure. In later years, Ash's death — only three weeks before the bridge opened in the spring of 1930 — was attributed by his friends and colleagues to the strains of the descent to inspect the caisson.

(right) Like many other large bridges of the period, the Vicksburg Bridge was designed to pay for itself as a toll facility. The firm quickly became an expert in calculating projected traffic and income for the bridges it designed. This expertise helped the firm win financial backing on Wall Street for many large revenue bond projects. The chart to the left is taken from Ernest Howard's final report on the Vicksburg Bridge.

29

set of plans or files, it was always on a bridge that Harrington had. He'd call me in and want to know why the hell we hadn't selected that one."

The Vicksburg Bridge

The choice of the Vicksburg Bridge — a pet project of Louis Ash — proved to be a mixed blessing. The project was a large one. Henry Tammen was the engineer-in-charge. Harry G. Hunter, Robert Sailer, and C.M. Greer completed the preliminary design work. R.N. Bergendoff was chief designer. Jim Exum was chief draftsman. Ellis Paul and four others were assistant designers. Future HNTB partner Ted Cambern and Jake Fast were among the 21 draftsmen assigned to the project. Until his departure to Harrington's new quarters in the summer of 1928, Frank Cortelyou served as resident engineer.

The bridge had received congressional blessing in May 1926. Preliminary surveys and site location work on the banks of the Mississippi River took about a year. The Chief of U.S. Engineers approved final plans in December 1927. Construction began the following year.

All went like clockwork until trouble developed with pier #4. The Mississippi had flooded in April 1928 forcing the construction crew to stop work. Because of problems with settlement, the first caisson for pier #4 had to be scuttled the following December. Work resumed eight months later in August 1929 when a second caisson for that location was launched. Three months later the caisson for pier #4 was sealed. On April 28, 1930, the Vicksburg Bridge opened to traffic.

Louis Ash did not live to see his bridge open. He died on April 7, only three weeks before the opening ceremony. Although Ash's death was never officially deemed a result of his work on the bridge, his contemporaries came to believe that his insistence upon personal inspection of the troubled pier #4 the previous year had taken its toll. Ellis Paul remembered:

> "Mr. Ash, in my book, was one of the nicest gentlemen I have ever run into. Lovely family man, good church man, very quiet, and I thought very, very clever. He was responsible for the Vicksburg Bridge, and of course, that pier #4 is what killed him — going down in the air. Ash felt that since it was his job, he had to go down and look at that pier for the final inspection and he had no business going down under 40 some pounds of pressure, climbing down all those ladders and that, but he went down."

The loss of Ash was a tragedy which was felt by the entire firm. But other events were soon to have an even greater impact on Ash-Howard-Needles & Tammen. Six months before the opening of the Vicksburg Bridge, the nation's financial structure collapsed on Black Tuesday, October 29, 1929. The Great Depression had begun.

The Great Depression

When bad news of the stock market crash hit, the new partnership was only a year old. The firm was busy finishing up projects which it had secured before the split with Harrington. The series of Welland Canal bridges was still ongoing. Three bascule bridges for Miami, Florida were underway. Vicksburg was nearly completed. The majestic and record-breaking Burlington-Bristol Bridge over the Delaware River between Pennsylvania and New Jersey was almost finished. It would be the longest vertical lift bridge in the world when opened. At least a dozen other bridges were in various stages of design and construction.

The pinch, however, of the national financial panic was soon felt. New work trickled in. A few Ocean Highway bridges in New Jersey around Ocean City, Longport, and Cape May and small projects elsewhere kept chief designer Bergendoff and his staff partially occupied. Bridge inspections became an important sideline.

It wasn't enough. The three remaining partners faced tough decisions about the future. There simply wasn't sufficient work to keep everyone on the payroll. Even chief draftsman Exum and chief designer Bergendoff — next in command after the partners — were let go, a sure sign that work had almost come to a standstill. Bergendoff and Exum tried to make the best of it:

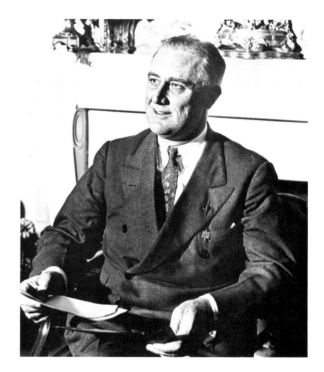

(above) In response to the increasing numbers of able-bodied unemployed during the Depression, Franklin Delano Roosevelt persuaded Congress in 1933 to increase funding tenfold for the ERFC and to create the Public Works Administration. Although some questioned the long-term benefits of FDR's "make-work" programs, for many the projects funded by the federal government were the only means of survival.

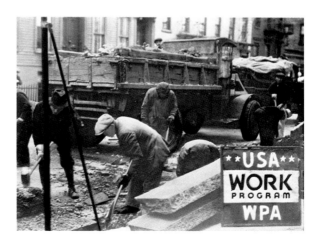

(above) The PWA, and later the Works Progress Administration, oversaw millions of dollars' worth of public works projects during the 1930s. Enoch Needles' knowledge of governmental processes helped the firm land its share of PWA assignments.

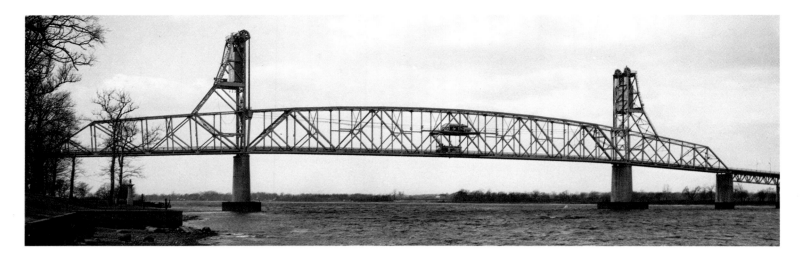

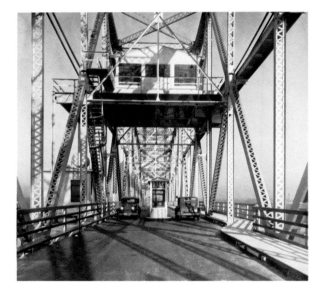

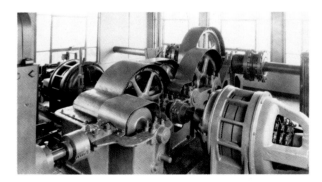

(this page) The Burlington-Bristol Bridge spanning the Delaware River was the longest lift span in the world when the bridge opened in 1930. The length of the lift span was 534 feet with a vertical clearance of 135 feet and weighed 1,300 tons. (facing page) Fifty-nine years later, the Burlington-Bristol Bridge is still operational and forms a vital link between Burlington, New Jersey, and Bristol, Pennsylvania.

> "Mr. Exum and I were both laid off. It was a rough time. I sold my car, rented my house, went home and lived off of my father-in-law. Jim Exum and I tried to sell insurance. We had a fraternity brother who was a businessman in an insurance company. We tried to sell insurance on commission. It was a struggle."

The market for insurance was disappointing. Both Exum and Bergendoff were fortunate enough to find other jobs. Exum returned to the Texas Highway Department, where he had worked as a young man. Bergendoff landed a temporary job in the Montana State Highway Department with the help of a former Harrington, Howard & Ash colleague.

The future of the fledgling partnership hung in the balance. Between the unexpected death of Ash — at 57, the oldest partner — and the economic adversity of the Depression, the firm might easily have folded. Ellis Paul, who weathered part of the Depression in New York City with Enoch Needles, 50 years later credited Ernest Howard with the firm's survival:

> "In the early 1930s, during the height of the Depression there were Howard and Tammen in the West and Needles and [I] in the East. There was no work and little prospect of any except possibly the Triborough bridges [in NYC]. There were many talks about folding, but Howard agreed to hang on and financed the operation."

The decision was far-sighted. The nation's economic recovery was slow and painful, but the firm would stand ready to take advantage of the opportunities.

A Slow Recovery

Tentative federal measures toward recovery surfaced in January 1930. President Herbert Hoover met with congressional leaders to discuss the advisability of developing a public works program as part of a solution to economic woes. In April, Congress responded by appropriating $300 million for highways. In December, it earmarked another $116 million for public works.

These gestures were necessary, but too limited to be of any significant use. In his annual message at the end of 1931, Hoover finally asked Congress to establish the Emergency Reconstruction Finance Corporation (ERFC or RFC), the "primary goal" of which

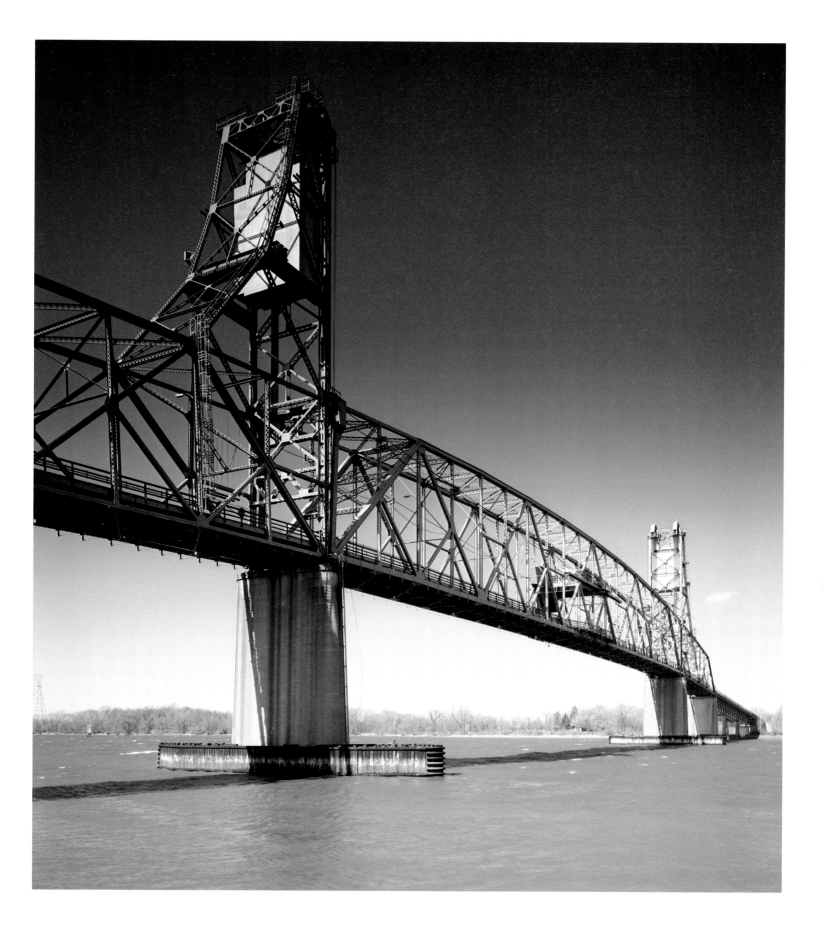

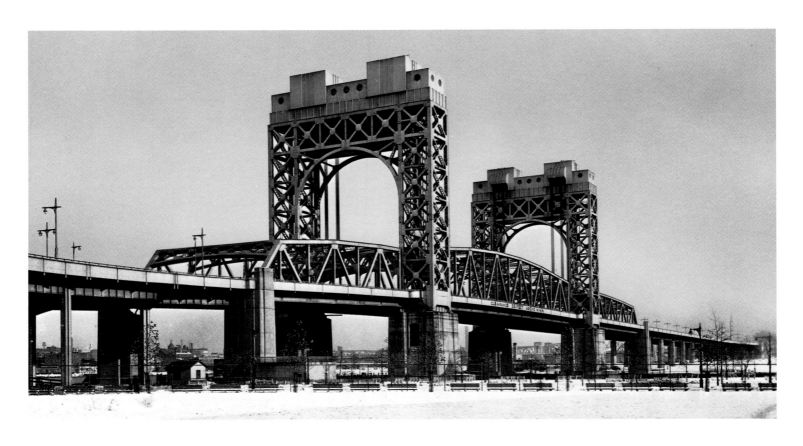

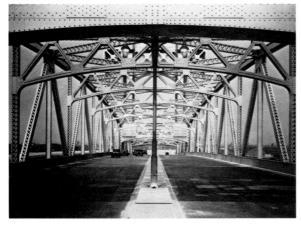

(top, above) The first major project obtained by the firm under the ERFC/PWA was the massive Harlem River Bridge in New York City. The bridge has a 310-foot lift span that rises 80 feet. Henry Tammen moved to New York to assist Enoch Needles with finding staff to handle the project, the first to be designed in the New York City office.

(facing page) Still in use today, the Harlem River Bridge was a critical turning point for the firm in 1933 at the height of the Great Depression.

"would be to provide money to lend to banks, insurance companies and other bodies that would then lend the money to the nation's industries." Congress agreed.

When Franklin Delano Roosevelt swept into office in March 1933, one of his first acts was to increase the ERFC's pocketbook tenfold, to the tune of $3 billion. He also persuaded Congress to establish the Public Works Administration (PWA), which was "authorized to supervise the construction of roads, public buildings, and other projects."

Money — and actual work — were not simply handed out by the two agencies. Competition for the limited funds was fierce. Success in landing new projects depended upon the perseverance and savvy of the seeker.

If AHN&T was going to get its share of the work, someone would have to learn how the programs worked. Enoch Needles, by now well-versed in the financial world of Wall Street, was the best-equipped of the three partners to develop overnight expertise in dealing with the new, overwhelming bureaucracy in the nation's capitol. Needles spent a lot of time in Washington, D.C., during the next few years, following papers through the various offices while waiting for the money to materialize. While in Washington, D.C., Needles might have crossed paths with his old boss, John Lyle Harrington: Harrington had been appointed in 1932 by President Hoover to the Engineers Advisory Board of the ERFC.

Needles' efforts paid off in 1933. Ellis Paul recalled the flush of success when the firm landed its first ERFC/PWA projects:

> *"I recall seeing the first list of projects which were awarded by the RFC, and I think the firm had about half of them, because they had been foresighted enough to get together with clients and get permits and plans."*

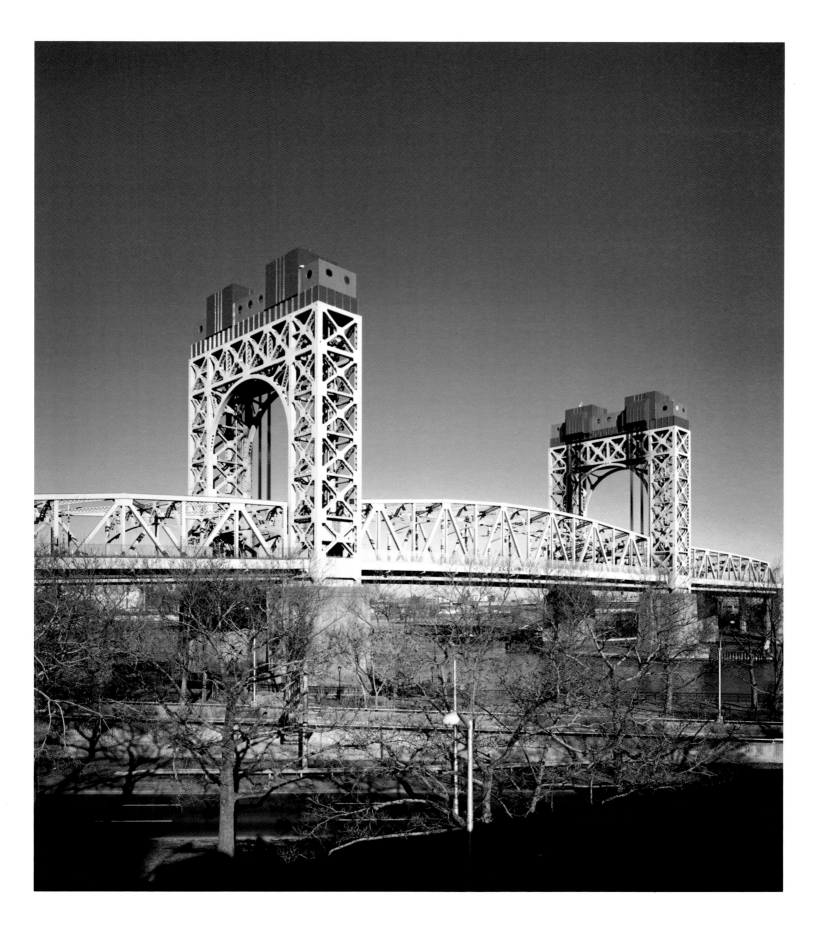

34

The Triborough Bridge Authority

One ERFC/PWA project was especially gratifying to Needles: a lift span over the Harlem River for the Triborough Bridge Authority in New York City. Needles' youngest daughter, Sally Needles Toffey, recalls a family story about her father's satisfaction in being able to turn down financial aid for his eldest daughter Elma's education:

> *"... it was not only a success for the New York office but he happily tore up the scholarship papers and took great pride in being able to send his daughter to college."*

The Triborough Bridge Authority project was unquestionably a turning point in the firm's immediate survival. The work also had another revolutionary effect. After a dozen years as a small outpost for the Kansas City office, the "small room and an entryway" at 55 Liberty Street had finally come into its own.

The Harlem span was to be designed in New York City. Enoch Needles might have insisted, feeling it only right that the important job which he had helped to secure for the firm should be handled in his bailiwick. Howard and Tammen agreed. Henry Tammen, after 24 years in Kansas City, packed his bags and moved to New York City to staff and equip a design office, leaving Howard to handle business at home. "Enoch and Harry were a perfect combination," recalled Ellis Paul. Paul had moved to the New York City office a few years earlier in conjunction with the supervision of the magnificent Burlington-Bristol span. He was actively involved in the process of staffing up the new design operation. "[We] had the selection of the best designers in New York City — we were the only firm that had any work at the time."

Soon after securing the bridge assignment, it became clear that the office needed more room. In June 1934, a drafting room became necessary and the firm moved its offices to 111 Eighth Avenue, the Port Authority Building. The firm remained there until May 1937, after completion of the bridge. The staff moved back to 55 Liberty Street, but this time to more spacious quarters on the 12th floor. The days of living out of his hat in New York City were over for Enoch Needles.

The South Omaha Bridge

The Kansas City office, in the meantime, was also basking in the glow of an ERFC/PWA project. Funding had come through at last for a toll bridge over the Missouri River at South Omaha, Nebraska. Irving (Ike) Watkins, whose father was active in promoting the bridge, remembers the firm's very early involvement in the project:

> *"... while I was still at Cornell, Mr. Ash came to Omaha and tried to work with my father and some other people in promoting a bridge in South Omaha. In fact, Mr. Ash put up $15,000 of his own money in order to finance the site survey, which was rather a practice in those days. It was something like building railroads ... it was a gamble."*

According to Watkins, who joined AHN&T as a result of working on the bridge, the site survey was completed in 1929. Ash's death and the Crash put a temporary end to plans.

Local businessmen who felt certain that the bridge would bring economic prosperity were not willing to give up. It was not long before the South Omaha Bridge Association was formed to try to secure PWA funding for the project. Ike Watkins' father, a

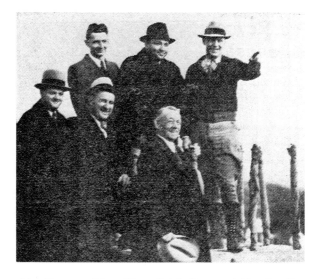

35

The Kansas City office of Ash-Howard-Needles & Tammen also won its share of projects under the federal government's economic recovery programs during the Great Depression. The design of the South Omaha Bridge in Nebraska was awarded to the firm in 1933. R.N. Bergendoff returned from Montana to take charge of the project. Built over dry land, construction of the bridge was a marvel to local citizens watching its progress. The Corps of Engineers rechanneled the Missouri River to flow under the span. (top) Five thousand pedestrians braved icy winds to stroll across the new bridge when it opened in January 1936.
(above) Clad in high boots, Chief Designer R.N. Bergendoff explains a technical point of construction on the South Omaha Bridge to a group of local civic leaders.

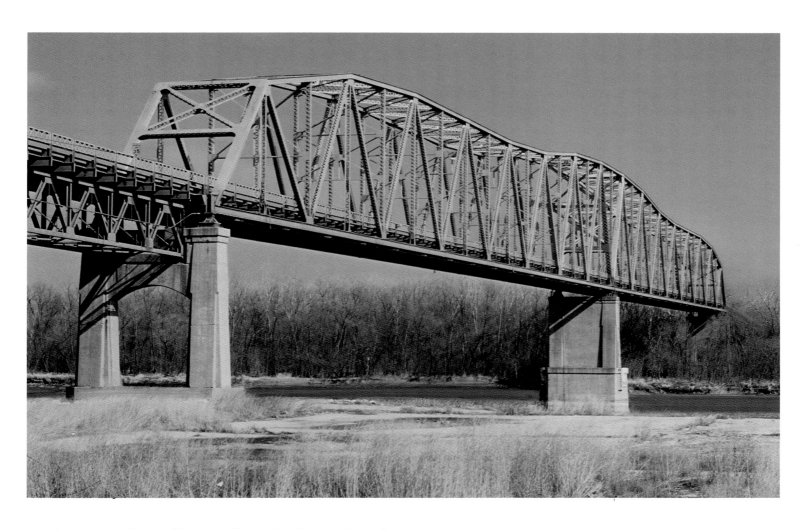

lumberman and the director of the local chamber of commerce from 1934 until 1936, was one of a small group of men who "camped at PWA headquarters in Washington and came home with the grant known as PWA Project No. 22 with $1,740,000 pinned to it." AHN&T was retained in early 1933. R.N. Bergendoff returned to the firm to take charge of design. By October 1933, plans were prepared and approved and bids for construction had been let.

Local papers breathlessly followed the progress of the bridge. Half-page photographs of major steps in its construction dominated the photogravure sections on Sundays. The bridge attracted special attention because it was not actually being built over a river, but over completely dry land. During the final phases of construction, the Corps of Engineers worked methodically to shift the course of the Missouri River 1,800 feet to flow under the bridge. The townspeople marvelled at the engineering feat taking place in their backyard. "Despite temperatures near zero and a biting wind," according to one local newspaper, 5,000 pedestrians crossed the bridge when it opened on January 19, 1936.

Just when both the Harlem River span and the South Omaha Bridge projects were drawing to a close, AHN&T received more good news. Another set of ERFC/PWA projects had been announced. The firm had seven bridges up for approval. When the list came out, remembered Ellis Paul, "all seven were included, with special mention of four which were to go forward immediately." The worst years were over. ■

(top) The two-lane highway bridge in South Omaha was designed as a continuous-truss, with two 525-foot spans over the Missouri River. The bridge continues to serve today as vital river crossing.

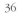

CHAPTER FOUR

Howard Needles Tammen & Bergendoff: World War II (1940-1945)

ASH-HOWARD-NEEDLES & TAMMEN
CONSULTING ENGINEERS

LOUIS R. ASH
ERNEST E. HOWARD
ENOCH R. NEEDLES
HENRY C. TAMMEN

1012 BALTIMORE AVE.
KANSAS CITY, MO.
55 LIBERTY STREET
NEW YORK

HOWARD, NEEDLES, TAMMEN & BERGENDOFF
CONSULTING ENGINEERS

ERNEST E. HOWARD
ENOCH R. NEEDLES
HENRY C. TAMMEN
RUBEN N. BERGENDOFF

921 WALNUT STREET
KANSAS CITY 6, MO.
55 LIBERTY STREET
NEW YORK 5, N. Y.

(above) With the death of Louis Ash and the subsequent appointment of R.N. Bergendoff as a partner, the firm's name changed for the last time in 1941.

In 1941, the firm changed its name for the last time. Louis Ash had been dead for nearly 11 years. R. N. Bergendoff had been named a partner the previous year. The time was right. As if to celebrate the rebirth of the firm after the lean days of the Great Depression, on January 1, 1941, Ash-Howard-Needles & Tammen became Howard, Needles, Tammen & Bergendoff.

Ernest Howard had now been in practice for 40 years. His name had been in the firm's name for a quarter of a century. Since 1934, after Henry Tammen moved to New York City, Howard had been the sole partner in the Kansas City office. When Howard and Waddell took their cruise on the Staten Island Ferry in 1936, Howard was in a position to understand the burdens of being a senior partner. The promotion of Chief Designer Bergendoff into the partnership took a bit of the weight of day-to-day business cares off Howard's shoulders.

Howard was as fascinated as ever by bridge design. The last batch of ERFC/PWA bridge assignments in 1937 had given him the opportunity to apply his interest in history to engineering. One of the projects which received ERFC funding provided financing for a toll bridge across the Mississippi River at Natchez, Mississippi. Howard seized on the theme of history and pilgrimages to the old mansions of Natchez. He had long fancied the idea of designing a bridge with colonnades as a primary visual motif. Natchez was the ideal setting to justify the artist. Howard put pen to paper and created an approach to the bridge's toll booths which made use of a graceful curve of columns.

Howard's outside interests had not diminished over time. In fact, he pursued them with increasing vigor as he got older. Howard quietly revelled in his large library, archaeology, historical research, frequent travel, and work with tools. Over the years he delved into such esoteric topics as tracing the use of asphalt and other building materials from early historical and Biblical references and archaeology. He also came up with the idea of inscribed plates for bridges and slaved over the resounding themes for the inscriptions.

While AHN&T had been keeping its staff busy with ERFC/WPA projects, political tempers were building to a fury in Europe and Asia. The outbreak of the second world war was imminent. Ike Watkins, whose father had been a key player in the firm's South Omaha Bridge project in the early 1930s, recalls the atmosphere of the time:

> *"In 1940, the writing was on the wall. You could see it when Hitler went into Austria in the fall of 1939, you could see that something was going to happen. So we got busy to see where we were going to fit into the picture."*

The firm, in fact, had begun to restaff in the mid-1930s, when Roosevelt's public works programs took effect. R.N. Bergendoff had come back for the South Omaha Bridge project. Other AHN&T

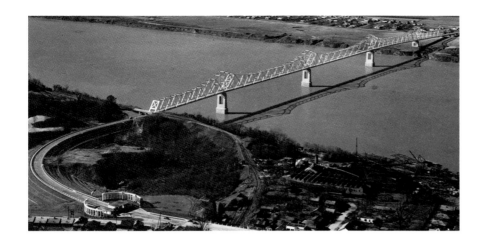

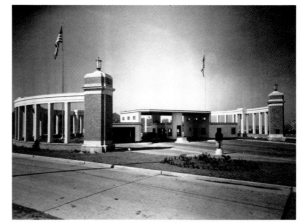

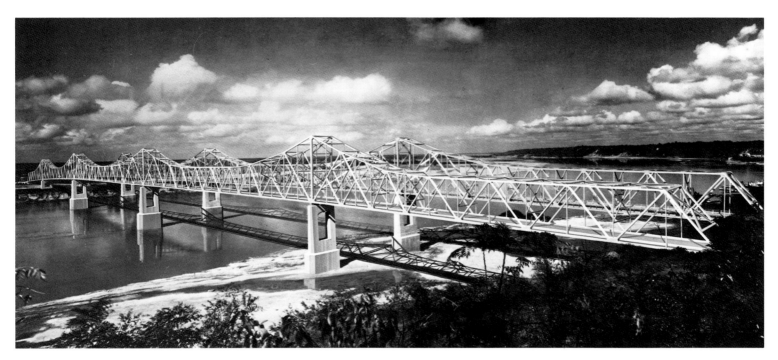

employees had returned to the fold. War meant the loss of many of those men to military service or other war-related operations. To survive, HNTB was going to have to find its niche in the country's war effort.

Staff, indeed, quickly disappeared. A small group stayed behind in the two offices and took care of odds and ends in connection with unfinished civilian jobs which had been started before the war. Howard and Bergendoff kept an eye on Kansas City matters. The New York City office lost nearly everyone, according to Josef Sorkin, who spent part of the war there. Sorkin transferred east from Kansas City in 1942 to work with the "rubber reserve … which was being organized to produce synthetic rubber on account of the Philippine Islands being occupied by the Japanese":

> *"Tammen was just about the only guy in the office — that's when I met Henry Tammen for the first time. I was there when Enoch Needles got his physical exam. They certified him as able to serve. Enoch's comment was 'Nice*

(top left and right) Another major river crossing designed by Ash-Howard-Needles & Tammen in 1937 was the three-quarter mile Mississippi River Bridge at Natchez, Mississippi. A project of Ernest Howard, he drew on his love of history in designing the elaborate toll plaza in the spirit of old southern mansions. (above) HNTB designed the new Natchez Bridge along side of the old bridge nearly 50 years later.

Southwestern Proving Grounds

When Sorkin ran into Needles in the New York City office, the latter had just been ordered to active duty effective December 2, 1942. By that time, HNTB had already completed two major projects for the War Department. The first was the Southwestern Proving Grounds at Hope, Arkansas. The project was a $12 million facility situated on 49,500 acres of hills, creek bottoms and swamps for the testing of heavy ordnance ammunition, including aerial bombs.

Under peacetime conditions, the magnitude of the undertaking would have been mind-boggling. During a wartime emergency, no one had a spare moment to let the awesome size of the task sink in. The project encompassed no less than 93 miles of highway, 13 miles of railway, 402 drainage structures, and 112 buildings. A 2,300-acre airport complete with 18,500 feet of concrete paved runways and eight buildings was also part of the assignment. Supporting the entire facility was a sewage disposal system, water supply, gas and electrical distribution systems, and communications systems. HNTB selected the site. On July 4, 1941, the firm set up offices in the high school. Recalled Needles, "We finished that winter."

HNTB, of course, couldn't handle the assignment alone. Dozens of people were needed to complete the work. HNTB was to oversee the entire operation, drawing together teams of experts to handle every technical area. Josef Sorkin recalls the extraordinary financial arrangements for the enterprise:

> *"... the firm took that job for a fee of $50,000 including cost. Cost, NO plus, just cost! On that first job, the firm furnished Ted Cambern, myself, Eddie Kuhn, Dick Wakefield ... for all practical purposes that was the staff. With that nucleus, we expanded into an office, into a staff in excess of a hundred. Ted Cambern was chief engineer and I was office engineer. The whole thing was virtually completed by the end of the year."*

Sorkin emphasized the speed with which the firm was expected to complete the work:

> *"... a great deal of that work was adapting buildings and facilities that the Quartermaster Corps already had. All throughout much of the work, we could see out the window the buildings being constructed — we were still working on the plans. The real task we had was managing the thing. We had to have the plans, the field personnel, and had to have it done at the right time."*

Bluebonnet Ordnance Plant

The firm didn't have a chance to catch its breath before plunging into a second project for the War Department: the Bluebonnet Ordnance Plant, near Waco, Texas. Josef Sorkin remembers:

> *"Almost immediately after Hope, Arkansas was finished, we went into the Bluebonnet Ordnance Plant, and again our total staff from HNTB was the same — Cambern, myself, Eddie Kuhn. Elmer Timby joined us later to write specifications on the job. On Bluebonnet,*

39

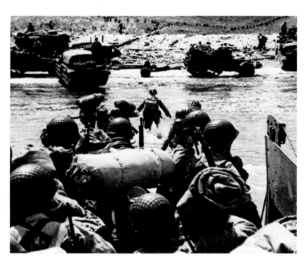

(above) Although the war scattered HNTB's staff to military service, it also brought the firm new and valuable project management experience. Partners and staff found themselves overseeing large-scale defense projects which laid the groundwork for the firm's later ventures into airport design, environmental work, and architecture.

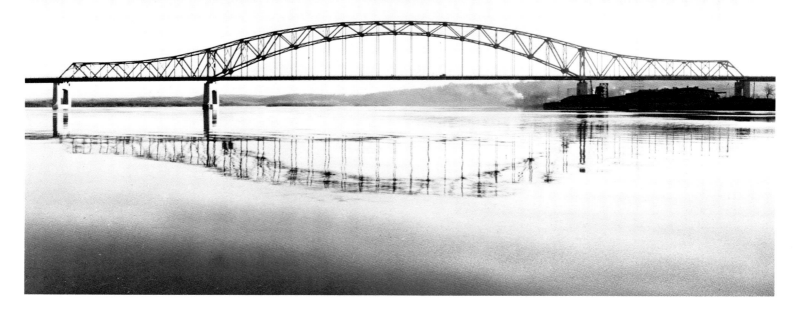

the organization expanded into 400 personnel. That project was completed before Thanksgiving that year."

Enoch Needles, who was resident engineer on the project, recalled that early in 1942 he and his staff "were given one year and a budget of $30 million for the project. Six weeks later, we were told to hurry — finish in six months if possible. By keeping work going night and day, we made it and came out under budget."

Bluebonnet consisted principally of a $17 million explosives and bomb loading plant. HNTB's responsibilities on the project included design and supervision of construction of the complete 18,000 acre facility, including industrial and residential buildings, storage magazines, railways, highways, a sewage system, a water supply and distribution system, gas and electrical power distribution systems, and steam generating and distribution systems. Like the Southwestern Proving Grounds, Bluebonnet was no paint-by-number project.

Settling in for the Duration

As the Bluebonnet assignment drew to a frenzied close, Enoch Needles received word that his services were required in Washington, D.C. Ellis Paul had also been drafted. Just before Thanksgiving in 1942, they drove east in the Buick which Needles had purchased for the Bluebonnet job. Paul was soon on his way to Miami, Florida, for officers training school, followed by a tedious three-year stint at Wright Field (Ohio) as procurement officer. After passing his physical in New York City, Needles headed for a desk assignment in the nation's capital.

Like many HNTB partners and employees who served in World War II, Needles was quickly exposed to engineering projects of enormous scale. The Southwestern Proving Grounds and the Bluebonnet plant had been excellent preparation for the task that lay ahead of Needles for the next two years. His assignment in Washington, D.C. consisted of nothing less than trying to keep

(above) Few domestic bridges were designed or constructed during the war years. One exception was the Mississippi River Bridge at Dubuque, Iowa. Faced with wartime rationing of steel, future partner Ellis Paul struggled to obtain reinforcing steel for the bridge's deck. Completed in 1943, the bridge won the major American Institute of Steel Construction award for that year.

40

The construction of the Bluebonnet Ordnance Plant near Waco, Texas, during World War II included more than 60 miles of highways, 60 miles of railroads and a large electrical power distribution system. HNTB quickly learned to coordinate and supervise teams of specialty firms to design and build huge wartime projects like Bluebonnet. (right) A newsletter published by the contractors reported the status of the project. (below) As a co-partner of the Bluebonnet Constructors, with the W.E. Callahan Construction Company and under the supervision of the U.S. Army Engineers, Enoch Needles served as resident project director.

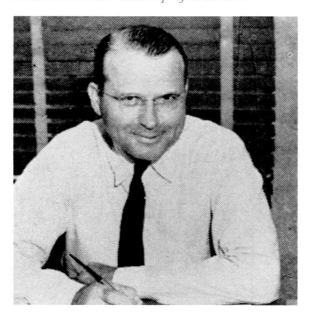

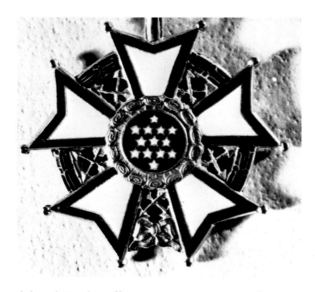

(above) For his efforts in inventorying and distributing some 100,000 pieces of heavy construction equipment for the domestic war effort during World War II, Needles was awarded the Legion of Merit in 1945.

Nearing the End

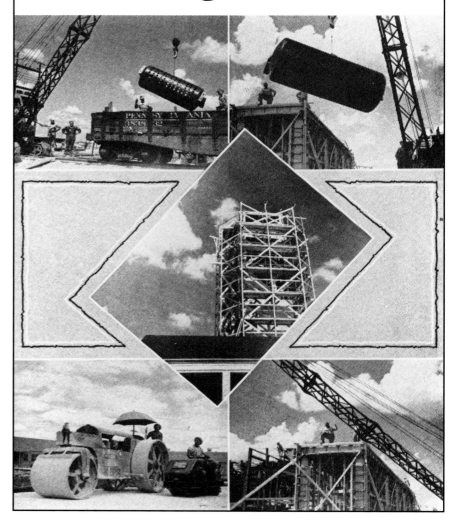

track of "some 100,000 pieces of heavy construction equipment valued at probably $200 million" which the Corps of Engineers had gathered for the war effort. Needles and his immediate colleagues were in charge of the distribution of this incredible inventory of equipment when and where it was needed. For his efforts, Needles was awarded the prestigious Legion of Merit in September 1945.

While Needles carried out his role as "desk-soldier ... in the vast Battle of Papers at Washington," his fellow partners and employees kept busy with projects closer to home. One assignment involved the conversion of historic Fort Riley, Kansas, from a cavalry to a mechanized base. The project was ultimately scaled back considerably from its original outline, but HNTB handled a piece of the facility's expansion, including the construction of a number of barracks. A larger project was the construction of a new prisoner-of-war camp at Concordia, Kansas. Josef Sorkin recalls that the government's decision to build the facility created a small local stir:

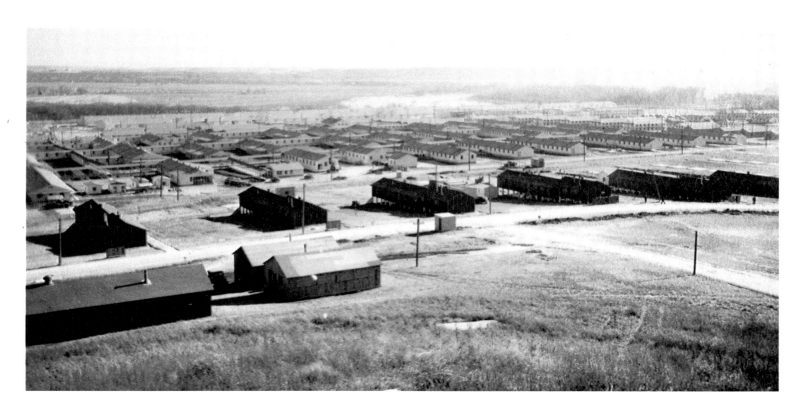

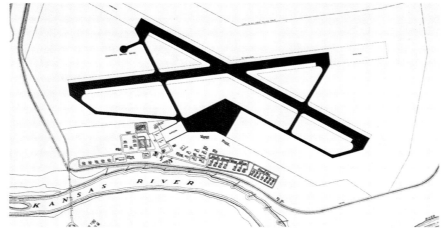

(this page) Another important wartime assignment involved the conversion of historic Ft. Riley, Kansas from horse cavalry to mechanized cavalry. HNTB managed a comprehensive program to overhaul and expand roads, buildings and utilities at the military post.

Part of the conversion of Ft. Riley included the design and construction of two 4,500-foot paved runways at Marshall Field. This airport and another at Southwestern Proving Grounds in Arkansas were HNTB's earliest airfield projects.

42

HNTB designed a 157-acre POW facility at Concordia, Kansas in 1944. The internment camp provided housing, mess facilities, recreation, and hospitalization for up to 4,000 internees. Its modern hospital and refrigeration facilities created a stir among Kansans whose own communities lacked such up-to-date amenities.

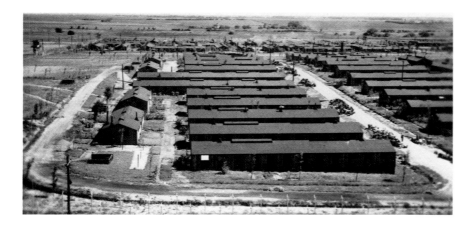

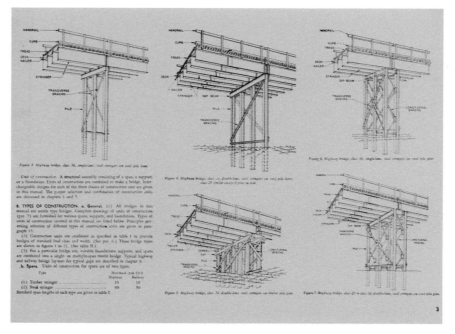

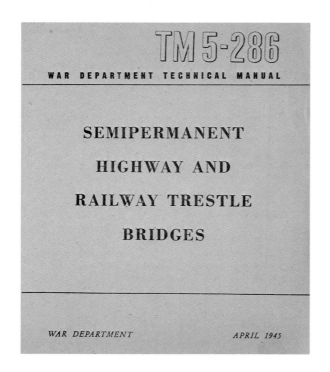

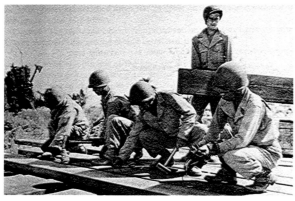

(above and right) During the war, the firm was requested to prepare a manual on bridge construction that would allow "a sergeant with an elementary education" to construct bridges up to 90 feet in length out of steel, concrete or wood for any kind of situation. Seventy HNTB engineers spent a year developing the book.

43

"... the hospital facilities and the refrigeration facilities for meat and the like at the camp were better than any community in Kansas had. Even at the time it seemed absolutely ridiculous that the government would proceed with the great expense to provide for war prisoners things that the native communities did not have. It was a full, complete community, with living facilities, kitchen facilities, storage for food — all up to date."

One more major war assignment followed on the heels of the Concordia camp project. This time the project involved a subject area in which HNTB was extremely well-versed: bridges. The Army wanted a manual which would show a sergeant exactly how to build a temporary bridge or trestle for any kind of situation.

Ernest Howard took up the challenge and put the Kansas City office to work on the project. By the time of its publication, more than 70 engineers had spent a year on it. Pulling together a staff large enough to handle the assignment proved to be tough. Don Stevens, then a very young employee of the firm, remembers:

"They were hiring everybody. They put ads in the paper — 'If you can write, we'll teach you the rest.' Women would come to work because there wasn't much manpower around. We did this work on linen tracing cloth. During the war, linen was really hard to come by. The women would make mistakes, take the linen home, wash it out and make scarves and things like that."

In spite of a suspiciously high number of tracing "mistakes" which left the firm's male engineers consternated, the office managed to get the job done. The result was a beautifully illustrated 350-page book as detailed and almost as simple as the instructions that come with a child's building set. The book was christened with the unwieldy title: *War Department Technical Manual 5-286, Semipermanent Highway and Railway Trestle Bridges.* In April 1945, the huge epistle was published. A month later, V-E Day signalled the beginning of the end of the war. ■

PART THREE

Growth Years

"On the heels of the Maine Turnpike came a flood of requests for HNTB's services on other turnpikes. ... Almost overnight, turnpike authorities were established, bond issues floated, and work begun."

CHAPTER FIVE

The Turnpike Era: A Decade of Expansion (1945-1955)

World War II brought changes to many lives. An entire generation had set aside the business of daily life for almost five years to focus singlemindedly on the goals of victory and peace. When the country came home from the battles abroad, many Americans realized that their world would never be as it had been before the war.

Among the most deeply felt and long-lasting changes wrought by World War II were developments in technology. Some had been put to devastating use. At Hiroshima and Nagasaki, humanity witnessed the first use of atomic power. Other technological advances had more benign applications. The first "electronic brain" was unveiled in 1942, hailing the beginning of the computer revolution. The future of American aviation changed overnight after Bell Aircraft successfully tested the first U.S. jet plane during the war. And, Americans who had served in the military or in industry on the home front carried with them into peacetime employment technical education and a battery of skills second to none.

The employees of HNTB were no exception. As the firm's staff began to rebuild after the war, many of HNTB's engineers returned from their military assignments equipped with experience in every sort of engineering project imaginable. The urgency of wartime conditions had taught them that no project was impossible if everyone were willing to learn the ropes quickly and buckle down to get the job done. On jobs like the Southwestern Proving Ground and the Bluebonnet Ordnance Plant, Needles, Sorkin, Paul, Timby, and dozens of others had gotten a first-hand look at what sheer determination and a lot of hard work could accomplish.

Many of the engineers who joined HNTB for the first time following the war also brought confidence and experience from their own time in the military. Dozens came to the firm either straight out of the service or a few years after their discharge. Others came from school or jobs where they had gotten a civilian's eye view of the impact of the war on the engineering field. Several future HNTB partners were among those who arrived on the firm's doorstep after the war. Frank Bleistein and Chris Lamberton arrived in 1946. Dan Watkins joined the firm in 1947. Paul Heineman, Bob Drange, Don Harper, Gerard Fox and Browning Crow all came in 1948. Bernard Rottinghaus came the next year. Ed Johnson joined in 1951 and Bill Meredith in 1952. The fresh faces on HNTB's staff after the war came on board at the beginning of one of the most exciting periods in the firm's history.

The Maine Turnpike

On July 25, 1945 — a month before the Japanese surrender brought World War II to an end — HNTB secured an assignment which launched a major extension of the firm's practice: the Maine Turnpike.

Turnpikes in the United States were not a new idea in the 1940s. Toll roads under private ownership had flourished in New England

45

(below) Advances in military technology spawned the domestic computer and jet aircraft industries in the 1940s, two developments which profoundly altered HNTB's practice after the war.

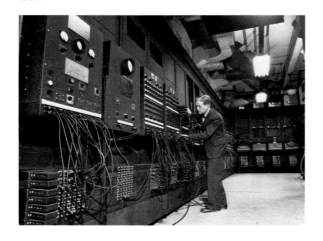

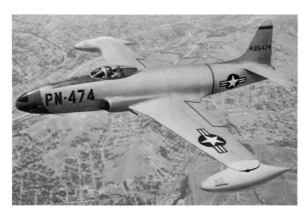

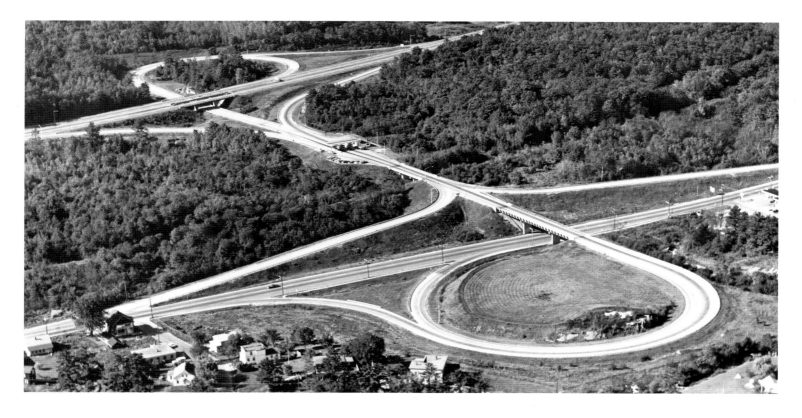

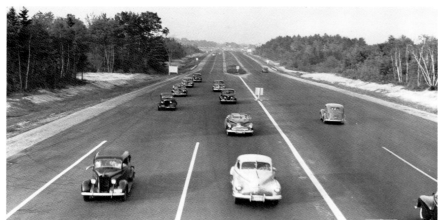

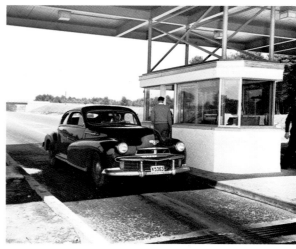

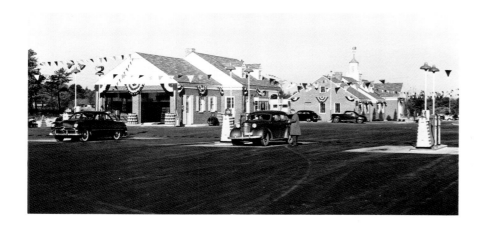

(this page) The Maine Turnpike was the first of the modern turnpikes, financed entirely with private funds. Because of the firm's extensive experience in toll bridges, HNTB was retained as consulting engineer on the project in 1945. The first 47-mile section of the Maine Turnpike extended from Kittery to Portland and opened to traffic in December, 1947. The dual roadway turnpike was considered a model for other toll highways both in its design and financing.

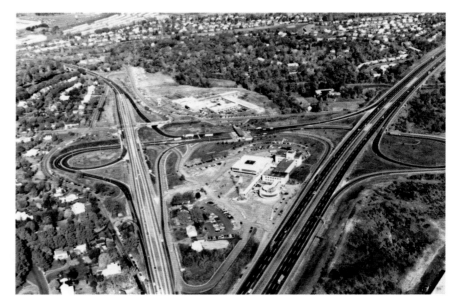

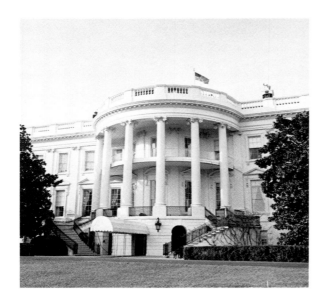

47

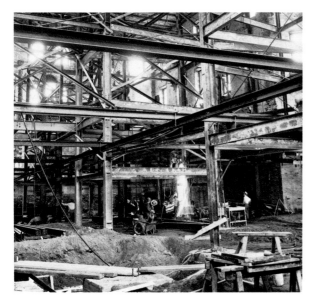

and elsewhere in the eighteenth and early nineteenth centuries. By the mid-nineteenth century, a rudimentary network of free public roads began to develop as the country grew in population and settlers started to move west across the mountains. Toll roads slowly diminished in importance. The idea was not revived until a century later, when the Pennsylvania Turnpike was built in the late 1930s. Even then, the Pennsylvania toll road was not wholly of the old tradition. The turnpikes of the eighteenth century had been privately built and owned. The original section of the Pennsylvania Turnpike was partly financed with $47 million in federal funds.

The seeds of the Maine Turnpike were planted in 1941, when Maine state legislator Joseph T. Sayward saw the new Pennsylvania Turnpike first-hand. He was impressed. Sayward thought that the coastal region of Maine, in the southeastern corner of the state, could benefit by a similar road. Traffic in the area had been becoming more and more congested over the years. The new road could alleviate the problem.

The new road, unlike its Pennsylvania predecessor, would also pay for itself — without dipping into state or federal coffers. For the first time in more than a century, a major toll road was going to be built that would be entirely privately financed. The turnpike would be paid for with revenue bonds, the debt to be liquidated wholly by tolls collected for the use of the road. Legislation was duly offered, and in August 1941 the Maine Turnpike Authority met for the first time in Augusta.

Progress on the turnpike was slow. The outbreak of World War II put a halt to most civilian public works. The only thing that the Authority managed to accomplish during the war years was to arrange financing and completion of a feasibility study. The study was finished in April 1945. Three months later, HNTB was retained as consulting engineer for the project.

Although the Maine Turnpike has come to be remembered as a pet project of Enoch Needles, R.N. Bergendoff also played an important role in keeping tabs on the status of the prospective turnpike while Needles was absent from the firm during the war. Ellis Paul recalled:

> *"If I remember, Enoch had made contacts with the Maine people — then he was in the service and then [the*

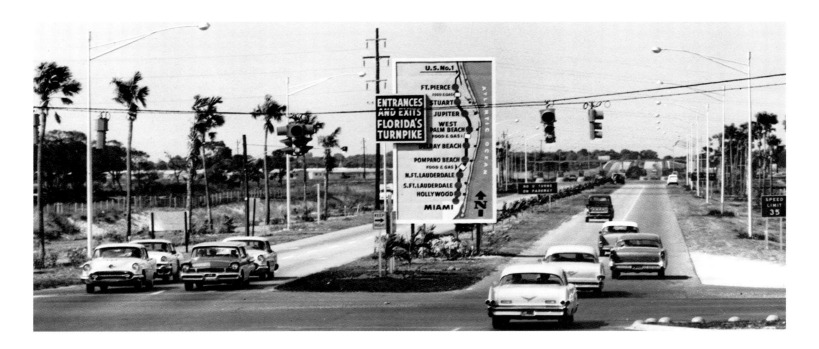

project] became active before Enoch got out. [During that time], it's my understanding, Bergie had gone up there and kept it active. Then when Enoch got out [of the service], he went back on [the turnpike]."

When Needles was separated from the service in November 1945 he headed straight for Maine. He lived in a local inn during the first months of the project. Soon he bought a house in Kennebunk-Beach — one still used every summer by the Needles family. Needles "felt it was very important for us as a family to go there and show that we weren't outsiders," recalls his daughter, Sally Needles Toffey.

Not everyone thought that the new toll road in Maine was a sound idea. The American Automobile Association and the Federal Public Roads Administration both were sure that the stretch would be "a financial white elephant." Despite their skepticism, the Maine Turnpike opened on December 13, 1947. Mrs. Joseph Sayward cut the ribbon, and the first cars rolled down the new 47-mile road between Portland and Kittery. Soon, traffic on the turnpike exceeded the most optimistic predictions. Within a year, even the cynics were satisfied. The first modern turnpike designed to pay for itself was a resounding success.

Opening the Floodgates

On the heels of the Maine Turnpike came a flood of requests for HNTB's services on other turnpikes. States and bankers had been keeping an eye on developments in Maine. If Maine could do it, other states could, too. Almost overnight, turnpike authorities were established, bond issues floated, and work begun.

HNTB was ideally situated to take the lead in the modern turnpike field. The firm's reputation in the nation's bond markets had been established during the toll bridge era of the 1920s and 1930s. The addition of toll roads to HNTB's repertoire in the 1940s and 1950s was well-received on Wall Street. HNTB's experience during the war in the supervision of large projects gave the firm additional qualifications. Because of its expertise in managing

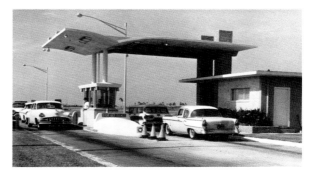

(top and above) HNTB's initial work on the Florida Turnpike began in 1952. The original four-lane section ran for 109 miles and boasted 89 bridges. The firm also worked on several extensions.

48

teams of specialists, the firm was often asked to take the role of general consultant for a state's turnpike program.

Every turnpike was an opportunity for the firm to hone its expertise, break into a new market, and develop new business relationships. Before the turnpike era came to a close in the mid-1950s, HNTB had sent staff to New Jersey, Delaware, Ohio, West Virginia, Colorado, Texas, Kansas, Florida, Massachusetts, and nearly a half dozen other turnpike states. One turnpike, in particular, became almost legendary for its scope and long-term significance to HNTB: the New Jersey Turnpike.

Like some other turnpikes — notably the one in Massachusetts — the New Jersey Turnpike had to be built in an already heavily populated area. The magnitude of the task impressed even Enoch Needles, whose wartime job of overseeing $200 million of construction equipment for the federal government might have jaded his view of civilian-scale projects. Needles had played a major role in securing the turnpike assignment for HNTB. He revelled in the engineering challenges it presented. "Never before," explained Needles in a 1954 article in the *Daily Bond Buyer*, "had the problem been presented of carrying an 118-mile expressway with a 60-mile speed limit directly into the central portion of the greatest metropolitan area in the world, greater NYC and environs."

The New Jersey Turnpike was launched in October 1948 when the state legislature formally approved the project. Ground for the four-lane, 117.5 mile main stem was broken in January 1950 and completed in a record 23 months. The first section between Deepwater and Bordentown, New Jersey, opened on November 5, 1951. Many subsequent additions of lanes and extensions to the original road have been designed by HNTB. Thirty-five years after Needles' comments in the *Daily Bond Buyer*, the New Jersey Turnpike continues to supply enough challenges to keep the HNTB's Fairfield, New Jersey, office busy year-round.

The Delaware Memorial Bridge

In spite of the firm's overnight popularity as a toll road designer, bridges were not forgotten during HNTB's turnpike heyday. One of the firm's most important bridge projects came just prior to the New Jersey Turnpike assignment: the Delaware Memorial Bridge.

During World War II, a small amount of civilian bridge work had continued to come through HNTB's doors in Kansas City and New York City. Design and construction of the new bridges progressed slowly because of limited engineering staff and the wartime strictures put on the use of materials for civilian projects. Despite the constraints, HNTB won five of nine awards given in 1946 by the American Institute of Steel Construction for the most beautiful bridge designs.

As the New Jersey Turnpike assignment was getting underway in the late 1940s, HNTB began designs for the Delaware Memorial Bridge. The new toll bridge would connect Delaware and New Jersey over a wide channel of the Delaware River near Wilmington. The proposed six-lane span had the blessing of President Harry Truman, who emerged from World War II as convinced as his World War I predecessors had been that the United States needed to secure its home front with a good network of roads and bridges. The Delaware Memorial Bridge was a vitally needed link in East Coast transportation routes.

As the bridge design neared completion, HNTB's plans hit a snag. The bridge commission suddenly was not sure that it could afford a six-lane bridge based on the traffic projections it had been

(below) Designed in the early 1950s, the West Virginia Turnpike winds for 88 miles through some of the East's most mountainous terrain. The project included the design of one of the firm's first major tunnels.

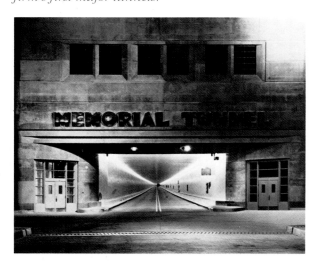

49

(facing page) Enoch Needles was instrumental in obtaining the design of the $35 million Delaware Memorial Bridge in 1948. This was one of the first post-war projects for the firm. The Delaware Memorial Bridge replaced the New Castle-Pennsville Ferry. The bridge ultimately formed a vital link with another major HNTB project — the New Jersey Turnpike. Originally designed as a six-lane bridge, HNTB scaled down the design when funding became a problem. Working with the contractor, the redesign was built with the available funds and the bridge was opened to traffic in August 1951. With a channel span of 2,150 feet, it was the fifth longest span in the world when constructed. The magnificent suspension bridge won the AISC's Most Beautiful Bridge award in 1951.

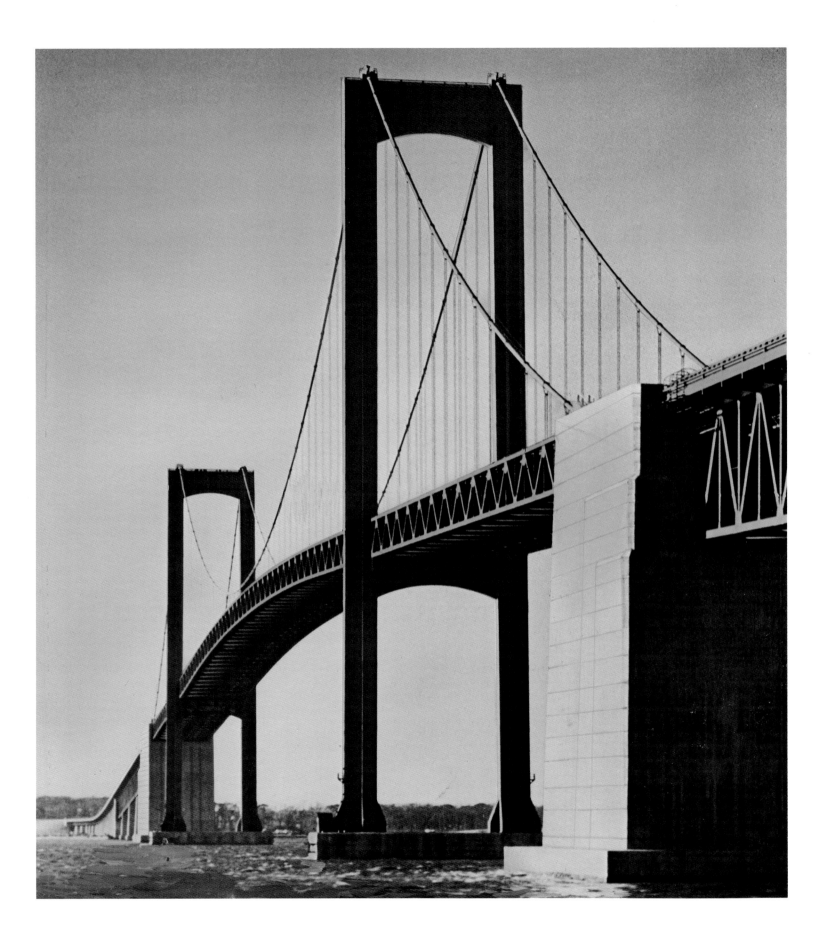

50

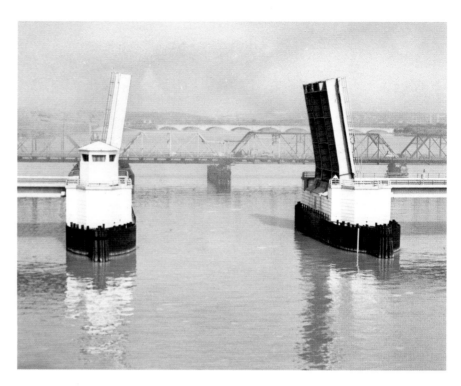

(right) Even during the turnpike era, HNTB's expertise in movable bridges thrived. The Fourteenth Street Bridge with a double leaf bascule span over the Potomac River in Washington, D.C. was awarded first place for its design by the National Commission of Fine Arts and District of Columbia governmental agencies.

Highway needs during the 1950s included more than turnpikes. Millions of automobiles were being manufactured each year to meet the demand of an exploding population. HNTB found a rapidly expanding market in urban expressways such as the Southern State Parkway, New York (below), and Kansas City's Southwest Trafficway (bottom).

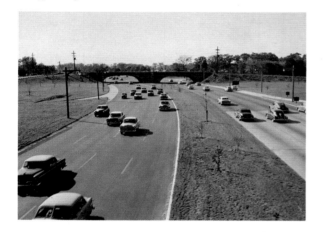

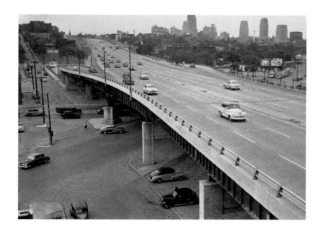

provided; it wanted to cancel the project. Enoch Needles and his staff worked feverishly to save it:

> *"By then the Delaware Highway Department owed us $400,000. In desperation, we worked over the plans to show a 4-lane bridge, cooperating with the prospective contractors to bring the bridge within available funds. When they paid us, Warren Mack, of the bridge commission, commented that he got more satisfaction out of writing this check than any he had ever written."*

Despite the frantic, last-minute redesign, the bridge was completed and ready to open on August 15, 1951 — right on time. The opening was of special satisfaction to Needles. He had been listening for a full decade to discussions about building a bridge at that site. And, he had made a bet with his neighbor, Frank duPont, that the bridge — once committed to — would open on time. Frank duPont duly paid Needles the $500 the two men had wagered. With his winnings, Needles had two dozen small silver cups inscribed in commemoration of the bridge opening. He gave a dozen cups to duPont and a pair to each of his own six children as souvenirs of one of HNTB's most memorable projects.

Enoch Needles wasn't the only one who'd made a wager related to the opening of the Delaware Memorial Bridge. His wife, Ethel, had guessed that 20,000 cars would use the new bridge on opening day. The final tally was 20,024. Homer Seely, HNTB's construction project engineer on the Delaware bridge, good-humoredly sent Mrs. Needles a $4.00 check to settle their bet.

New Partners

The avalanche of turnpike projects after World War II caught the firm short of staff. HNTB needed lots of good engineers and technicians, and it needed them fast. "The work load was building up," remembers now-retired HNTB partner Bob Drange, who

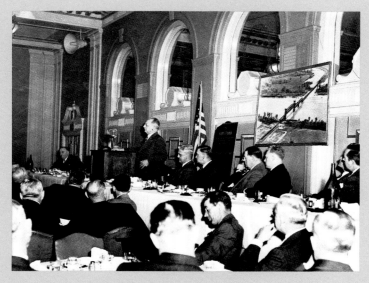

HNTB and Service to the Professions

The second half of the nineteenth century and first half of the twentieth saw the establishment of assorted discipline-based professional societies in architecture and engineering. These societies were organized to help secure the professional status of practitioners and to promote common interests of members. Over the years, HNTB has maintained close ties to the societies, contributing time, energy and resources at the local, state, and national levels.

The first U.S. professional engineering society was established in Massachusetts in 1848: the Boston Society of Civil Engineers. National organizations soon blossomed. In 1852, the American Society of Civil and Architectural Engineers was formed. Five years later, the architects split with the engineers to form the American Institute of Architects. In 1880, the League of American Wheelmen, a bicyclists' group organized to promote good roads, was founded; a century later, after several name and membership changes, the group is now called the American Road and Transportation Builders Association. In 1910, the American Institute of Consulting Engineers was established. Twenty-four years later, the National Society of Professional Engineers was formed. By the time that the Consulting Engineers Council was organized in 1947, architecture and nearly every discipline of engineering — mechanical, electrical, chemical, metallurgical, etc. — had organized its members into national organizations. Other groups with more highly specialized interests have also developed as the need for their services became apparent.

Through the years, HNTB has won many cherished awards from the various societies and organizations in which it participates. Every HNTB office boasts its share of local, state, and national prizes. In return for the professional honors bestowed on the firm's people and projects, HNTB has tried to shoulder some of the leadership responsibilities of the societies. Since 1914, scores of HNTB employees and partners have held elected offices or appointments in local chapters of various membership organizations. A few have held the highest posts at the national level. The earliest was John Lyle Harrington, who in 1923 was president of the American Society of Mechanical Engineers. In 1946, Enoch Needles held the presidency of the American Institute of Consulting

Engineers. Three years later, he began his term as president of the American Road Builders Association, while Ernest Howard prepared to take the helm of the American Society of Civil Engineers in 1950. While Howard was president of ASCE, he had the honor of bestowing the society's prestigious Thomas Rowland Fitch Award on R.N. Bergendoff and Josef Sorkin for their paper on a bridge at Dubuque, Iowa. Howard had won the same award in 1921 for a paper on vertical lift bridges. Five years after Howard's term, Enoch Needles was elected to the presidency of ASCE. While Needles was in office, President Eisenhower signed the legislation finally kicking off the long-delayed Interstate Highway Program. Two years later, Needles was at the helm of the Engineers Joint Council, an umbrella group of 17 engineering organizations with 250,000 members. As president of the group he testified before Congress on the merits of creating a Cabinet-level Department of Science and Engineering. In 1960, Jim Exum was elected to the presidency of the American Institute of Consulting Engineers, a post which Needles had held 14 years earlier. In 1971, Carl Erb was at the head of the AICE when he died of cancer, age 58.

HNTB has on occasion also been involved in the work of international organizations. Ernest Howard devoted time to the activities of the International Association for Bridge and Structural Engineering (IABSE), service which allowed him to combine his love of travel with professional obligations. Following Howard's example, Elmer Timby and, later, Gerry Fox, served as president of the USA Group of the IABSE. Timby also represented IABSE at various United Nations activities designed to facilitate transfer of technology to developing countries. The most recent HNTB partner to hold a national office with a professional society is Dan Spigai, who spent 1988 at the helm of the American Road and Transportation Builders Association. Enoch Needles held the same post 39 years earlier in 1949 with ARTBA's predecessor, the American Road Builders Association.

"By serving in our professional organizations," says HNTB partner Frank Hall of Spigai and the many other HNTB partners and employees who have held offices, "maybe we're giving something back to the profession that's been so generous to us."

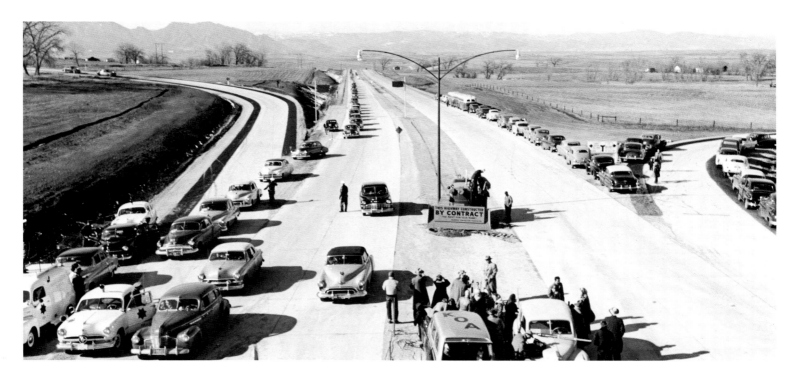

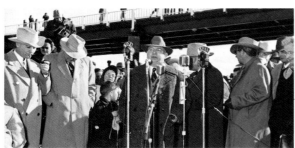

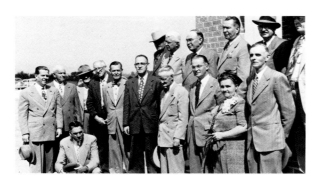

(top) The 17-mile Denver-Boulder Turnpike, the first modern toll road west of the Mississippi, provided an early training ground in roadway design for an entire generation of HNTB engineers. By the early 1950's, HNTB's days as a bridges-only firm were over. (middle) Ernest Howard (center) addresses officials and dignitaries at the opening of the Denver-Boulder toll road in January, 1952. (above) R.N. Bergendoff (far left) joins dignitaries in celebrating completion of the Denver-Boulder Turnpike.

joined the firm in 1948, "so they were adding new college graduates. All the engineers who were hired began their careers as draftsmen on the boards. My first full day was spent reading the drafting room standards."

Many of the future HNTB partners who joined the firm in the late 1940s and early 1950s got their start on the board or in the field on the designs of one or more of the new toll roads. Others came to HNTB with plans to make a career in bridge design, only to find that their talents were badly needed on the new turnpikes. Now-retired HNTB partner Dan Watkins, who joined the firm in 1947, spent his first three years designing bridges. Then he was suddenly asked if he would like to work on the first toll road to be built west of the Mississippi: the Denver-Boulder Turnpike. The challenge appealed to him; four decades later he was still working in highway design.

The sudden influx of turnpike business after the war put its share of strains on HNTB's small partnership, as well as the firm's staff.

The firm's two offices — Kansas City and New York City — each had two partners in residence. Howard and Bergendoff were in the Midwest; Needles and Tammen were in the East. The pairings worked well. Bergendoff and Needles were generally thought of as the "outside" partners, who enjoyed the more entrepreneurial aspects of the firm's business. Public presentations and meetings with prospective clients appealed to both men. Howard and especially Tammen, on the other hand, were viewed more as the "inside" partners, by nature fascinated by the technical intricacies of design work. Both delighted in their regular strolls — pencil in hand — through the firm's drafting rooms to review projects currently on the boards.

As business picked up to an almost frantic pace during the late 1940s, the time and energy of the four partners were stretched to the breaking point. Seventy-year old Ernest Howard was about to begin his term as president of the American Society of Civil

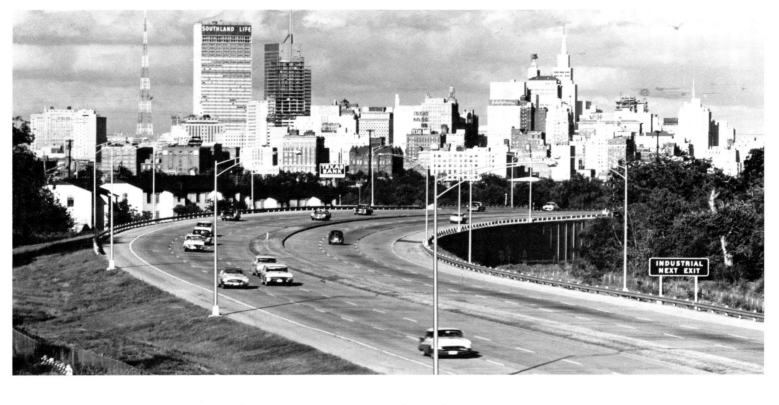

Urban highways built within the confines of highly developed areas presented new design complexities. An example was the Dallas-Fort Worth Turnpike, (top) a major expressway connecting a number of major arterials in the congested metropolitan area.

Engineers (1950) and Enoch Needles was serving as president of the American Road Builders Association (1949-1950). Both positions carried professional responsibilities which neither Howard nor Needles took lightly. But their obligations to the professional societies also meant being away from the office, at least part of the time, just when the new turnpikes were being launched.

The temporary absences of Howard and Needles from the daily life of the firm during their society presidencies might have been manageable in the short run. Bergendoff and Tammen, the two partners who would be left in charge, certainly were not new to the business of being partners. Between the two of them, they could shoulder a little more responsibility for the duration. One critical development stood in the way of such an easy, short-term solution: Henry Tammen had decided to retire from the firm at the end of 1949.

Tammen's decision caught many people off guard. Never before had a partner in the firm retired. The loss of a partner had always been for other reasons. Louis Ash had died. Waddell, Hedrick, and Harrington had each withdrawn to move on to other firms. No one had really thought about what the current generation of partners might do. It was assumed that hard-driving Henry Tammen would be at his desk until the day he died. To those who knew him well, retirement did not seem like a state of mind that Tammen would get used to. Josef Sorkin remembers:

> "When Henry retired, everyone thought it would be the end of him because he was so involved in his work. He was always the first one to arrive in the morning and the last one to leave — always carrying a large portfolio with him home. But he surprised everyone ... his personality changed somewhat — he was relaxed, more affable, and in every way, he was a happier person."

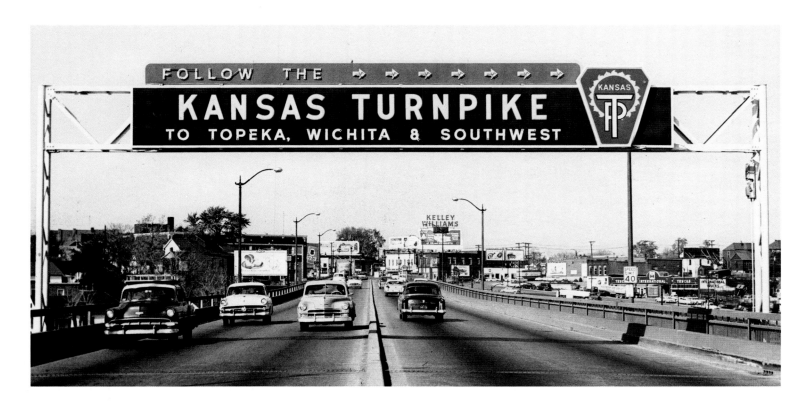

(top) The 236-mile Kansas Turnpike was completed in a fast-paced 24 months, opening to traffic in October 1956. In addition to acting as general consultant to the Kansas Turnpike Authority, HNTB designed and supervised construction of a 57-mile segment of the road.

55

(facing page) The Kansas Turnpike today remains an important segment of a nationwide network of roadways that have been maintained by user revenue.

Of the four HNTB partners, Henry Tammen had been the least public-oriented. Not a salesman by temperament, Tammen savored his in-house role in the technical end of business in the New York City office. Precision was his hallmark; he was a stickler for perfection, even if it meant doing work over and over again until it was right. Elmer Timby, who was hired by Tammen on a part-time basis in the 1930s and became a partner upon Tammen's retirement, remembers his first impression of his new boss:

> "It was Tammen who hired me, and when I first came to work for the firm, he put me at a desk in his office and for some time I had a firsthand view of the way he did things ... Dave Hall ... I can remember he came in there once with the design of a vertical lift tower ... Dave was a brilliant mathematician, but you couldn't read his handwriting. I remember seeing Harry look through these calcs — he looked up at Hall — he looked at the computations — then he turned around, threw the whole bunch in the wastebasket and told him to go back and do it over again and do it so he could read it."

Tammen's decision to retire posed a dilemma for his partners. Ernest Howard and Enoch Needles, in particular, could readily remember the tensions that the partnership had faced in the late 1920s when John Lyle Harrington had tried to juggle too many responsibilities. A bitter partnership split had resulted. Now, with such a bright future ahead in turnpike design, Howard, Needles, and Bergendoff must have thought twice about allowing a similar scenario to develop from the stress of trying to manage more business than the three of them could reasonably handle. With Tammen gone, plus Howard and Needles on the road, and a veritable tidal wave of new work coming through the doors, the time had come for the partnership to grow. Howard, Needles, and Bergendoff agreed to take on five new partners.

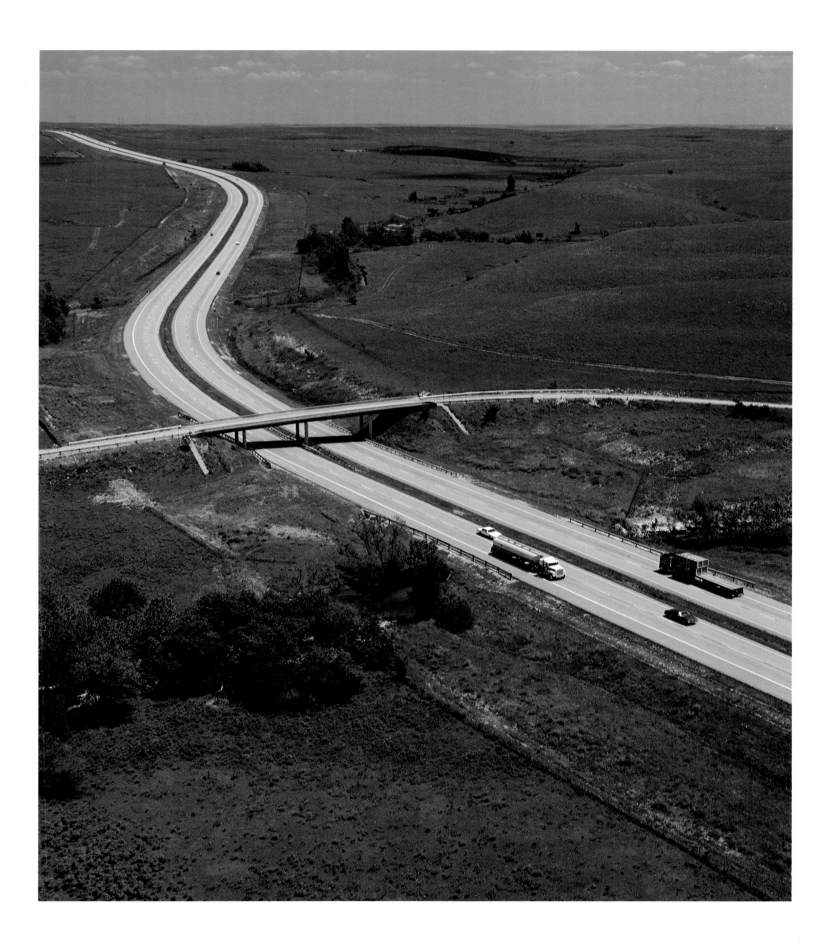

56

(right) R.N. Bergendoff and Hal Sours were instrumental in obtaining an assignment to design two portions (33 miles) of the Ohio Turnpike in the early 1950s.

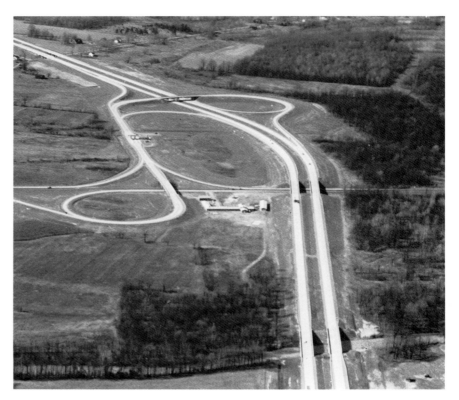

(below) As HNTB prospered in the post-war years, the idea of opening another permanent office arose. R.N. Bergendoff persuaded his partners to establish a branch operation to handle the firm's work in Ohio. In 1954, future partner Carl Erb and a handful of Kansas City staff moved to Cleveland. Soon, local HNTB offices blossomed across the country.

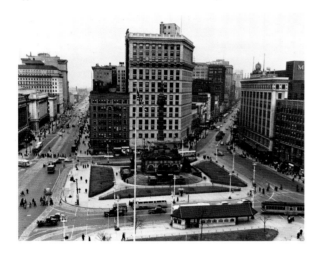

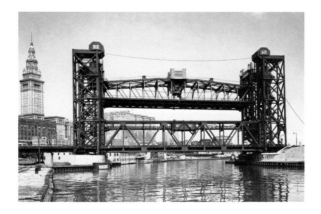

(above) Cuyahoga River Bridge No. 1, Cleveland, Ohio.

On December 31, 1949, during the annual ASCE meeting in New York City, Henry Tammen formally retired. The next day — January 1, 1950 — Ted Cambern, Jim Exum, Ellis Paul, Josef Sorkin, and Elmer Timby became partners. Exum, Paul, and Timby were located in the New York City office. Cambern and Sorkin were in Kansas City. HNTB's two offices each now had four partners in residence. The numbers maintained the East-West balance that had been in place since 1940 when R. N. Bergendoff joined Ernest Howard as partner in the Kansas City office.

The five men who became partners in 1950 were hardly strangers to the firm. Ellis Paul and Jim Exum had first joined HNTB in 1922, in the same year as R.N. Bergendoff. Paul had been with the firm without interruption for nearly three decades. Exum had twice left to work in the Texas Highway Department, but returned to HNTB permanently in 1948. Theodore (Ted) J. Cambern had joined the firm in 1925, immediately after graduating from the University of Kansas with a B.S. degree in civil engineering. He left three years later at the time of the split with Harrington, working for Harrington & Cortelyou until 1940, when he returned to the HNTB fold. All three men — Paul, Exum and Cambern — had common roots going back to Harrington, Howard & Ash days.

Elmer Knowles Timby came to HNTB by a different route. In the tradition of J.A.L. Waddell, Ernest Howard, and Louis Ash, Timby spent part of his early engineering career as an academic. After graduating from Ohio State with a B.C.E. degree in 1928, he taught for one year at his alma mater. Timby then moved to Princeton University where he rose from instructor to chairman of the Department of Civil Engineering. While at Princeton he was associated with HNTB on a part-time basis, working in the New York City office beginning in 1938. In 1949 he left Princeton to join HNTB full-time.

Josef Sorkin, the fifth man to be named as a new partner in 1950, also came from an unusual background. Russian by birth, Sorkin arrived in the United States in 1923, sponsored by an American family. Despite an initial lack of English, Sorkin made his way through the University of Nebraska, graduating in the summer of 1929, only a few months before the stock market crash. Following a decade of work in Nebraska and Montana, Sorkin joined HNTB's Kansas City office in 1939 and quickly made himself at home.

Loss of a Partner

The addition of five more partners in 1950 was better-timed than those making the decision perhaps realized. Just as the partnership was adjusting to its new, larger size, Ernest Howard died. On August 19, 1953, while at his desk in the firm's new Kansas City office at 1805 Grand Avenue, Howard suffered a heart attack. He died within hours at Kansas City's Research Hospital. He was 73.

Howard had never completely unpacked his boxes from the move to the new office two months earlier. In the years after his death, this uncharacteristic behavior was interpreted by some as a sign that Howard had perhaps sensed that his time was short. In a letter to Enoch Needles only three months before he died, Howard hinted at just that:

> "Bergie has proposed another idea inspired by what seems to be going on in certain large organizations. He suggests, for instance, that the firm should have a 'business' conference of all partners with wives for a week or at least several days. I have long been convinced that we are the hardest working firm that could be found, and have been so intense that we seem to have a guilty feeling if we take an ordinary vacation. We may be overlooking the fact that our lives are going on and we are living today, and will not be living at some future distant time."

Ernest Howard's funeral was a major event for the city. He had been active in civic and local business matters since his first days in Kansas City. His personal friendship with President Harry Truman had helped the city and his 24-year tenure as the chairman of the board of trustees and founder of the University of Kansas City had endeared him to many. The list of honorary pallbearers ran to 39, including his seven partners.

Only a year after he died, Howard's widow, Josephine Tiernan Howard, endowed the Ernest E. Howard Award of the American Society of Civil Engineers. This annual award recognizes advances in structural engineering. In 1980, HNTB partner Gerard Fox, at the time of Howard's death a young engineer in the New York City office, won the Howard award for his innovative work in bridge design.

New Offices

In the 1950s, while HNTB's partnership adjusted to its new size and coped with the loss of Ernest Howard, critical decisions about the firm's future also needed to be made. One issue in particular required attention: Should HNTB open another permanent branch office?

Since 1922, the New York City office had been the firm's only effort to establish a permanent presence for HNTB outside Kansas City. The experiment had been successful, but not easy. The

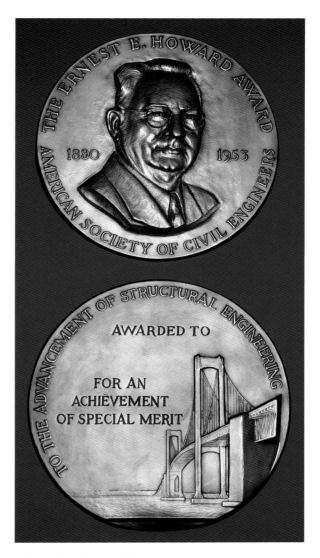

(above) In honor of Ernest Howard's contributions to the profession, the ASCE in 1954 instituted the Ernest E. Howard Award to be conferred annually for advancements in structural engineering. HNTB partner Gerry Fox won the award in 1980. Kansas City artist Thomas Hart Benton designed the medal.

58

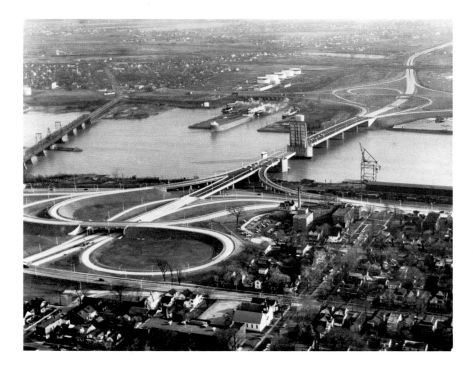

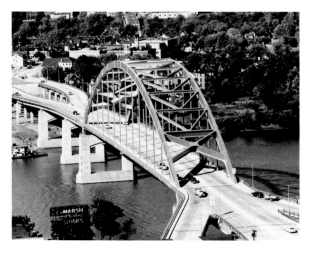

(above) Bridge design continued to be the main focus of the firm's business, even at the height of the turnpike boom in the mid-1950s. The Fort Henry Bridge over the Ohio River at Wheeling, West Virginia is a four-lane highway bridge with a 580-foot arch span. Completed in 1955, it was awarded an honorable mention in AISC's Most Beautiful Bridges Competition that year.

59

Depression, of course, had not helped matters; a dozen years had passed before the new office was able to land a project sizeable enough to free the New York City office of its dependence on Kansas City's largesse. Only after securing the Triborough Bridge Authority project in 1934 did Enoch Needles breathe easily.

Since then, small project offices had continued to open and close in locations from Maine to Colorado in connection with work on bridges and the new turnpikes. HNTB was well-known and well-respected in dozens of cities, counties, and states around the country. But change was in the air, change which large, old firms like HNTB could not ignore. There was new competition afoot. World War II had spawned hundreds of new, small engineering firms across the landscape. Many of these enterprises felt that local projects should fall to local firms. They argued that an outside firm would only take hard-earned tax dollars out of the community's economy. Furthermore, an outsider couldn't possibly grasp the needs of a particular community as well as a firm whose staff had grown up in the area. Their arguments held great appeal for local politicians and taxpayers.

HNTB could readily appreciate the arguments. The firm itself had always had a strong local presence in Kansas City. Many of the major bridges in the city had been designed by HNTB and its predecessor firms. And the firm fully expected to play a major role in transportation developments in the metropolitan area well into the future.

Unlike the vocal new firms which were struggling to get established in their own backyards, however, HNTB had also been doing design work all over the country for decades. The firm had worked hard to develop close client relationships from the East Coast to the West. To give up a well-established national practice in the face of increased local competition was not even a consideration. Instead, HNTB decided to adjust to changing times and bolster its ability to serve clients on a local basis.

HNTB's first new permanent office in more than 30 years opened in Cleveland, Ohio, in 1954. Ohio was a natural choice.

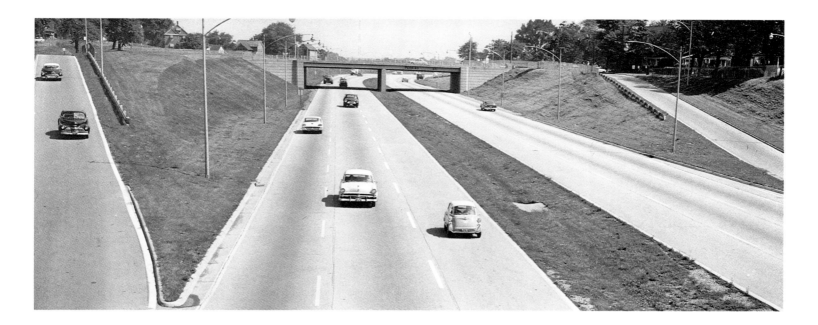

HNTB had designed many bridges in the state, including a large number in Cuyahoga County. Ohio was also quite interested in developing modern expressway systems in its major metropolitan areas, and, of course, in building a turnpike across the state. The potential for steady work in the future was very good.

Three years before the Cleveland office formally opened, R. N. Bergendoff took it upon himself to investigate setting up a local operation in Ohio. Not all of his fellow partners were as convinced as he that branch offices were a good idea. But Bergendoff thought that Ohio was too good an opportunity to pass up. In February 1951 he suggested to Enoch Needles that the firm add an Ohio office address to its letterhead:

> *"As you know, we now have work in Toledo, Akron, Columbus, and Marietta. We hope, also, of course, to secure some of the turnpike work. I mentioned to Hal [Sours] that it might add to establishing us locally in Ohio if we had a local Ohio address."*

Hal Sours had been Director of Highways in the state of Ohio. Two years after his retirement from that post in 1945, he joined HNTB as an associate and was given a free hand to develop work for the firm. His insight into the transportation needs of Ohio was second to none. Now-retired HNTB partner Joe Looper describes Sours as "the key ingredient in the development and growth of the Cleveland office … He played a significant part in our securing work" in the state. It was partly Sours' success in Ohio that helped to sell R.N. Bergendoff's fellow partners on the Cleveland office experiment.

An Ohio address was added to the firm's stationery, for Hal Sours' use in business correspondence. Within three years, the partners were ready to take the next critical step: to make the Cleveland office a full-fledged design operation. Carl Erb, chief draftsman in the Kansas City office, packed his bags and headed for Cleveland with a half dozen of his staff. It would be up to Erb and his staff to make the new office work. Under Erb's guidance, the Cleveland operation took off. The seeds sown by R.N. Bergendoff and Hal Sours — and watered by Carl Erb — had blossomed into HNTB's first branch office in more than 30 years. ∎

Carl Erb and his staff in the new Cleveland office had plenty of work to keep them busy in the late 1950s and early 1960s. Cities like Akron, Cleveland and Toledo, among others, wanted expressways to ease growing traffic congestion. (top) Akron Expressway, Akron, Ohio.

60

CHAPTER SIX

Branching Out: More Decentralization (1955-1970)

T he decision to open HNTB's Cleveland office in 1954 soon proved to be as farsighted as the opening of the firm's New York City office in 1922 had been. Enoch Needles' fledgling operation near Wall Street in the 1920s had put the firm squarely where it needed to be: close to the bankers who could make or break the toll projects upon which the firm's business had been built. Similarly, the opening of a small branch office in Ohio 30 years later gave HNTB the bonafide local presence it needed to compete with an increasing number of aggressive, homegrown firms.

Soon other HNTB branch offices opened. By 1956, HNTB had added design offices in Boston, Miami, Orlando, and Milwaukee.

HNTB's Boston office opened in 1954 with a dozen employees, led by Henry Leon. Like most other offices which eventually became permanent operations, Boston began as an office associated with a single project. The original assignment for Leon and his staff was the Massachusetts Turnpike. In the 1960s, when HNTB secured an additional assignment to design the Boston Extension of the turnpike, the office became permanent.

The firm's Miami office got its start in 1954 with the assignment to handle a few financial matters for Miami International Airport. In April 1955 design services were added and the office became permanent. Another office, in Orlando, Florida, opened a few months later under the direction of now-retired HNTB partner Carl Peterson. The Florida Turnpike kept the second Florida design office busy.

HNTB's Milwaukee office opened in March 1956 when now-retired HNTB partner Joe Looper moved to Wisconsin in the dead of winter to handle the design of the new interchange near the

(below) In the 1950s HNTB began to explore the field of airport design. The firm's earliest civilian aviation project involved the expansion of Miami International Airport, Dade County, Florida. HNTB was able to apply runway design expertise gained during the war to the enormous paving requirements of Florida's largest airport.

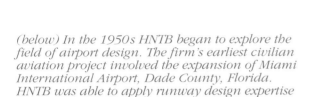
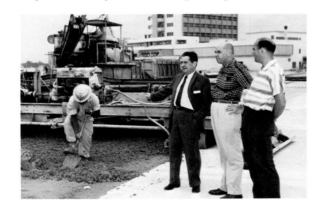

(right) Because of HNTB's revenue bond experience, the Dade County Port Authority selected HNTB as general consultant to oversee a $21 million bond issue for airfield improvements and a new terminal at Miami International Airport in 1954, four years before the first scheduled jet passenger flight from the airport.

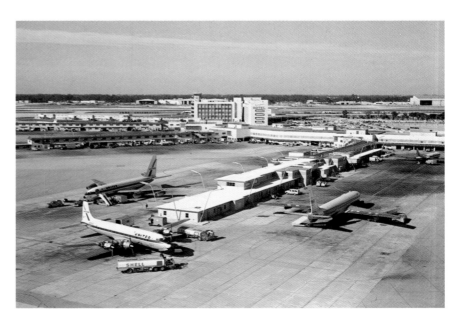

(facing page) HNTB continues to serve Miami International Airport as general consultant, providing comprehensive design services for both landside and airside areas of the facility.

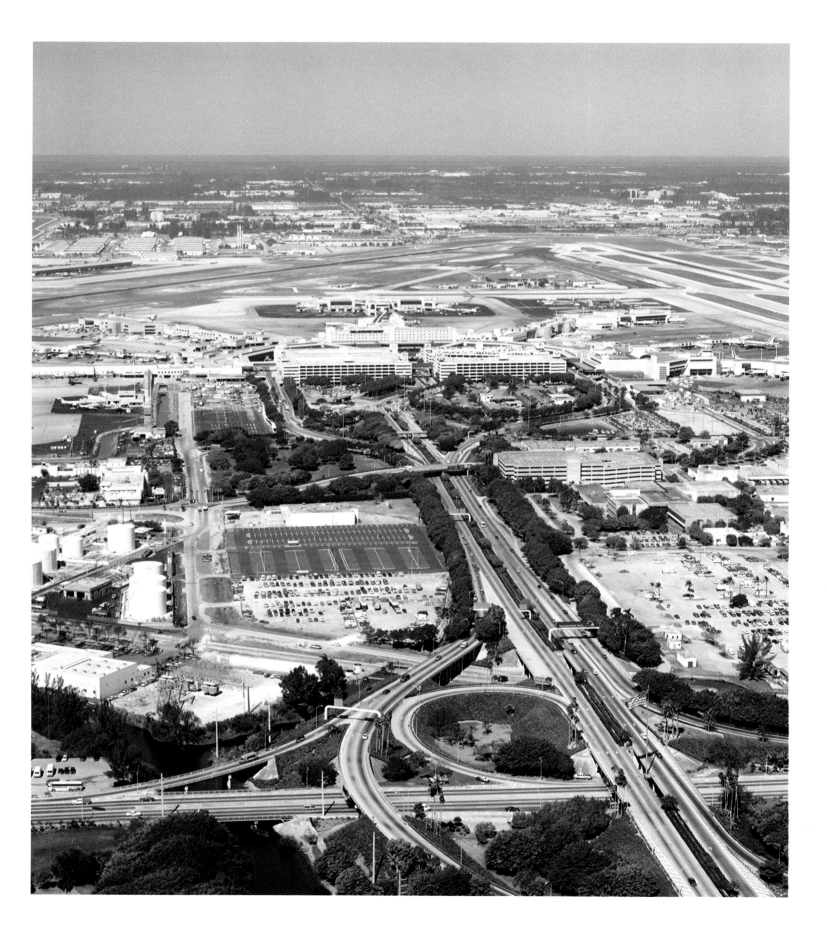

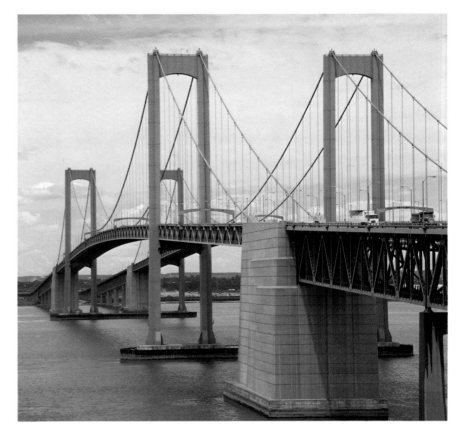

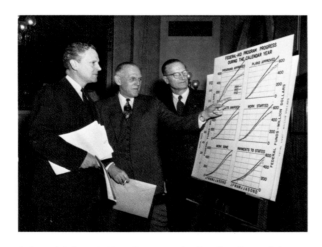

63

(above) The 1950s also saw the beginning of the boom in interstate highways. A national network of roads had been called for almost annually since 1916. Two world wars and the Great Depression had delayed most progress until funding and materials were plentiful. Francis duPont (left), a friend and neighbor of Enoch Needles since the latter's pioneering days in the East in the 1920s, was a prominent leader after World War II in the development of the federal highway program.

city's stadium. Looper had been with HNTB's Kansas City office only two years when R.N. Bergendoff offered him the Milwaukee assignment:

> *"Bergie called me into his office in the late fall of 1955. He said, 'How would you like to go to Milwaukee?' I hardly knew where Milwaukee was. I came up in February to find an apartment and locate an office. We moved in March. First thing was to find an office, buy furniture. I was only 30. So it was a lot of fun. As Bergie gave me more rope and more leeway, I began to do more things. We added a part-time draftsman. Began to do some of the studies up here instead of in Kansas City and one thing led to another."*

The prospect of having "more rope and more leeway" to "do more things" appealed to Looper and many of the men who pioneered in HNTB's branch offices in the 1950s and 1960s. Some, like Looper, were natural organizers who thrived on the challenge of creating a full-fledged local design office from scratch. Others, like now-retired HNTB partner Browning Crow, simply enjoyed the chance to work in a smaller office that offered "more opportunity, less competition" than the larger Kansas City and New York City offices.

Soon, an additional reason for young HNTB engineers to look forward to life in one of the firm's fledgling branch offices developed: election to partnership. Some of the men who had been sent out to open branch offices in the late 1950s and early 1960s were being named partners after a few years out in the field. At first, the connection between an assignment to open a new office and the path to partnership was not particularly clear —

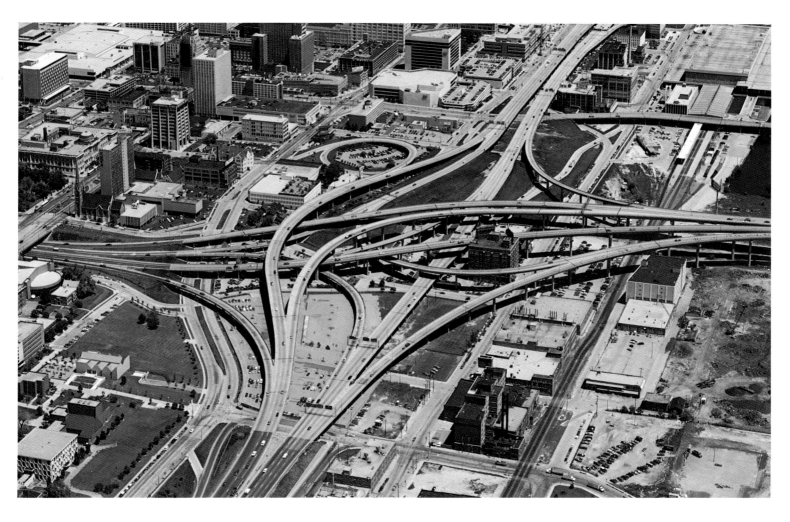

possibly not even to the partners who were giving out the marching orders. In the eyes of many HNTB employees, a branch office "tour of duty" was simply a detour from a successful career in Kansas City or New York City. Eventually, however, an interesting pattern emerged in the election of new partners. People began to take notice. Joe Looper, who became a partner in 1965, nine years after opening the Milwaukee office, explains:

> "It wasn't until later years that the whole business of being out and running a branch office assumed a quite different image in the eyes of all the key people in the home offices. They suddenly saw that [the firm was] putting these young guys out there, and, because they were very visible and the results of their work very easy to measure and identify, they were the ones rising to the top of the heap and being elected partners."

There was another important reason for electing men from the firm's branch offices to the partnership. Clients often preferred to deal with principals who could give authoritative answers to questions and requests about their projects. With an HNTB partner just across town or down the street, clients wouldn't have to wait for strangers in far-off Kansas City or New York City to give them what they needed.

Carl Erb had been at the helm of the Cleveland office for three years when his election to the partnership was announced. He was

(top) Not surprisingly, HNTB's experience in both bridges and roadway design naturally blended on such projects as the complex Marquette Interchange in Milwaukee, Wisconsin. Sixty-five bridge units and a variety of structures ranging from one-lane ramps to four-lane main-line roadways were required. The interchange, completed in 1969, is the critical link between the east-west and north-south freeways on I-94 and I-794.

64

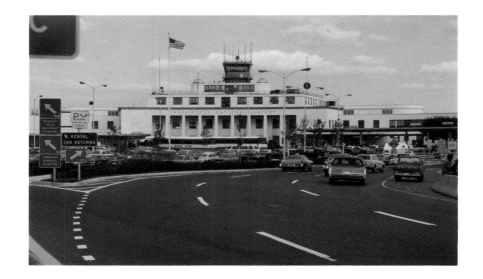

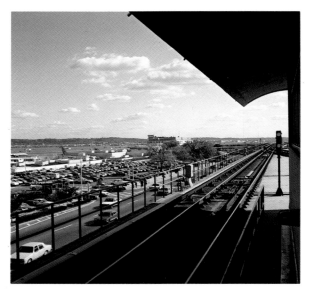

(top and above) By the mid-1960's HNTB had established a solid reputation in airport planning and design. In 1964, the firm was selected to design runway rehabilitation at National Airport in Washington, D.C. The metropolitan area's airport authority became one of HNTB's many long-term clients, putting the firm's complete planning services to use over the years.

65

the first new partner since 1950, when Howard, Needles, and Bergendoff had offered shares in the partnership to Cambern, Exum, Paul, Sorkin, and Timby. Erb was generally viewed as so talented and well-respected that his election to HNTB's partnership was perhaps inevitable, but the successful Cleveland office highlighted his leadership abilities.

Opening a branch office for the firm was not an easy assignment for anyone. Now-retired HNTB partner Edgar Johnson helped to get the firm's Seattle, Washington, office off the ground in the early 1960s. Like their counterparts in other cities, Johnson and now-deceased HNTB partner Frank Bleistein had a "tough row to hoe" in the Northwest:

> *"When we came out here nobody knew HNTB, nobody knew who we were. I always said that the partners back in the established offices didn't understand the difficulties of trying to get work where nobody knew you."*

The same comment might have been made by Enoch Needles in 1922 when he hung up his hat in the "little room with an entryway" at 55 Liberty Street in New York City. The opening of a new office for the firm was a personal and professional challenge to the man who had been given the assignment to make it work. The road to success was rarely an easy one. Local circumstances dictated the ground rules. The Seattle operation faced vigorous, vocal and organized opposition from local engineering firms who weren't anxious to share their market with an "outsider." In order to turn local conditions in Wisconsin to its advantage, the Milwaukee office under Joe Looper found that it needed to diversify its operations and develop expertise in engineering projects other than bridges and roads. Other offices faced other problems unique to their locales.

HNTB's campaign to open branch offices in the mid-1950s served at least two important purposes. Each new office gave the firm a toehold in a city or state; with perseverance, the right leadership, and a favorable economic scenario, an office could really "dig in" and become a part of the community. Once the office was established, it could offer its prospective clients the best of a small, local operation, backed by the long experience record of a national firm.

In addition, branch offices gave bright, ambitious employees

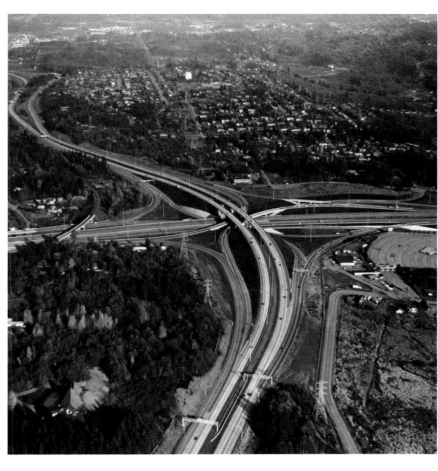

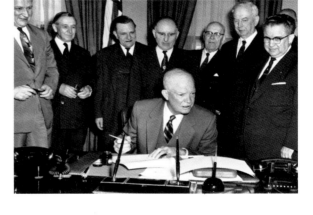

(left) After helping to redesign portions of Seattle's Hood Canal floating bridge in the early 1960s, HNTB landed an assignment on I-90 for the State of Washington. A permanent branch office in Seattle was soon established.

(below) President Dwight D. Eisenhower signed legislation creating the interstate highway system in 1956. This legislation catalyzed nearly 30 years of highway construction activity.

more opportunities to move up the career ladder into positions of responsibility. Kansas City and New York City could tap only a limited number of employees for leadership spots. But every branch office boasted its own cadre of section heads and project managers. Even if an assignment in a branch office didn't lead to partnership, it certainly offered plenty of chances to demonstrate executive talent.

Those two reasons alone — local competitive edge and career mobility for talented employees — might have been enough to persuade HNTB to open small offices in a handful of key market areas in the 1950s and 1960s. But another, compelling reason sealed the decision to plant HNTB "seeds" in dozens of locations across the nation: the Interstate Highway Act of 1956.

The Interstate System

The first Federal Road Aid Act was signed by President Woodrow Wilson in 1916. The Act called for "an integrated, nationwide system of interstate highways." Part of the impetus behind the Federal Road Aid Act was much the same reason that President Harry Truman gave 30 years later for the Delaware Memorial Bridge: the nation's defense. The country needed good roads to transport people and weapons in case the nation was ever attacked by foreign military forces. The 1916 Act, and the many editions of it which followed during the next 40 years, was also promoted by such civilian groups as the American Road Builders Association (formerly the American Road Makers, now the

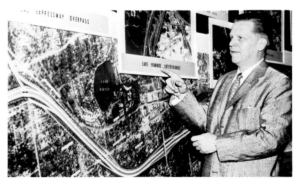

(above) R.N. Bergendoff was especially instrumental in developing HNTB's expertise in highway planning during the 1960s. As urban expressways and the interstate system began to appear across the landscape, Bergendoff stressed the value and importance of a comprehensive approach to design.

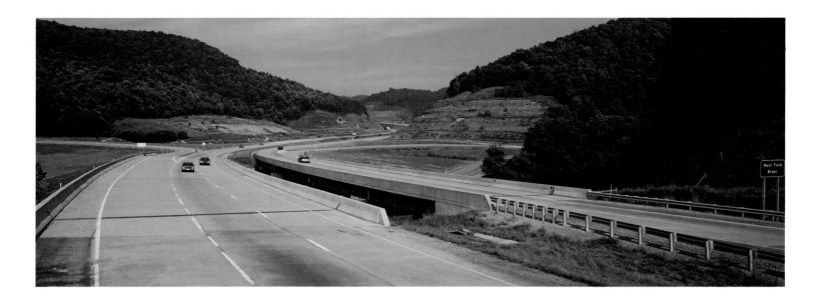

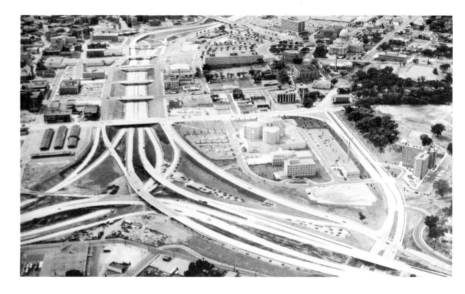

(top) The West Virginia Department of Highways selected HNTB to design 7.3 miles of I-79 in Lewis County, near Weston, West Virginia. Completed in 1973, this rural interstate project cuts through some of the most rugged terrain in the East. The firm also worked on sections of I-77 and I-64 in West Virginia.

67

(right) Completed in 1968, the graceful lines of this three-level directional interchange were designed to complement the State Capitol Complex in St. Paul, Minnesota.

American Road and Transportation Builders Association) and the American Automobile Association. Demographics in the late 1910s and 1920s underscored the need for a good national system of roads for domestic use: the country's population was booming and more and more Americans were reaching into their pockets to buy one of Mr. Ford's very affordable Model T's.

Not much happened with the 1916 Act — or with most of the nearly annual calls for an interstate highway system that followed. The reasons for delay were understandable. The Great Depression and two world wars diverted attention, money, and material away from any sustained roadbuilding program. In 1956, however, during Enoch Needles' tenure as president of the American Society of Civil Engineers, President Dwight D. Eisenhower signed legislation to fund a national system of interstate and defense highways. The 1956 legislation finally gave real muscle to a federal assistance program aimed at helping the states build a 42,500 mile network of freeways designed to connect every city in the country with a population above 50,000. This time Congress appropriated

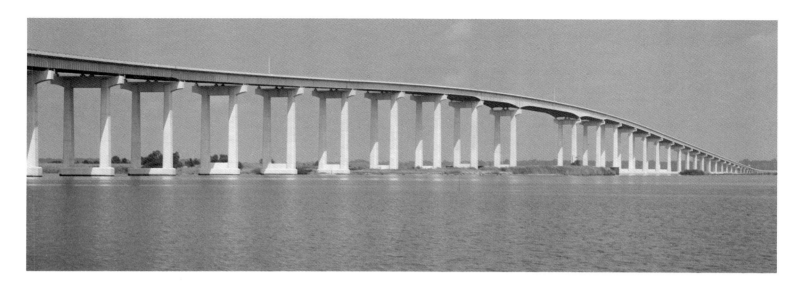

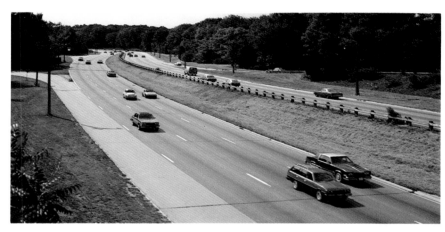

68

the level of funding necessary to get the program rolling.

With eight years of experience in the financing and design of a dozen turnpikes all over the country, HNTB was in an ideal position to offer its services on the new interstates. Not every state was looking for help. Several states built up their own highway departments to a size which did not require using outside consultants on their sections of the interstate system. But many states were delighted to contract with specialists to handle the complicated tasks of road location and design. There was one important condition to be met, however, before an assignment as a consultant on an interstate could be secured. "The Bureau of Public Roads," says now-retired HNTB partner Elmer Timby, "suddenly made the states use engineers which did not require out-of-state travel by government engineers supervising designs." If HNTB wanted its share of the interstate "pie," it would have to play by the program's rules. Branch offices were the answer.

The interstate program got off to a slow start, but HNTB soon was busy: assignments included locating and estimating costs for more than 1,000 miles of the interstate system in two states as well as designing nearly 1,500 miles of the new system — significant mileage for a single consultant to contribute to the program. More than a dozen HNTB branch offices popped up across the country in the late 1950s and early 1960s, with one or two offices opening almost every year. In many cases a state's interstate work was the initial reason for choosing a particular location for an office, but many branch offices soon found that their future depended upon securing other kinds of projects as well. Most took in stride the challenge of finding new work. In the course of just a few years, what had begun as a wary experiment in Cleveland in the early 1950s had become an accepted — indeed, expected — way of HNTB life.

Aviation

HNTB was in a position to try new things in the 1950s. Riding high on its success in the turnpike field, the firm had proven to itself that it could take on the challenge of mastering an entirely different engineering field — and do quite nicely. The opening of

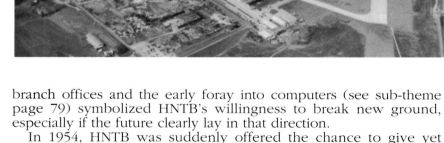

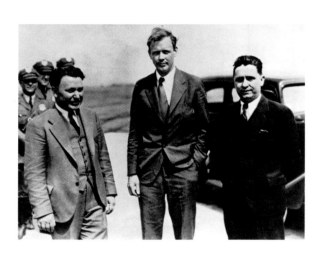

(above) HNTB's success in adding roadway design to its portfolio prompted the firm to expand into other fields. Encouraged by its success on the original Miami International Airport assignment in 1954, HNTB looked for more airport work. In 1958, Colonel Bennett H. Griffin (right) became a special aviation consultant to HNTB. Griffin was a pioneer of the aviation industry and almost as well-known in his day as Charles Lindbergh (center) and Wiley Post (left).

(above right) Lunken Field, Cincinnati, Ohio.

branch offices and the early foray into computers (see sub-theme page 79) symbolized HNTB's willingness to break new ground, especially if the future clearly lay in that direction.

In 1954, HNTB was suddenly offered the chance to give yet another new idea a try: civilian airport planning and design.

Miami International Airport in Miami, Florida, had decided to expand its facilities. The expansion included a new terminal. In 1954, just as the project's bond sale was about to go forward, a problem developed with the local engineering firm that was handling the assignment. Dade County Port Authority, into whose jurisdiction the airport fell, needed to replace the engineering firm quickly, or risk jeopardizing the bond sale and the entire expansion project. HNTB's long experience in project financing fit the bill. The firm was asked to come in for an interview. Elmer Timby, who promptly hurried to Florida with some of his staff from the West Virginia Turnpike, remembers:

"They'd gone quite a ways with this engineer preparing a feasibility report to support the bond issue. They needed a new director and new engineers. They

69

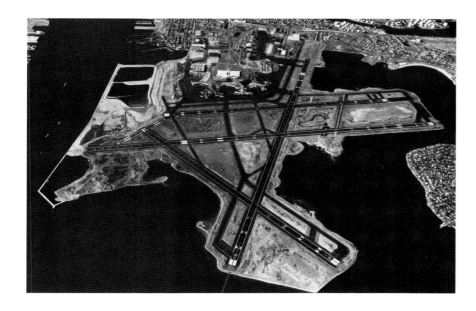

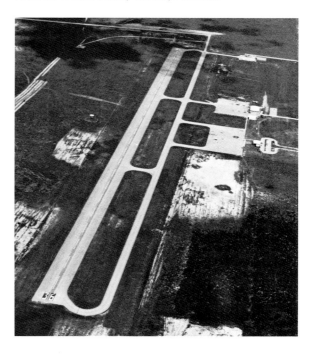

had no staff of their own — no engineering staff — so we took over one of the temporary buildings there as our office, and our first work was to check over and get out this feasibility report and then to provide services as their staff on a cost-plus basis."

With HNTB's help, the bond sale for the airport was a success. Not everyone was thrilled with HNTB's pinch-hit role in the project. Several Florida engineering firms were not happy that out-of-state engineers had been hired by the Port Authority to handle such an important local assignment. HNTB soon found that if it wanted to stay on the Miami International Airport job, the firm would have to prove its mettle. Now-retired HNTB partner Chris Lamberton remembers:

"On one point we were very vulnerable. We had no civilian airport experience. The fact was that none of the other local firms had any either, but that would have been irrelevant. Our response was to bring in someone who was experienced. There was no one in the firm who could qualify, so someone from outside the firm was brought in — Benny Griffin, by Elmer Timby. Benny was a well-known and liked old barnstorming aviator who had flown the Atlantic post-Lindbergh. Franklin Roosevelt had appointed him Director of Washington National Airport, where he remained until the Republicans appointed someone else. Practically everyone in aviation anywhere was Benny's friend."

Griffin saved the day. With his help, HNTB was able to offer the Dade County Port Authority the advice and experience it needed to complete its expansion project. Thirty-five years later, the firm's Miami office is still deeply involved in assignments for the Miami International Airport, now under the aegis of the Dade County Department of Aviation.

The Miami International Airport project in 1954 could have faded into the background as a one-of-a-kind experience for HNTB. But Chris Lamberton, who helped to review the feasibility report for the airport's bond sale, had been inspired by the idea that HNTB could get into airport planning and design. A pilot himself, Lamberton collected and read everything he "could get his

70

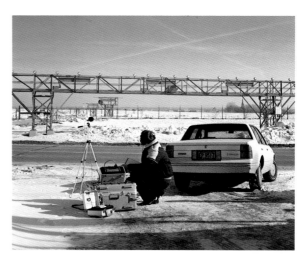

(above) Noise testing was just one of the many highly specialized aspects of airport design that HNTB had to master to become competitive in the post-World War II domestic airport boom.

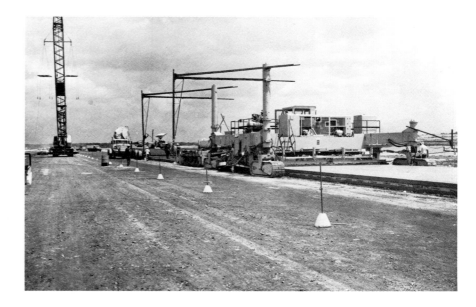

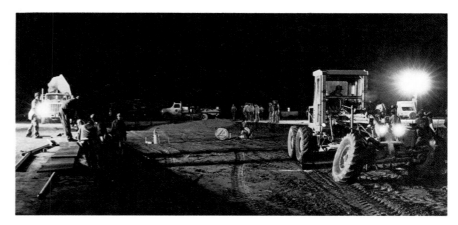

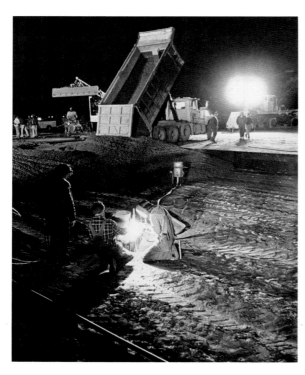

(this page) HNTB was part of a unique effort in 1969 to replace 10,000 feet of runway and parallel taxiway at Atlanta Airport in only 40 days — ordinarily a 10-month job. Working around the clock, 500 workers and $9 million worth of equipment removed the deteriorating 12-inch runway and replaced it.

(facing page) One of the busiest air transportation hubs in the world, Hartsfield-Atlanta has been served by HNTB through a joint venture since 1968.

hands on concerning airports" with the thought that the New York City office could take the lead in developing aviation business for the firm. With the help of Benny Griffin, Lamberton pursued assignments. Small airport projects popped up in Minnesota, Ohio, Wisconsin, and elsewhere. These early airport projects were learning experiences for the firm; HNTB lost money on a number of them, absorbing the cost as the price of establishing its credentials in the aviation field.

Those small assignments — successful, if not profitable — soon turned into a major commitment by HNTB to offer full-fledged airport services. In 1964, HNTB developed its first airport marketing brochure. Five years later, at Chris Lamberton's suggestion, the firm consolidated its aviation staff into one office in Alexandria, Virginia. Coincidentally, the HNTB Atlanta project office for Atlanta Airport helped to pull off a minor engineering miracle that same year: the fastest runway paving job in peacetime history. In exactly 40 days and 40 nights — without interruption of air traffic — around-the-clock construction crews laid the equivalent of 45 miles of two-lane highway to replace one of the airport's main runways. By the end of the 1960s, HNTB had worked on nearly 300 aviation assignments, with many more to come in the future.

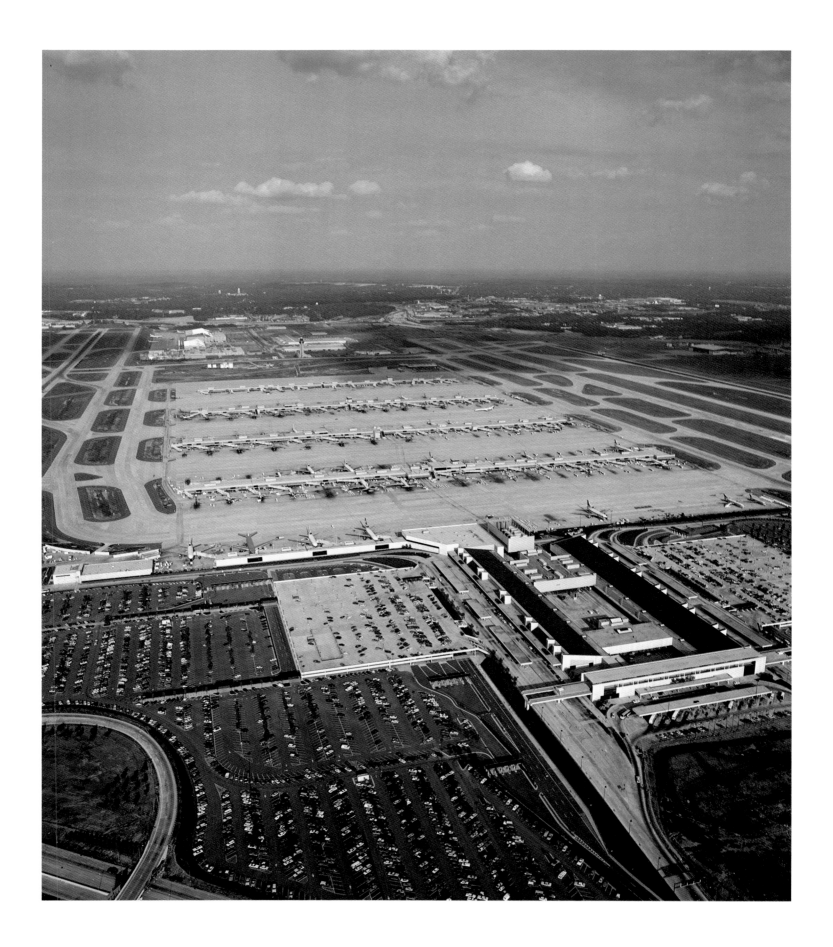

The Environmental Movement

In the 1960s, HNTB's plate was full. New bridges, the interstate system, urban expressways, airports, as well as continuing work on many of the turnpikes which the firm had designed 10 years earlier kept the firm's large, far-flung staff busy. From two design offices in 1953, the firm spread to 19 by 1970. A staff of about 700 in 1958 nearly doubled to 1,300 one decade later. A dozen partners were constantly on the road or the telephone, talking to clients, overseeing projects, and trying to keep track of the firm's whirlwind growth. A half century after the founding of Harrington, Howard & Ash in 1914, HNTB was no longer a small Kansas City firm specializing in railroad and highway bridges, but a national leader in roadway design and a new force in the aviation field.

Like other old, established civil engineering firms, HNTB was proud of its contributions to the country's transportation system. The firm had changed with new developments, offering services to fit the times. When the country's general prosperity in the years after World War II gave the green light to long-delayed public works, HNTB was delighted to be among those busily designing bridges, roads and airports to meet the demand. In 1968, HNTB headed *Engineering News-Record's* annual list of leading U.S. engineering firms; the firm was on top of the world.

Not everyone thought that the boom in new bridges, roads and airports in the 1950s and 1960s was for the best. A small, but vocal, movement had taken root across the country to combat what it felt was a cavalier disregard by developers for the natural environment. There was some truth to their assertions that new projects were often planned without taking into consideration the long-term or broad environmental impact on the surrounding area. Sometimes the damage *was* the result of a cavalier attitude on the part of an irresponsible designer. But more often the lack of attention to the environmental dimension of a project was an innocent lack of knowledge; government agencies and the engineers they hired had never before been asked or expected to do more than to get whatever was needed built. Taxpayers after the war had wanted progress in a hurry: faster routes to work and play, fewer traffic

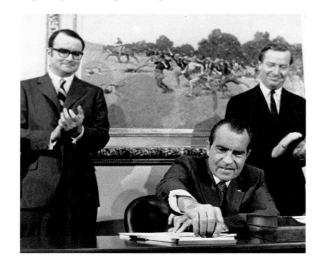

(below) In 1969, President Richard Nixon signed the National Environmental Protection Act, formalizing the federal government's response to the burgeoning environmental movement. Firms like HNTB suddenly found themselves caught up in heated public debates over the impact of proposed bridges and highways on neighboring areas.

73

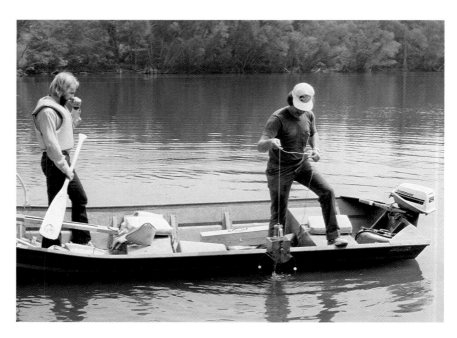

(right) In response to public concerns, HNTB added environmental specialists to its staff who could assist project engineers in avoiding or mitigating environmental damage.

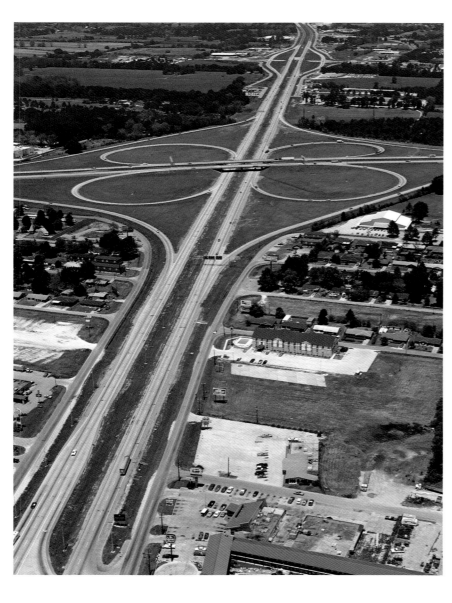

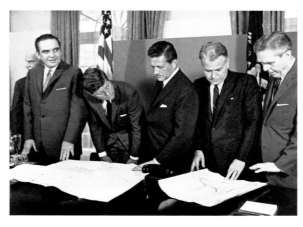

74

jams, and better roads. "For about fifteen years," says now-retired HNTB partner Joe Looper, "the big question was how fast can you get these freeways designed and built?"

Suddenly, engineers who believed that they were helping to improve the quality of life for taxpayers were being accused of despoiling the landscape and destroying neighborhoods. Much worse, concern for the environment quickly became a cover for other, less altruistic motives to stop or hinder a project. Engineers could find themselves cast in the role of villain in a public fight that had very little to do with environmental issues and everything to do with local politics. With the passage of the National Environmental Protection Act in 1969, HNTB engineers frequently occupied the hot seat in mandatory public hearings across the country, trying to read between the political lines and figure out how to balance everyone's needs. The engineers soon discovered that the noisy, emotional hearings at the local high school were a far cry from the calm order of the drafting room.

In January 1967, Rex Whitton, former head of the Federal Highway Administration, joined HNTB. While at the FHWA,

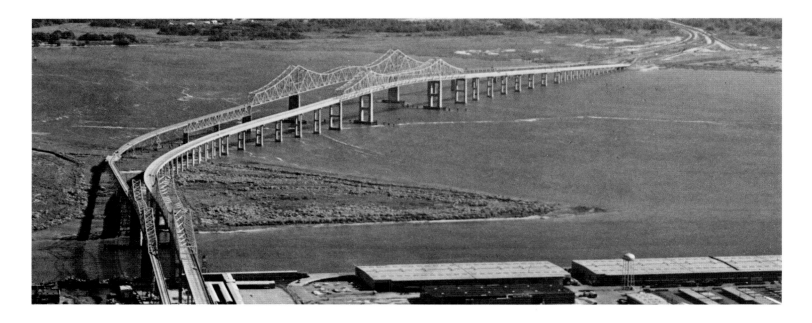

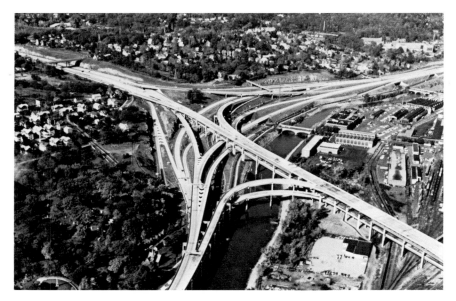

(top) The Silas N. Pearman Bridge (right in photo) was the second long span bridge over the Cooper River at Charleston, South Carolina. The bridge stretches for nearly two miles and was opened to traffic in 1966. Twenty years later, HNTB would design yet another bridge over the Cooper River.

(right) The need for additional highways in urbanized areas made design more and more complex. An example of the challenge was the I-84/Route 8 interchange in Waterbury, Connecticut. The interchange, with eight miles of controlled-access expressway, includes 6,700 feet of double-deck spans over the Naugatuck River and the tracks of a railroad classification yard.

Whitton had promoted a team approach to expressway planning. He brought his philosophy to HNTB. By the spring of 1967, the firm's new Urban & Regional Planning Department had completed its first "comprehensive metropolitan plan" for Shreveport, Louisiana. At about the same time the firm finished its first highway beautification study. To top it off, in November 1967 Elmer Timby and Rex Whitton both testified in front of the public works committee of the U.S. Senate on the merits of a multidisciplinary approach to urban highways. By the time the National Environmental Protection Act was passed by Congress two years later, HNTB had already forged a role for itself in the new environmental movement.

Although the activities of the national environmental movement sometimes seemed to bring more that was negative than positive to the process of meeting public needs in the 1960s and early 1970s, HNTB didn't hide its head in the sand. Like the firm's early

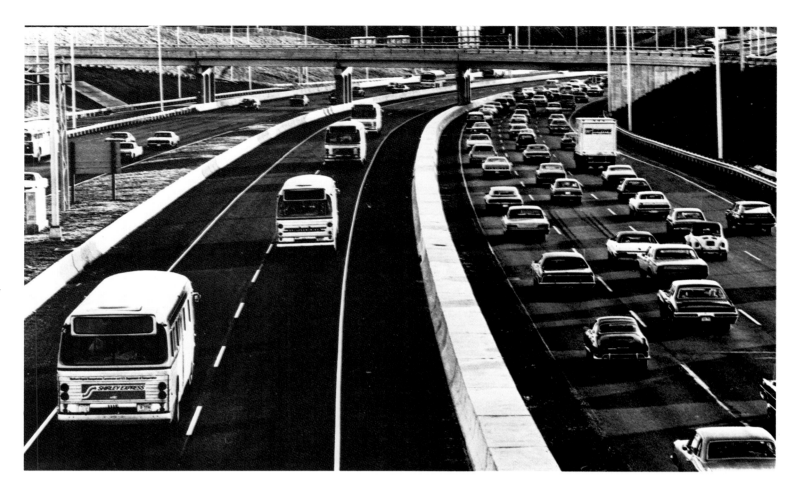

experiments in branch offices and computers, HNTB intended to meet the future on its own terms — and succeed.

Changing of the Guard

On December 30, 1969, HNTB partner Josef Sorkin retired. Sorkin had been a member of the firm for more than 30 years and had spent the last 19 of those as a partner. At the time of his retirement he was the firm's senior partner and the last of the "class of 1950" to step down. His farewell marked the end of an era of leadership which had shepherded the firm through the Depression and two wars into the prosperity of the 1950s and 1960s. The old generation of partners had passed the baton to the new.

The transition between old and new leadership had taken place throughout the 1960s. The four men whose surnames graced the firm's name had all retired or died by the time of Sorkin's retirement. Howard had died in 1953. Henry Tammen, already retired in 1950, died on July 6, 1961, aged 76, while playing golf near his home in Short Hills, New Jersey. Enoch Needles retired in 1962, slowed down by heart ailments. He died ten years later on January 5, 1972, aged 83. R. N. Bergendoff was the last of the four to step down. He retired in 1968, dying eight years later at age 77 on November 14, 1976.

Sorkin's fellow partners had begun to retire in 1965. The retirements of the five men who had become partners in 1950 came quickly, each a year apart. Younger men were immediately elected to pick up the reins of leadership. In 1962, the year of

(top) The early 1960s also brought HNTB one of its earliest mass transit-related assignments: the conversion of four-lane interstate, Shirley Highway, outside of Washington, D.C., to an eight-lane route with bus and car-pool-only lanes. The 3-2-3 system with reversible center roadway runs 17.5 miles and is one of the most heavily traveled segments of the I-95 corridor on the East Coast.

76

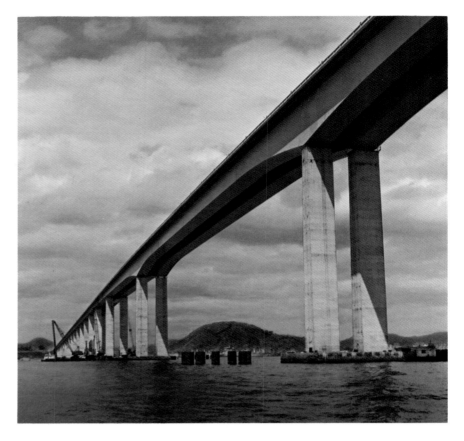

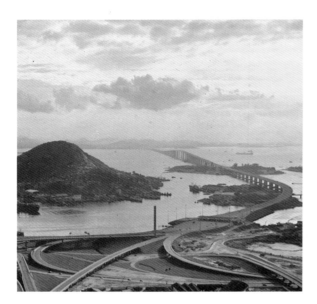

(top, above and facing page) International work beckoned in the mid-1960s. In 1968, HNTB began work on the Rio-Niteroi Bridge across Guanabara Bay between the cities of Rio de Janeiro and Niteroi, Brazil. The eight-mile long structure includes a world record steel box girder span of 984 feet. The bridge garnered the ACEC Grand Conceptor Award in 1975.

Enoch Needles' retirement, Carl Peterson was elected to the partnership, the first new partner since Carl Erb's elevation in 1957. Chris Lamberton and Frank Bleistein followed in 1964. When Jim Exum retired at the end of that year, Jim Finn, Paul Heineman and Joe Looper joined the partnership ranks. The next year, Ellis Paul retired and Bob Drange, Don Harper and Bernie Rottinghaus were elected. Ted Cambern, as well as Carl Peterson, retired in 1966, bringing Gerry Fox and Bill Wachter into the fold. Elmer Timby retired in 1968 along with R. N. Bergendoff. Chuck Hennigan and Browning Crow shortly joined the firm's inner circle. When Josef Sorkin stepped down at the close of 1969, Dan Watkins and Ed Johnson were welcomed into the partnership ranks. With the exceptions of Carl Peterson and Carl Erb, who had joined the firm in 1939 and 1941, respectively, HNTB was now entirely in the hands of a group of men who had arrived on the firm's doorstep only after the close of World War II.

The transition between the old and new generation of partners was complete, but not entirely smooth. In 1969 and 1971, two of the more senior partners of the younger generation died unexpectedly. Frank Bleistein, a partner since 1964, passed away on April 20, 1969, at the age of 54. Carl Erb, whose election in 1957 marked the first selection of a new branch office head to the partnership, died on December 5, 1971. The two deaths, combined with Carl Peterson's early retirement in 1967, took from the partnership some of its most experienced leaders. "You suddenly had men in their early 40s responsible for one of the largest engineering firms in the country," remembers now-retired HNTB partner Paul Heineman. In spite of — or because of — their relative youth, this small circle of men took up the challenge and transformed HNTB into the firm it is today. ■

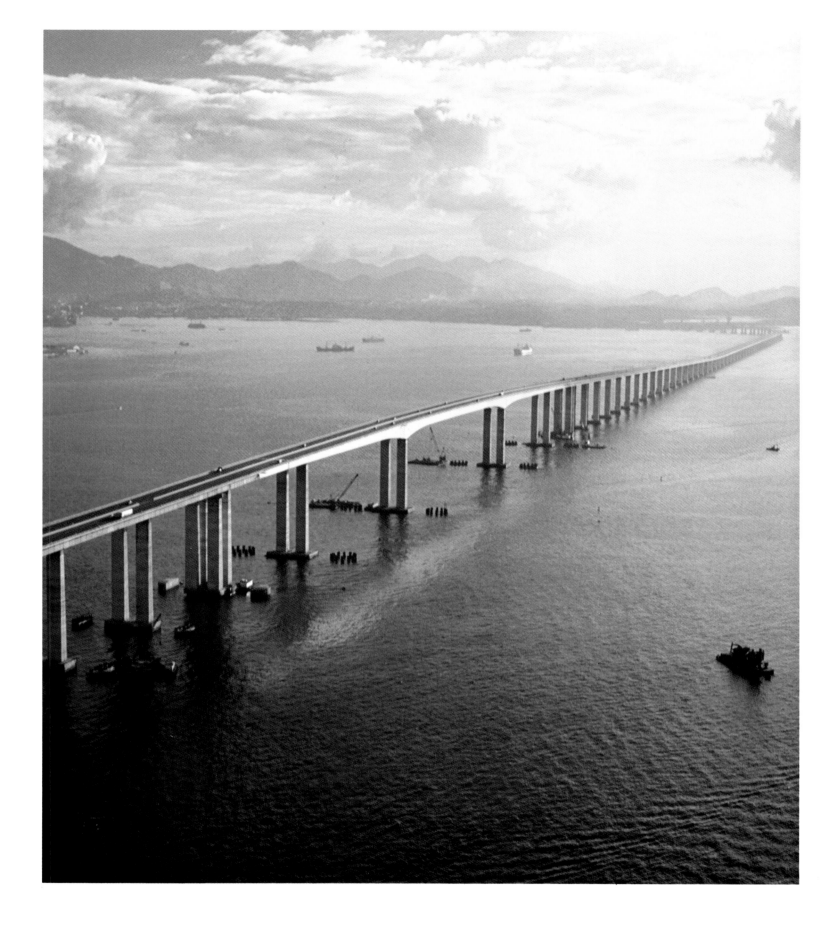

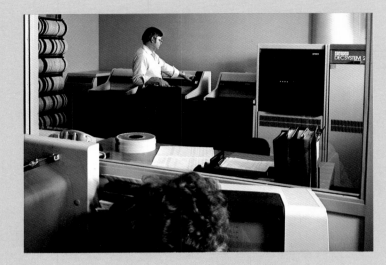

The Computer Revolution at HNTB

"I remember spending most of one whole summer just doing the calculations ... for a bridge in Shreveport, Louisiana. It was awful ... I didn't think too much about it at the time. I didn't know any better ... [We had] this huge old thing that we used to have to set and push buttons and crank it to get the answers and after that was all done, someone had to check it, so it just took forever to get anything done."

Gil Cole, Kansas City Central Services

Computers at HNTB have come a long way since the mid-1950s when the firm pioneered in applications of the new "electronic brain" to common engineering problems. The days of meticulously punched cards and waits of a week or more for calculations to be returned by mail from the mainframes in Kansas City or New York City are no more. Today, every HNTB office can communicate instantly through the firm's central computer network. CADD stations abound.

HNTB's earliest forays into computers were encouraged by former Princeton University professor and now-retired HNTB partner Elmer Timby. The firm's New York City office took the lead, first leasing time on equipment off-site, then leasing and finally purchasing a machine for use in HNTB's office on Church Street. "Access to the Computer Room," says now-retired HNTB Associate Robert W. Richards, "was controlled much like the gold vaults at Fort Knox ... not even the partners had keys!"

While the New York City office began to play with program development on its IBM equipment, the Kansas City office tried its hand with a General Electric. At first, the two offices kept their computer operations independent of one another. But it soon became apparent that there were long-term advantages to joint program development. The Kansas City office's General Electric 225 included software which allowed the machine to simulate an IBM 650. Kansas City reprogrammed the IBM 650 geometry programs of the New York City office in Fortran for use on the GE, leading to the beginnings of the firm's unique in-house H.I.S. (HNTB Integrated System) problem-solving software.

In 1967, the New York City office purchased an IBM 360. "It was like going from the Dark Ages to the Nuclear Age," says

engineer Victor Ho Sang. The second computer actually caused some problems. If the 360 and 650 were run at the same time, the 650 would sometimes "knock out" the newer computer. The office began to phase out the 650 and convert old programs to the more powerful 360. While programs were being changed and tested, the 360 was used for payroll and accounting as part of a firmwide effort to computerize financial operations. Within two years, the Kansas City office upgraded its punch-card GE 225 to a magnetic tape GE 415. At the same time, the New York City office donated its computer to Columbia University and switched to less-expensive remote processing through the McDonnell Douglas McAuto library in St. Louis. After a decade of using McAuto's services, HNTB decided to get back into in-house computer systems, purchasing its first VAX 11/780 in 1979. The next year a DEC System 20 was purchased and earmarked for the firm's centralized financial operations in the Kansas City office. It marked the first time that an HNTB computer was dedicated specifically to business applications. Early efforts in the 1960s to use the firm's computers for financial housekeeping had been difficult on the "crude" GE 225. "We had limited hardware and software," says Gil Cole. "Most everything we had we had to develop ourselves and it wasn't too fancy. However, we were able to write paychecks and do the rudimentary things that were essential." The firm's sophisticated financial operations are now fully computerized.

Today, all of HNTB's offices are connected by an integrated Digital computer network, as well as by FAX. The instant communications system allows design work to be shifted easily from office to office. The firm owns 17 VAX machines, located in various branch offices across the country. HNTB has also made a major investment in CADD (Computer Aided Drafting and Design), beginning in 1983 with the purchase of two workstations. Today, 68 CADD workstations are distributed among the firm's offices. Now, in a matter of a few minutes or a few hours, engineers can test hundreds of alternatives that would once have taken months or years to investigate. "I'm sure the guys who are using CADD stations now would just throw up their arms if they were to see the way we used to do plan preparation," says Cole. "Many of the things that they're designing now we probably wouldn't even have been able to build just a few years ago because of the sheer effort to design them — even if we'd known how to do it."

PART FOUR

Managing Change

"As HNTB offices began to appear across the national landscape in the late 1950s and early 1960s in response to the interstate program and local competition, the day-to-day business of running a far-flung operation became more complicated."

CHAPTER SEVEN
Diversity by Design (1970-1989)

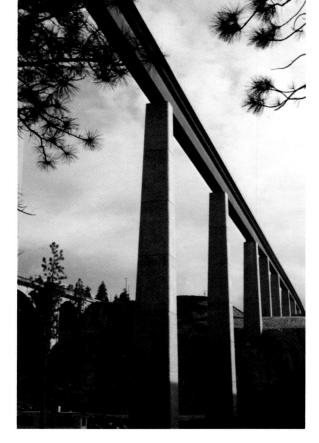

(above) Although the 1970s brought many changes to the firm's organization and practice, ties with tradition remained strong. HNTB's long history of railroad bridge design found fresh expression in the sleek and modern lines of such bridges as the Latah Creek Bridge, Spokane, Washington. Completed in 1973, the 3,730-foot single track bridge was designed for Burlington Northern Railroad.

(right) HNTB's decision to diversify its practice on a large scale in the 1970s was made easier by the example set more than a decade earlier of the firm's successful entry into the civilian airport design field. By the 1970s, the firm had developed a solid reputation in the aviation arena. The Tulsa Airport Authority of Tulsa, Oklahoma is just one of many airport clients for which HNTB has provided extensive planning and design services.

The retirement of "old guard" partners and the premature deaths of two others left the 13 young partners of HNTB facing the 1970s in charge of a firm with more than a thousand employees in two dozen offices. Only four of the men had more than five years' experience as partners — Lamberton, Finn, Looper and Heineman. Most of the others had been partners for only two or three years. Despite relatively limited partnership experience, the 13 men were far from ill-equipped for the job ahead. The young partners from Kansas City and New York City had "grown up" at the elbows of the older partners. Their counterparts from the branch offices were the pioneers who had set up the firm's new offices. Every partner had been with the firm for more than two decades.

The partners were not alone in facing the future. The retired partners were members of an advisory board to which the new partners could turn for guidance. Also, a large staff stood by to back them up. Dozens of the firm's engineers and support personnel had been on HNTB's payroll for as long or longer than the partners. They were astute, experienced, wise. They could be counted on to shoulder the day-to-day burden of getting the firm's work done.

Competitive Bidding

One of the biggest challenges faced by the new partnership in the 1970s was one shared by the entire civil engineering profession: competitive bidding. For the first two decades following World War II, private engineers had been granted a fairly free hand by many government agencies. Officials were anxious to catch up on the massive backlog of public roads and other infrastructure needs which had built up over the course of two world wars and the Great Depression. HNTB, like other firms that

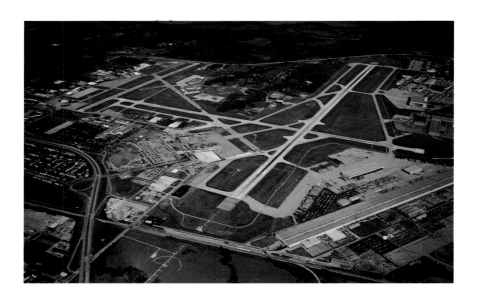

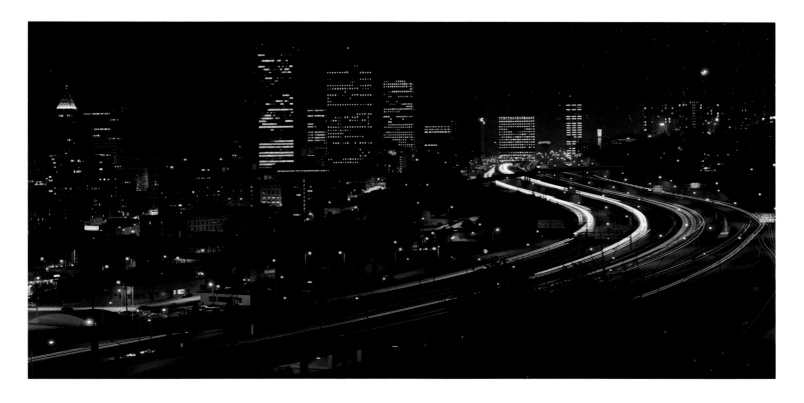

had survived hard times, was grateful for the burst of activity.

By the mid-1960s, the pendulum of public sentiment had begun to swing the other way. Not only was the environmental movement going full tilt, but governmental agencies were under mounting pressure to account for every public penny spent. The engineering profession, too, had changed since World War II. The proliferation of small, aggressive engineering firms after the war had stepped up competition among consultants. The newer firms often favored a bidding system which might favor them over the established firms claiming higher overheads.

Older firms viewed the proceedings with alarm. In their eyes, the high standards held by the engineering profession were at stake. Firms with limited track records would be tempted — understandably — to bid low in order to secure an assignment. Whether or not they would actually be able to handle the job was an entirely separate question. The bidding system also went against the older firms' professional self-image and, to their minds, against economic sense. Most had sealed more than one professional deal over the years with little more than an honor-bound handshake. Mountains of paperwork produced by teams of lawyers seemed likely only to make the whole process of getting the job done more expensive for everyone in the long run. Ernest Howard had deplored the earliest signs of the trend toward bidding when he wrote to Enoch Needles in the summer of 1953:

> *"... it is a great disappointment when we have been thinking that our profession was making some progress as a profession to have us put against our will in the position of being considered on a price basis ..."*

Just a few weeks earlier Howard had learned that at least one state had instituted bidding as part of its selection process:

> *"... Our first reaction is to condemn them as using improper methods and completely ignoring proper ethics*

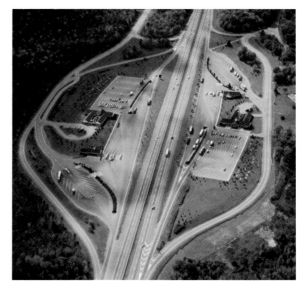

(above) Assignments such as the original Maine Turnpike project in the late 1940s often launched long-term client relationships that have lasted three decades or more. During the recession of the late 1960s and early 1970s, these valued relationships reinforced HNTB's commitment to survive and thrive in hard times.

(top) Although the 1950s and 1960s saw the beginning of HNTB's diversification into other areas, bridge and roadway design remained the cornerstone of the firm's business. The complex I-5 freeway near Seattle, Washington, is typical of HNTB's work for its traditional client base.

82

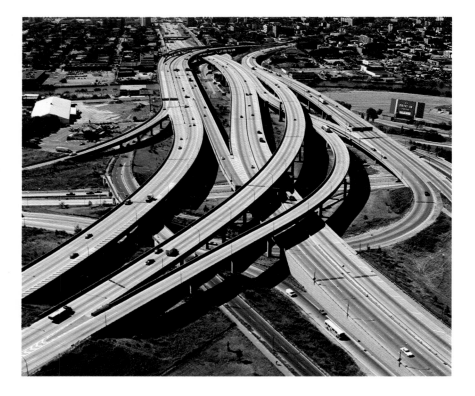

(right) The art of complex interchange design continued to be refined in the early 1970s in such projects as the Bruckner Expressway Interchange, an intricate three-level structure connecting no fewer than five major traffic arteries in the Bronx, New York. Completed in 1973, the $68 million multi-level interchange was the largest construction contract ever awarded by the New York State Department of Transportation.

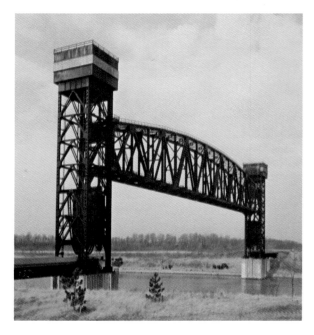

83

(above) The innovative vertical lift bridge which had given the firm its start at the turn of the century was still a part of HNTB's repertoire in 1965 when this span over the C&D Canal at Kirkland, Delaware, was built. Designed for the Corps of Engineers to carry the Pennsylvania Railroad, the 548-foot lift span is the world's second longest of its type.

in the selection of an engineer .... Certainly there is no satisfaction in being engaged wholly as a result of bidding."

The government agencies were not entirely to blame for the tenor of the times. After all, they had to be accountable to taxpayers who did not always understand that engineering firms needed to generate a profit like any other business. The engineering firms themselves sometimes didn't help their own cause. Two years before Howard's lamentations over bidding, Enoch Needles wrote to R.N. Bergendoff to complain of an unattractive tendency among some firms to advertise. A zealous salesman from a New York newspaper had approached Needles in an effort to persuade him of the merits of placing an advertisement to congratulate a client on the opening of a bridge. Needles was not charmed:

"Aside from the business angles, I took the position that such an advertisement was in poor taste ... I also pointed out that we did not consider it appropriate for a lawyer to advertise in the daily press, congratulating his client on having won a damage suit, nor did we consider it appropriate for a doctor to use paid space in the daily press for the purpose of congratulating his patient upon a successful operation."

The unhappiness of Howard and Needles over bidding and advertising was completely in character with their professional upbringing. Both men had devoted themselves to the enhancement of civil engineering as a profession. To watch considerations of the bottom line replace respect for qualifications and proven experience was disheartening to both men. Times were changing, however. Ernest Howard, Enoch Needles, and their partners could not turn back the clock. By the 1970s firms that wanted public work didn't have much choice except to throw their hats into the

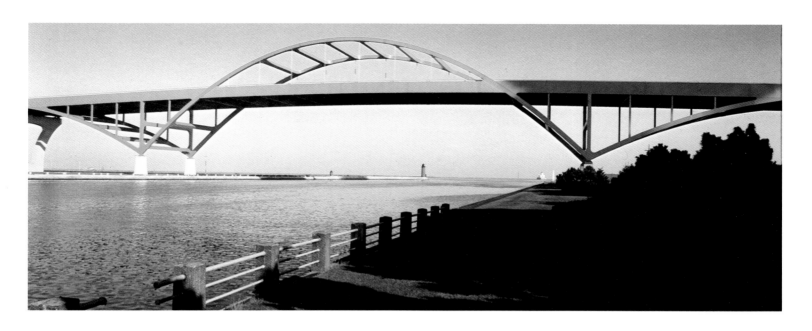

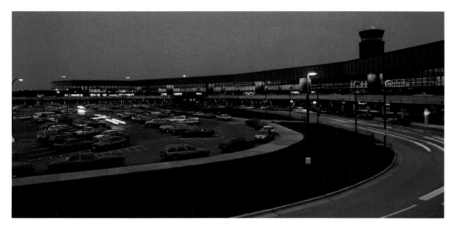

84

ring and hope that they would manage to come out in the black at the end of the job. For those engineers who prided themselves on high technical standards the new rules of the game were especially frustrating. That frustration eventually would lead many firms, including HNTB, to look to the private sector for new work.

Looking Within: Growth and Change

While HNTB and its sister firms learned to compete on new terms and explore new markets outside the public agencies, homefires needed tending. Management systems at HNTB had barely kept up with the fast-paced growth of the firm between the late 1950s and the late 1960s.

In terms of coping with its own burgeoning ranks, the partnership itself was in good shape. A formal partnership agreement which evolved in the late 1950s had put to rest the major source of tension and conflict that might have been a stumbling block to the firm's expansion. The document had been amended to include mechanisms to handle most potential individual conflicts within the partnership. For the peace of mind it offered the partners, the agreement had no equal. But it also had

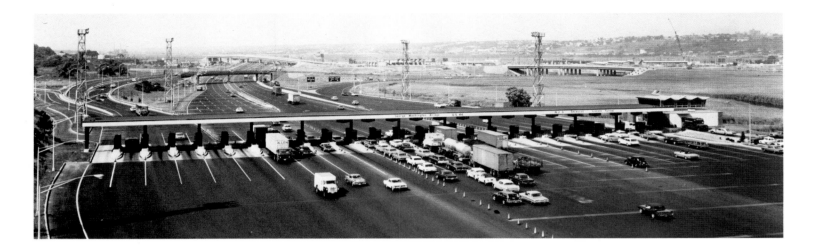

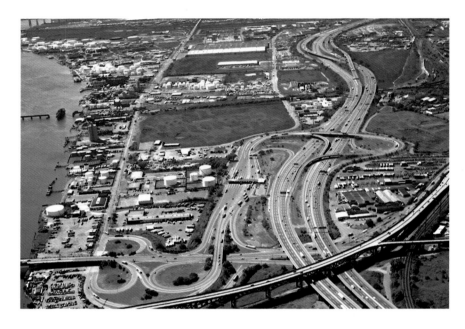

(top and right) The New Jersey Turnpike has remained one of HNTB's longest-running assignments over the years. The firm has been general consultant to the Turnpike Authority since 1948, advising the NJTA on operation, maintenance and expansion of this heavily-traveled corridor. Most visible of HNTB's roles has been the coordination of an ongoing program to widen portions of the tollroad from six to 12 lanes.

its limits. The agreement applied only to problems and procedures of the partnership, not to the daily routine of running the firm.

Professionally trained as engineers and not as managers, the partners had usually been content through the years to deal with internal personnel and financial management issues on an ad hoc basis. When a problem involving policy or procedure came up, it was dealt with and disposed of. Ernest Howard might pick up the telephone to chat with Enoch Needles before making a major decision. Josef Sorkin might consult with Ted Cambern by memo. As long as there were few partners and few offices, the approach worked quite well.

As HNTB offices began to appear across the national landscape in the late 1950s and early 1960s in response to the interstate program and local competition, the day-to-day business of running a far-flung operation became more complicated. By the late 1960s it was clear that some administrative changes were in order. Retirements of the "class of 1950" partners were imminent. Pressure was building from new partners in branch offices for more autonomy in their work for local clients and work without constant

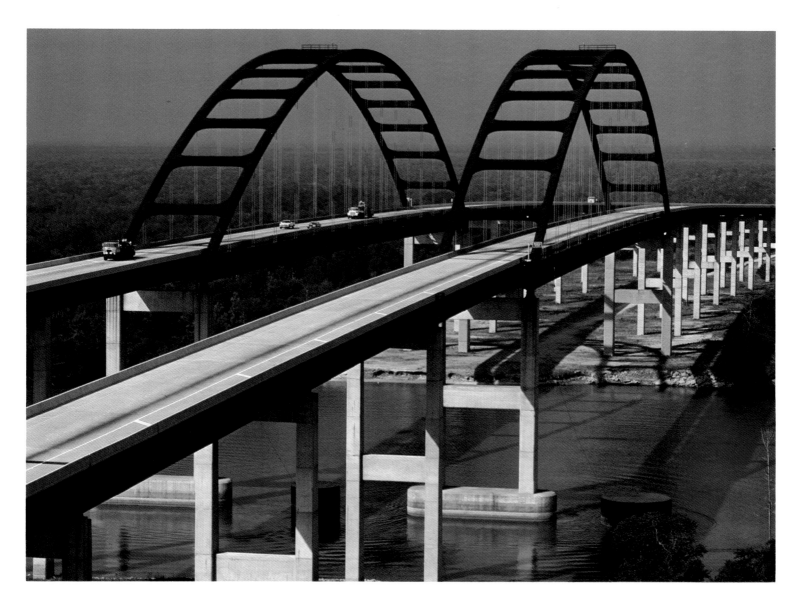

oversight from "headquarters." The complexity of the firm's finances threatened to overwhelm the organization's simple accounting systems. And the customary East-West division of the firm's offices had become not only irrelevant but frustrating.

The first order of business was to update the firm's financial systems. The son of a banker, Ted Cambern had long looked forward to the day when HNTB would put in place mechanisms that could grow as the firm grew. The centralization of accounting in Kansas City was the first step in the process. In 1967, a few months after Cambern's retirement, HNTB Associate Ken Lincoln implemented a computerized system to simplify the task of standardizing financial reports coming in from the firm's outlying offices. That change set the ball rolling. On the heels of computerization came the establishment of the eastern controller's office in Fairfield, New Jersey, in 1968. Soon the entire controller's operation was moved to Kansas City. Payroll for the whole firm was handled there, too, beginning in 1969. In 1971, Central Services was established in the Kansas City office, shortly taking under its umbrella the firm's personnel, financial, and information

(above) The twin tied-arches of the I-65 bridges near Mobile, Alabama carry interstate traffic over more than six miles of streams and swamps. The bridge was completed in 1979.

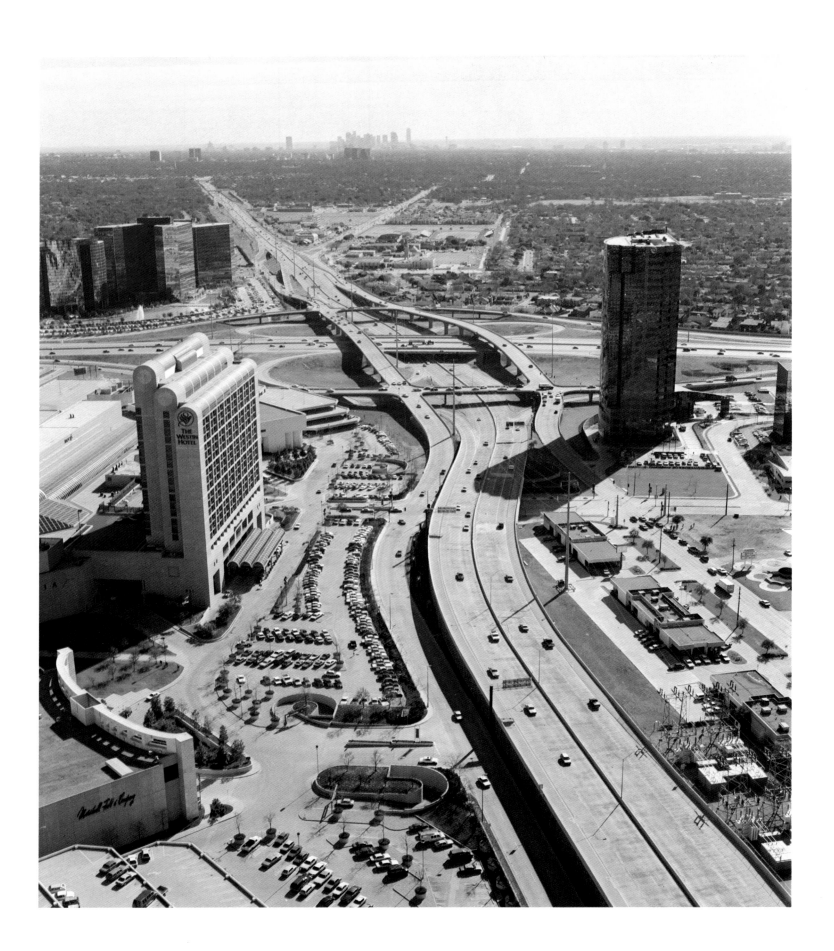

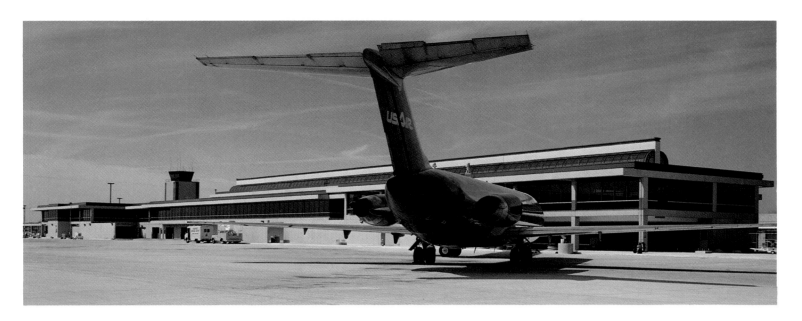

service functions. In short order, HNTB's administrative functions were pulled together into a single entity.

The centralization of administrative chores was more than a mere convenience or a matter of the bottom line. It served an important psychological purpose for HNTB. With a host of basic policies and procedures now applicable to all HNTB offices regardless of location, the individual offices operated more as a unified firm.

More importantly, centralization helped HNTB to get a grip on its own growth. Throughout the late 1950s and early 1960s the firm had experienced the potent *de-centralizing* impact of branch office openings. The new offices were a welcome addition to HNTB, but they also brought with them new organizational tensions. For the first time there were employees on the HNTB payroll for whom Kansas City and New York City were simply names on a map. Most of these new employees had never met, much less worked with, Ernest Howard or Henry Tammen or Enoch Needles or R.N. Bergendoff: the four names were simply that — names. Without ties to bind all of the offices, old and new, together, decentralization might eventually have destroyed any sense of common identity or common mission. Centralization of key administrative processes kept the balance tipped in favor of unity.

Change in the Ranks

Putting most of HNTB's assorted administrative systems under one roof wasn't the only answer to coping with the firm's growth. The time had come to think about formalizing another layer of management. In September 1970, the position of associate was introduced. The new rank was vested with less power than partnership, but with more than the post of engineer-in-charge or section head.

The decision to formalize the associate level was a big change in HNTB's traditions. Not surprisingly, agreement to the change was reached only after much soul-searching within the partnership. Not everyone was happy with the idea. Those who argued against it felt certain that valued employees who were not appointed to the associate level would leave. A few did so. But advocates of the idea argued that the size of the firm required a new level of

88

(top) HNTB's aviation capabilities had evolved into comprehensive services including master planning, site selection, design, special studies and terminal and facility planning, as was done for Evansville Dress Regional Airport, Evansville, Indiana.

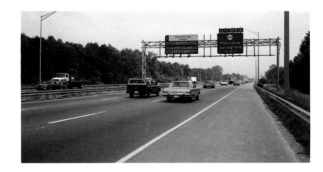

(above) Through the design of traffic management systems, or TMS, HNTB has continued its tradition of helping clients to evaluate and handle their traffic problems. The high-tech I-395/I-66 TMS in the western and southern suburbs of Washington, D.C., includes use of surveillance by closed-circuit television and incident detection via electronically-monitored loop detectors spaced at one-half mile intervals along roadways.

(facing page) The Dallas North Tollway is an example of the multi-disciplinary approach to urban design which HNTB refined in the late 1960s and early 1970s. Engineers, architects, planners, landscape architects, among others, joined forces to integrate a badly-needed trafficway into one of the city's most developed areas. HNTB has provided consulting services on the tollway for more than two decades.

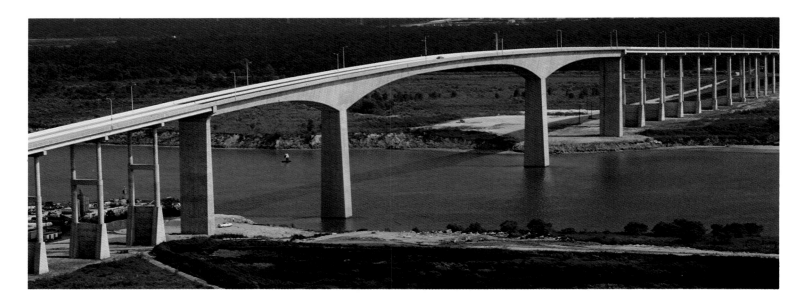

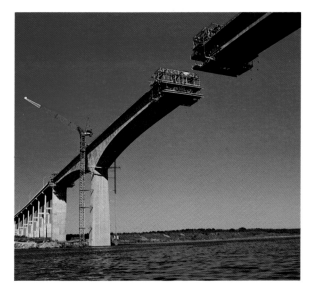

(top and above) The Jesse H. Jones Memorial Bridge over the Houston Ship Channel contains the longest pre-stressed segmental concrete box girder main span in the Americas (750 feet). Completed in 1982, the bridge carries Beltway 8 traffic on four lanes for 4.2 miles across this important navigation route.

management control just below partner rank. The reason was simple, if difficult to accept. As much as the partners might pride themselves on maintaining a "hands-on" involvement in projects under their direction, not even the most energetic partner could be all things to all people all of the time. It was simply a fact of life in any large organization. Furthermore, it was becoming more difficult to identify and prepare future partners to make the leap from the boards to the "boardroom." An informal mentoring system to produce partners had always existed, but associateship provided a formal proving ground for potential leaders. The associate level would also offer recognition to key technical or managerial staff who were not in line for partnership, but whose contributions to the firm were unique.

Proponents of the concept won. Dan Spigai and Dan Appel were immediately named as the first HNTB associates. Others followed quickly. Since 1971, the first year associates were appointed, most new HNTB partners have passed through the associate level on their way to partnership.

The Recession of the 1970s

HNTB's focus in the late 1960s on the firm's internal management could not have been better-timed. By the early 1970s the interstate highway program had begun to wind down and American engineering had entered a recession: the firm's future depended upon its ability to weather the downturn.

HNTB faced some difficult choices. Should the firm down-size while waiting out the recession? The firm had already dropped from a high of 1,300 in 1968 to just more than 1,000 employees in 1973, mostly by attrition. Further cuts wouldn't be so easy. Less-profitable offices would have to be closed and staff laid off. The partners could remember a similar economic slump in the mid-1950s between the turnpike era and the beginning of the interstates. The previous generation of partners — perhaps prompted by their own Depression era experiences — had bent over backwards during those tough days to avoid having to let someone go.

Another option was to get into other fields that were not affected by the recession. By diversifying the firm's practice

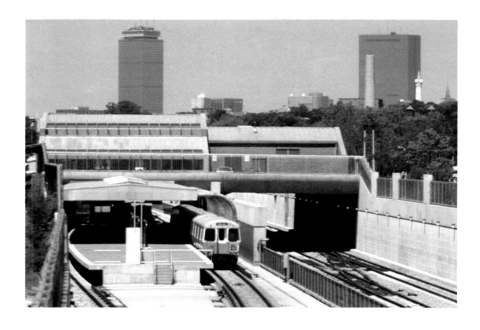

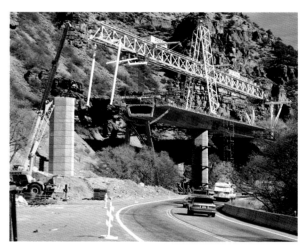

beyond bridges, roads and airports, HNTB might be able to hedge its bets against the natural vicissitudes of public works funding cycles. With the mounting frustrations and costs of competitive bidding for public work, the firm might do well to shift some of its energies to private sector projects. The idea of diversification seemed sound enough, but it also meant taking a few risks. It would require a collective commitment on the part of the partners.

Tightening the Reins

The strategy ultimately adopted by HNTB to cope with the recession of the 1970s was a pragmatic blend of retrenchment and diversification. First, the partnership agreed to take a harder look at the bottom line. The financial management controls which had been put in place beginning in 1967 had given the partners their first real tools to analyze and keep tabs on the firm's development. Numbers could be compared. Progress could be measured. This new ability carried with it a few unsettling revelations. Some offices were not living up to expected potential and a few partners were not focusing enough attention on developments in their assigned backyards. In better times, those problems were not too serious. But in bad times, they could not be taken lightly. Something had to be done.

Action by the partners came quickly, but not easily. Some tough decisions were made, including the imposition of a few management controls on the partnership's own members. Such self-imposed controls were foreign to a group of men who placed great stock in their independence. The autonomy granted to an individual partner to conduct business in his own bailiwick with a free hand is the most cherished element of HNTB's partnership. To surrender any of that independence was not an easy decision to make.

The prosperity of the firm, however, outweighed individual considerations. A number of critical changes were agreed to. A few voluntary retirements, the establishment of a small executive committee of partners to handle a range of management matters, and the creation of the post of Administrative Contact Partner were high on the list.

Learning at the Master's Knee: Passing Down HNTB's Values

"It may cost you money occasionally to hold fast to your ethics, but you cannot be honest in engineering and dishonest in business at the same time. The keystone of the engineering profession is integrity. We older men have a deep and great pride in our profession which we are anxious to pass on to you. We do not want to preach to you. We want to help you, to ask you to love your work as we have learned to love ours."

Enoch Needles, 1937

As HNTB has grown and diversified over the years, the question of how to pass down the firm's values to the next generation of employees has been answered in different ways. In the days of a single Kansas City office with a dozen employees, the problem didn't exist. Everyone knew everyone else; partners and employees worked elbow to elbow. New employees put in time as apprentices at the drafting tables, slowly working their way into more complex responsibilities. "The traditions and ethics of the firm were transmitted by example," says now-retired Josef Sorkin, who joined the firm in 1939. "Whenever it was convenient or to the point it was always pointed out ... 'This is the way the firm operates.'" In the 1950s and 1960s, when HNTB opened branch offices and doubled its staff, the task of transmitting the firm's traditions and principles became more difficult. In 1959, Robert W. Richards prefaced the New York City office's inaugural personnel manual with an acknowledgment of changing times:

"Ten years ago, when all personnel were working in close proximity, practically everyone knew everyone else. Personnel policies were flexible and informal, but generally understood. Today, however, as a result of rapid expansion and growth ... the number of employees has increased 300% from approximately 50 to more than 200. Because of the firm's present size, there is a need for statement of employment policies, so that all personnel are properly informed."

Informal mentoring continued in spite of the firm's expansion. HNTB partner Frank Hall vividly recalls an incident during his early days at HNTB with then-partner Ellis Paul. Hall was at work on a design for a new bridge over the Chesapeake and Delaware Canal. By extending the design an additional six feet, the bridge could have set a world's record for its type:

"What's another six feet and we've got the world's longest bridge? I suggested that to Mr. Paul one day and I got such a lecture and dressing down. To even think of doing something like that. Of spending the client's money to bring fame and honor to us professionally. I often look back at that and I think that sort of represents the philosophy of the firm."

HNTB partner Dan Spigai remembers a similar incident of a senior employee setting an example for a junior engineer:

"I had two primary mentors — Chris Lamberton and Jim Finn. I can recall, for instance, in my very early days trying to make an engineering drawing of a particularly complex shape and struggling with it pretty badly .... I found the next day when I came in early to work on it that Chris had gotten out the necessary textbooks and was right at the drafting table doing it."

In the late 1960s, the transfer of partnership experience to the new men elected to the firm's leadership was especially critical. In the space of a few short years, the older partners retired and a young group of men with relatively little experience as partners took over. Now-retired HNTB partner Paul Heineman remembers the process of trying to absorb as much as possible from Bergendoff, Cambern and Sorkin after his own election to the partnership in 1965:

"I had lunch with the three active partners in the Kansas City office .... When you suddenly have their confidence and are part of that intimate circle ... their 40 years' experience as partners was transferred very, very rapidly — not all of it, obviously, but much of it .... I didn't open my mouth, I just had big ears."

Today, as HNTB's employee roster exceeds 2,000, the problem of helping every new employee to feel at home and to understand the firm's traditions and its highly-valued ethics becomes an institutional challenge. "You can't do it verbally, one-on-one anymore," says HNTB partner Harvey Hammond. "There has to be a way to mentor whole groups of people. How do you convey what we are, how do you convey the values of the past, where we are today, and what we're trying to accomplish in the future? How do you pull all that together in a way that's communicated?"

Hammond and his partners have taken on the task of finding ways to accomplish those goals. An innovative series of management training seminars and other group functions are among the methods with which HNTB is experimenting as part of a firmwide quality control program. HNTB partner Gordon Slaney, serving as the quality control contact partner, neatly sums up today's challenge to transfer values, and its implications for the firm's commitment to maintain quality despite the pressures of diversification and expansion:

"As we grow and as we diversify, there needs to be a stronger awareness of the quality control issues .... That means that as we either absorb new folks into the firm, or acquire other firms, we need to recognize that these people may have different perspectives on operations. Part of the whole quality control program is to make sure that everyone has an understanding of what the firm's policies and procedures are. As we grow, we need to make sure that those are being passed on to others through formal training, on-the-job training, through mentors — there's certainly not a right way, there are various ways to do it. We just want to be sure that it is being accomplished one way or another."

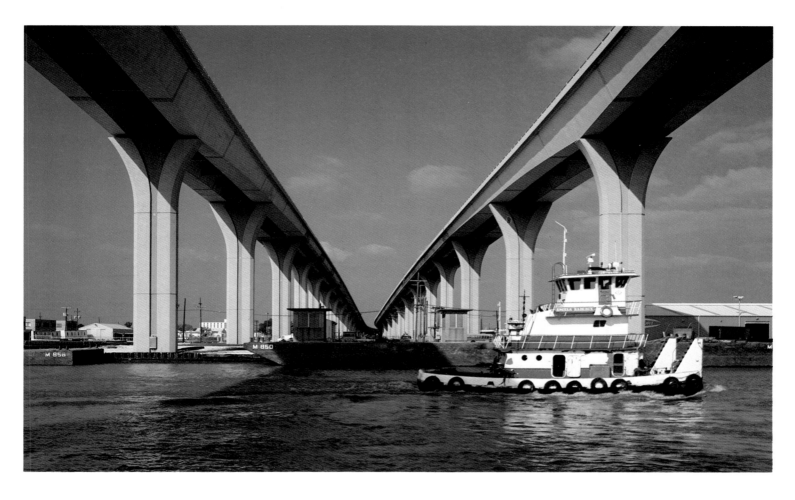

The appointment of an administrative contact partner in 1976 was an especially sensitive, but vital, decision. Someone needed to play the thankless role of fiscal watchdog. Partner Jim Finn, whose penchant for detailed financial analysis became a trademark, was elected by his peers for the post. Finn's influence was keenly felt during his decade as ACP. Joe Looper, whose advocacy of diversification was an equally potent force during this period, credits the now-retired Finn with having had an important impact on HNTB at a time when the firm was grappling with large questions about the future:

> *"I don't know that there's been a domination of a personality, but there's certainly been the impact of a personality on the partnership .... Of the personalities which affected the firm most, probably Jim Finn was the most dynamic partner. Jim's time as ACP was conservative, financially oriented, very strongly questioning of expenditures, whether it's for planning, diversification, or anything else; it certainly had to be justified before he would support it."*

Now-retired HNTB partner Dan Watkins observes that part of Finn's influence rested on his organizational savvy and on the wry recognition that "in a partnership of 15, 18 people ... you'd better damn well lead or get run over."

The ACP wasn't the only new leadership post to develop in response to the firm's growth in the 1970s. In addition to the establishment of the ACP and the powerful Executive Committee,

(top) The positive economic impact of adequate urban highways was the catalyst for the design and construction of the West Bank Expressway in New Orleans, Louisiana. The expressway was the largest state-funded project ever undertaken in the state.

92

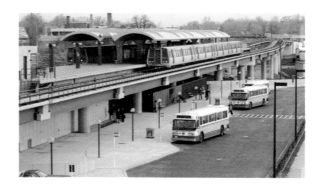

(above) The Rhode Island Avenue Station was the first aerial structure designed and built for the Washington, D.C. Metro rail transit system. The station's elevated center platform is sheltered by thin prestressed concrete shell gull wing canopies. The facility includes parking for 300 cars and a traction power substation.

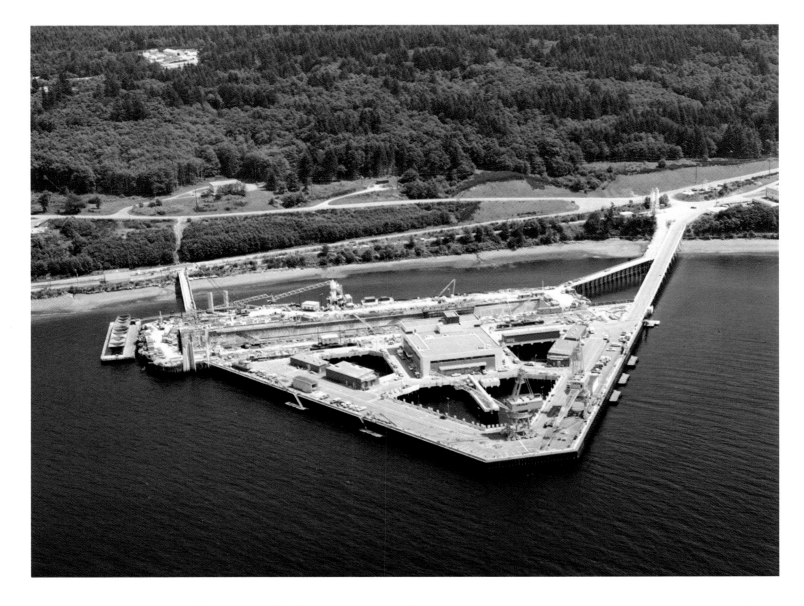

HNTB's involvement with military projects had continued since World War II. The firm provides design to all military services as well as the Corps of Engineers. (above) HNTB, as part of a joint venture, worked for the Naval Facilities Engineering Command in the early 1970s to plan and design the Trident class submarine refit and explosives-handling wharves at Bangor, Washington.

the partnership designated one of its members to be the firm's quality control partner. The QCP's role involved creating and refining internal mechanisms to ensure that HNTB's traditional attention to high technical standards kept pace with the increasing numbers and complexity of the firm's projects. More recently, the QCP's role has extended to the development of in-house management training programs.

Diversification

At the same time that HNTB's partners divided up some of the firm's internal management responsibilities among themselves, they also began to think about how to handle the second prong of their strategy to cope with the recession: diversification. Should HNTB get into new areas? If so, how should it proceed? Should the push be into the private sector, or into other public arenas? Which areas should the firm get into? How much risk was involved?

To help sort out potential avenues for diversification, interested partners split up into small groups to investigate the possibilities.

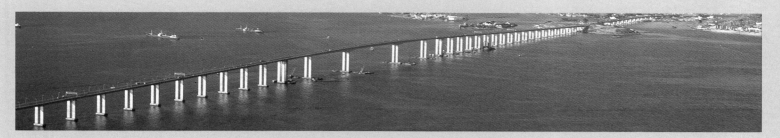

The International Scene

In September 1954, engineer Chris Lamberton wrote to HNTB partner Ellis Paul to let him know about the possibility of some bridge design work in Guatemala. Paul showed Lamberton's letter to Enoch Needles, who replied in the margin: "We are not in shape to take on foreign work for the present."

At the time of Lamberton's note, HNTB's dance card was filled to overflowing. The firm was barely keeping up with the influx of assignments to design new bridges and turnpikes after World War II. Within five years, however, the situation had begun to change. A slight recession had set in as states slowed their turnpike plans in the late 1950s in anticipation of receiving substantial federal assistance for their portions of the new interstate system. While waiting out the lull, HNTB decided to take a look at possibilities for work overseas.

One of the obvious places to start was Canada. HNTB could boast connections going back almost 70 years. Dr. J.A.L. Waddell and Ernest E. Howard both had been native Canadians. The firm had done a lot of work in Canada over the years, including 18 vertical lift bridges over the Welland Canal in the 1920s. In November 1959, HNTB set up a special firm in Woodstock, Ontario, with Canadians Dr. James A. Vance and Robert R. Smith, and the eight American partners of HNTB as principals. Vance, Needles, Bergendoff & Smith did not garner much work for the firm, but it helped to facilitate bureaucratic matters when HNTB needed a local hand in Canada.

The firm's interest in foreign work took a more aggressive turn in 1964 when HNTB International, Inc. was incorporated in New Jersey as a wholly owned subsidiary of the partnership. Ellis Paul was the first president, followed soon by Elmer Timby, and then by Bill Wachter. Slowly, opportunities began to develop. The year after HNTB International's incorporation, the firm formalized an agreement with the government of West Pakistan to perform general highway consulting services. In February 1965, an office was opened in Lahore. Closer to home, Josef Sorkin had been keeping his ear to the ground since 1962 for work in Mexico, Central and South America. His listening paid off in the form of the Rio-Niteroi box girder bridge in Brazil in the late 1960s, a world's record project which garnered the firm its first Grand Conceptor Award from the American Consulting Engineers Council in 1975.

Other assignments soon followed. The Kingdom of Jordan, for example, put HNTB's talents to work as an airport consultant in 1967. The possibility of other Middle East projects prompted the partnership to approve unanimously the opening of a marketing office in Beirut, Lebanon, in 1974. A contract for a major hotel chain resulted. Although political conditions in Lebanon forced HNTB to relocate its office to London, the chain's first hotel in Bahrain was successfully completed with HNTB's assistance. The Middle East also gave HNTB the firm's single largest professional engineering consulting contract of the time when the government in Iran awarded it an assignment for the management and control of a huge toll road project. When finished, the six-lane divided highway would have run 500 kilometers to connect the capital, Tehran, with the Persian Gulf. The overthrow of the Shah's government in 1979 precluded completion of the assignment, but the firm eventually received in 1986 its fee for services rendered.

Meanwhile, on the other side of the world, HNTB garnered a high-profile bridge project from the government of Malaysia. The country wanted to build a huge structure to link the city of Butterworth on the Malaysian mainland with Georgetown on Penang Island. HNTB accepted the assignment and in 1985 had the satisfaction of seeing its design of the longest span in Asia completed and opened for traffic.

Although HNTB enjoyed these and other notable successes overseas, international work presented some difficulties. Bill Wachter, HNTB International's president for 13 years, points out that political situations in Pakistan, Lebanon, and Iran, for example, caused problems in completing assignments successfully. He notes that some in the firm felt that HNTB didn't have the knowledge or grit to compete for significant assignments abroad, especially where business culture sometimes ran counter to the firm's practices.

Faced in the early 1980s with a choice between the pursuit of international work or the complex task of diversification on the home front, HNTB opted to focus solely on domestic work for the time being. That focus is about to change. Among the important issues with which the fourth generation of HNTB partners is wrestling is the firm's future role in the international arena. That there will be a role for HNTB seems guaranteed: the increasingly global dimensions of the markets in which HNTB moves and works will open opportunities that cannot be ignored. How soon and how aggressively HNTB will want to reenter the international scene are questions that thoughtful debate among the partners will answer. One thing is certain. When the firm once again looks actively abroad for new projects, HNTB will bring to its assignments a wealth of experience and a tradition of work overseas that spans the lifetime of the firm.

94

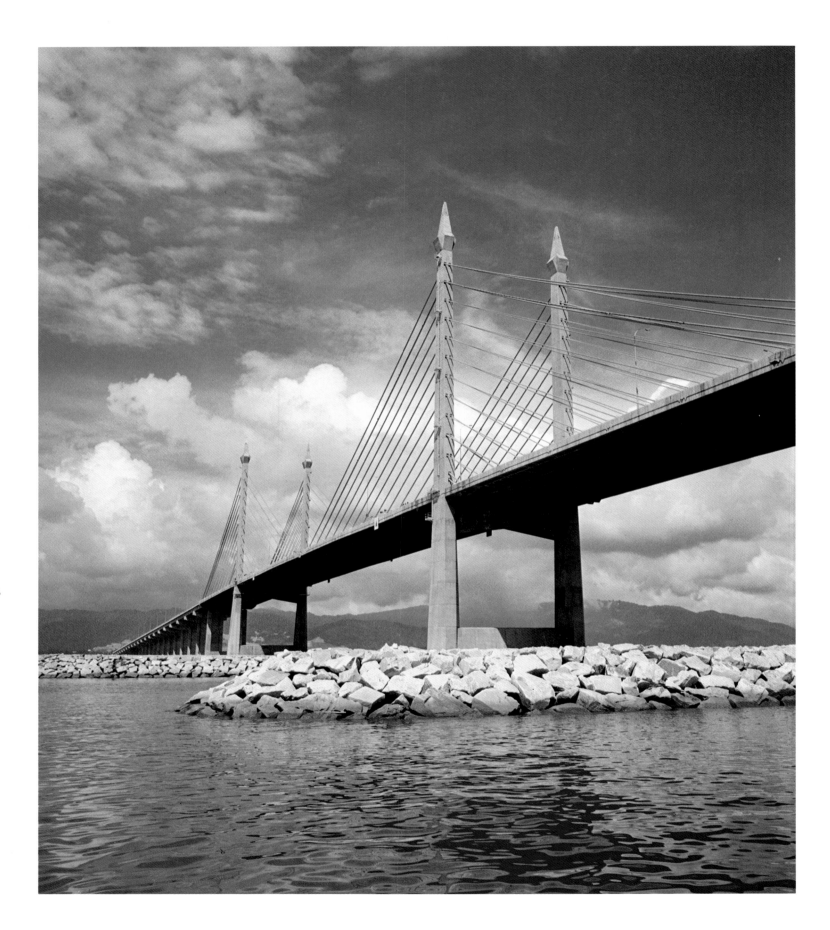

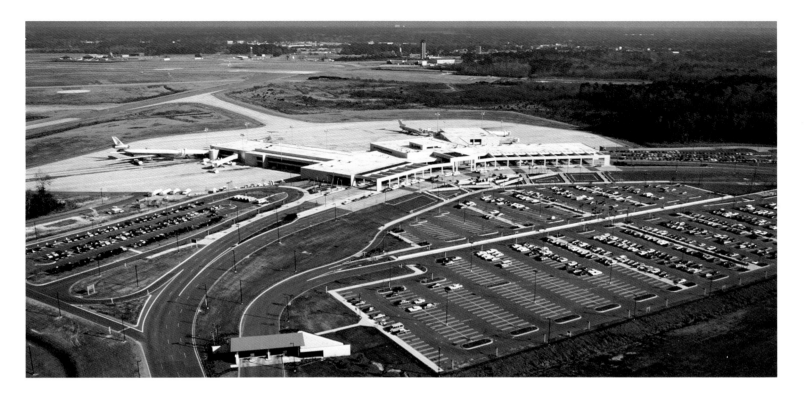

These groups eventually evolved into permanent committees, today called Professional Service Groups, charged with responsibility for overseeing the firm's different service lines. To start, however, the groups were informal in character and relatively limited in scope. Their main task was to identify new fields of potential business and develop strategies to help the firm break into those fields. They also faced the task of convincing skeptical fellow partners of the merits of diversification.

The concept of diversifying the firm's practice was not actually new. In a sense, HNTB had been slowly diversifying since its earliest days. Sometimes the "diversification" was simply one individual's mastery of unfamiliar knowledge. That individual became the firm's resident expert in that area. Ellis Paul's frantic introduction to mechanical engineering on the Welland Canal bridges in the 1920s was an early sink-or-swim leap into an unfamiliar discipline. Over the years, other HNTB engineers had learned new specialties as they arose. Manny Chafets, Frank Bleistein, and Gerry Fox plunged into computer applications with the encouragement of former Princeton professor Elmer Timby in the 1950s. Dan Watkins immersed himself in the intricacies of photogrammetry. At about the same time, Chris Lamberton and, later, Dan Spigai, took up the challenge of learning the aviation field from scratch. Bill Wachter, Orrin Riley, and others wrestled with the special problems of international work.

Diversification was also represented by firmwide shifts in focus over time. The firm's gradual switch from railroad bridges to highway bridges in the 1920s was the first broad change of emphasis. The Maine Turnpike in 1947 dramatically thrust HNTB into the roadway business almost overnight. The urban expressways and interstate system of the 1950s and 1960s were important variations on that new theme. Aviation further diversified the firm's focus beginning in the early 1950s. New branch offices such as Milwaukee under Joe Looper and Boston under Henry

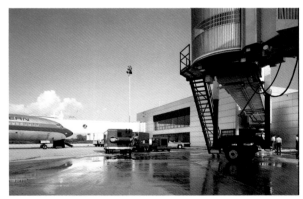

(top and above) In 1979 South Carolina's Charleston County Aviation Authority selected HNTB to assume overall responsibility for a new $48 million terminal complex at Charleston International Airport. The airport is one of the few joint-use facilities in the U.S., housing the 437th Wing of the Military Airlift Command of the U.S. Air Force and serving as a major commercial air hub.

(facing page) One of HNTB's most exciting overseas projects, the 8.4 mile long Penang Bridge in Malaysia includes a 738-foot cable-stayed, concrete segmental main span carrying six lanes of traffic. The national landmark structure boasts towers in the shape of minarets — a motif of Malay royalty — and serves as a vital link between the mainland and Penang Island, home of Georgetown, the country's second largest city.

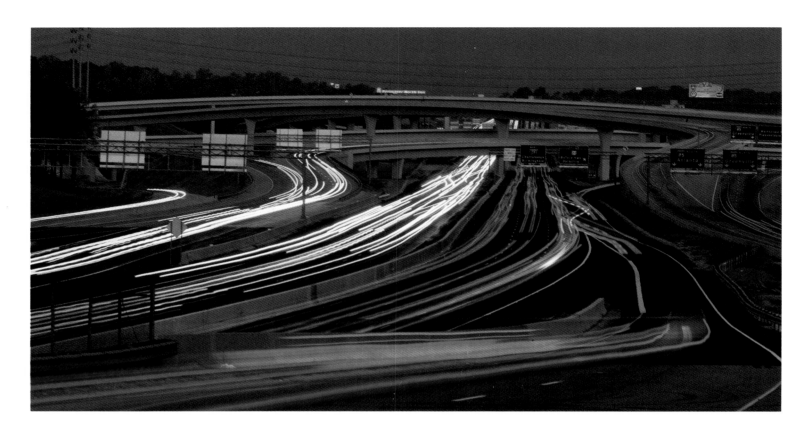

(top) HNTB's extensive experience in tollroad planning was put to use in the late 1980s on the long-awaited Georgia 400 extension connecting I-285 with I-85 in Atlanta. As part of this federal demonstration project, HNTB provided a complete traffic and revenue study as well as reviews, studies, and recommendations for the route's toll facilities.

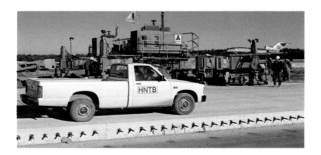

(above) By the 1980s, HNTB's aviation service line was in full flower. With more than three decades of experience to draw on, HNTB has been able to tackle an increasingly wide variety of airport projects. Here, construction is underway on an HNTB-designed runway at North Carolina's Raleigh-Durham Airport.

Leon eagerly experimented with expanding their own services locally as opportunities arose. And the environmental movement had nudged the whole engineering profession to learn to prepare environmental studies and to put together multidisciplinary teams to work with local citizens' groups.

In spite of these early, successful steps toward diversification, not everyone was readily persuaded that more diversification was the answer to the problems of the 1970s. Proponents of diversification, however, were ready with two key arguments. First, by taking a few figurative "eggs" from the bridge and highway "baskets" and putting them into other kinds of endeavors, the firm could dampen the impact of future recessions. Rarely would an economic downturn hit all sectors — private and public — at once or with the same intensity. If there was one thing that could be counted on, it was future recessions much like the current one. Why not take steps to shield the firm from the worst of the fallout?

Diversification advocates had another argument. By offering a wider range of services to clients, the firm could continue to serve the areas in which it was already established and at the same time expand into new markets. Valued clients would get the benefit of new services; new clients would get the benefit of HNTB's ability to pull together just the right mix of experts from its network of offices across the country.

Not all of the partners were convinced. Skeptics pointed to the bottom line. Serious diversification required not only up-front investment in putting together a team of experts in the new service line, but a great deal of time and marketing effort in trying to persuade clients — new and old — that the firm was a serious contender for projects outside its traditional disciplines. Yes, the firm's aviation line was a success. But the road to that success had been neither short nor easy. Nearly two decades after the establishment of the service, prospective clients were still occasionally surprised to hear that HNTB "did airports." The payoff from further diversification could be long in materializing; in the meantime, the firm might be risking its well-established reputation trying to break into fields in which it simply didn't have the recognized expertise to compete.

After long debate, diversification advocates won their point. In the early 1970s HNTB began to cautiously branch out into new disciplines.

The Acquisition of Expertise

In spite of the success of the firm's homegrown aviation service line, the idea of trying to diversify into other fields by starting from scratch in-house was not appealing. There was a consensus — especially among newer partners — according to retired HNTB partner Paul Heineman, that "if we were going to diversify in a significant way, and become strong in a particular field, we were going to have do something more than just hire a few young fellows and let them learn the ropes." A small number of carefully considered acquisitions seemed to be the logical route.

The methods for identifying a potential acquisition varied. Sometimes HNTB went looking for a match; sometimes the match came to HNTB. Often one of the partners would spot an opportunity to acquire a small specialty firm and put together a proposal for the full partnership's consideration. A sub-group of partners with a personal interest in the discipline represented by the small firm might come together to dig for details and open negotiations. The full partnership would then listen to the proposal, debate, ask for more details, debate again and finally vote. The whole process might take months, or even years, before a decision was reached and an offer-to-acquire made.

The cautious and methodical approach by the partnership to mergers was fueled by a deeply-rooted concern that the "fit" between HNTB and its new acquisitions be as close to ideal as possible. Acquisition for the sake of acquisition was simply not HNTB's style. According to Paul Heineman, who was involved in most of the firm's acquisitions, "many, many hours" were spent "just sitting down and visiting with the principals" of the prospective acquisition until all parties were fundamentally satisfied that the technical standards, ethics, and work styles of the two organizations could blend successfully.

"It's like a marriage," says now-retired HNTB partner Jim Finn, who served as ACP throughout the period of acquisitions. "You're going to live with a person and once you're in the partnership you don't have a chance to complain about his lifestyle, about how many hours he works and doesn't work or if he's doing things in a way that you don't like. In the case of a merger, you've got to decide if you're compatible before you shake hands. For example, we'd never 'marry' into another operation where the people aren't willing to work as hard as we do."

A Very Special Marriage: Architecture and Engineering

The strong emphasis on caution could easily have restricted HNTB's strategy to diversify to the acquisition of a handful of small engineering firms with specialties closely related to HNTB's traditional services. After all, with natural concern being expressed by many partners about not settling for less than the right "fit," the

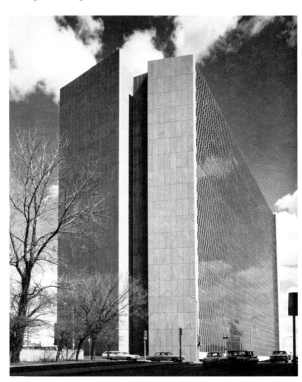

(below) Early architectural projects such as the Federal Office Building in Kansas City, Missouri, testify to the success of HNTB's decision to diversify into architecture in the mid-1970s. Today, architecture accounts for approximately one-fourth of HNTB's annual business.

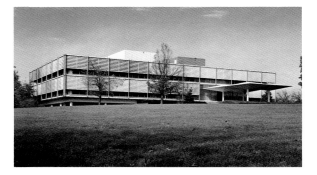

(above) HNTB acquired the talent and traditions of Kansas City architectural firm Kivett & Myers in 1975. K&M had designed such prestigious buildings as the Missouri Public Service Company headquarters (1958). Twenty-five years later HNTB remodeled and updated the interior of this Le Corbusier-inspired architectural gem.

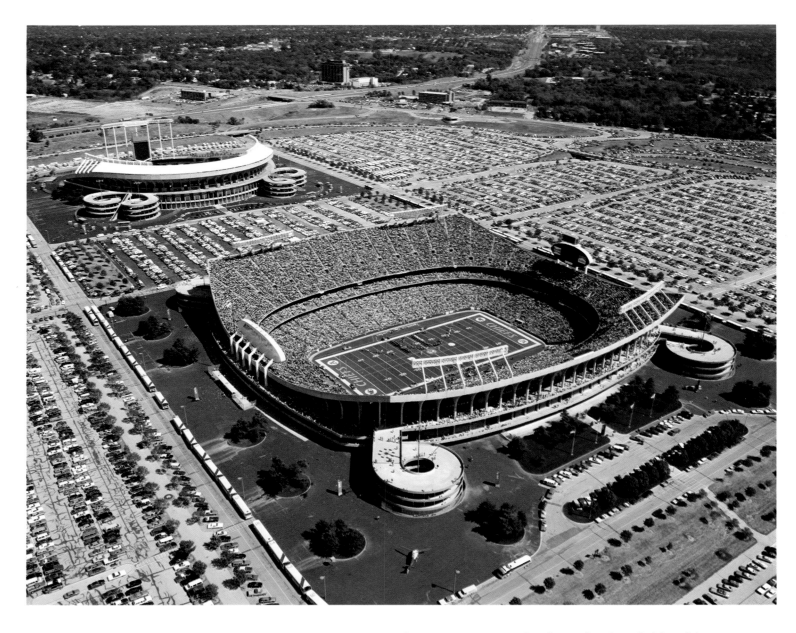

(above) The twin-stadium concept of the Harry S Truman Sports Complex in Kansas City helped to establish Kivett & Myers' reputation in sports facility design in the 1960s. As part of a joint venture with Charles Deaton, architect, design associate, K & M was responsible for the program and design of the total complex, including separate football and baseball stadiums with combined seating of nearly 120,000 and parking for 18,000 cars and 200 buses.

notion of not straying too far from familiar fields of business not only made sense, but might have been sorely tempting as well, to a group of engineers who were all fairly conservative by temperament.

Not surprisingly, about half of HNTB's acquisitions have been just such well-calculated forays into engineering disciplines which closely complement the firm's customary line of work. The other half, however, represent an extraordinary experiment that required one of the most revolutionary leaps of faith in the history of HNTB's partnership: architecture. With the acquisition of Kivett & Myers, a prestigious Kansas City architectural concern, in 1975, and two subsequent mergers, HNTB launched one of the most successful national architecture/engineering practices in the country.

The addition of architecture to HNTB's very traditional engineering practice was certainly not an impossible feat. But it was not an easy one either. More than anything else, it required a

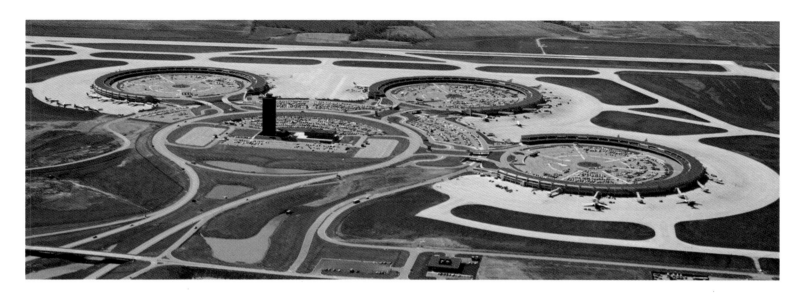

willingness by both sides to accommodate each other's styles. Communication, flexibility, and a measure of mutual faith were vital to success. Friction between the two groups could undermine the entire enterprise.

HNTB had dabbled on its own in architecture over the years, mostly on small buildings that were part of large transportation projects, and on giving the firm's bridges a more graceful look. Don Stevens in the Kansas City office had carved an enviable niche for himself in the firm through his talent for adding artistic touches to utilitarian structures.

In the early 1970s, a small in-house group was started in Kansas City with an eye to breaking into architecture. While this group was getting established, the senior partners were making nationwide inquiries to find an established architect or firm to join HNTB's fold. The search led straight to HNTB's own backyard: Ralph E. Myers, FAIA, and the Kansas City firm of Kivett & Myers. HNTB had worked on a few projects with Kivett & Myers and had always respected their work. Acquisition of the group could mean getting into architecture relatively quickly and on a large scale. The idea was tempting.

The idea was also a little unnerving. The acquisition of Kivett & Myers would be an unprecedented experiment by HNTB to put together under a single roof two groups of professionals with quite different professional visions, approaches, and personalities. Today, good-humored ribbing about each other's chosen field is traded back and forth between the architectural and engineering partners of HNTB. Behind the humor is a mutual recognition that architects and engineers as groups possess distinctive sets of characteristics. Architects describe themselves as more entrepreneurial by nature than engineers, and more flamboyant. Not surprisingly, their professional and personal emphases tend to be on the creative use of color, shape, texture and space. Engineers, on the other hand, acknowledge their generally more conservative bent and pride themselves on a rigorous devotion to finding practical, economical solutions to problems.

After much negotiation and at least one false start, HNTB acquired Kivett & Myers, effective January 1, 1975. Ralph Myers had bought out Clarence Kivett a few months earlier. Kivett had founded the firm in 1931. Myers joined Kivett in 1940 and five years later had become his partner. Ralph Myers made HNTB

(top) Opened in the mid-1970s, Kansas City International Airport utilized the concept of "drive to your gate" passenger handling. Three circular terminal buildings each contain 15 to 19 aircraft gates and provide capacity for 10.2 million passengers per year.

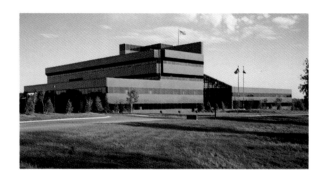

(above) HNTB was retained in late 1976 to design the corporate headquarters of the Employers Reinsurance Corporation in Overland Park, Kansas. The open atrium design of the 220,000 square foot building features a landscaped garden, pools and a waterfall.

(right) The Anaheim Convention Center, Anaheim, California, is a multi-purpose convention/sports/concert hall complex sited on 53 acres of land. In 1983, HNTB provided the master planning, schematic design, design development and construction administration for a 186,000 square-foot one-story and mezzanine addition to the main center. The facility includes an exhibition hall with more than 100,000 square feet of floor area, as well as 37,750 square feet for meeting rooms.

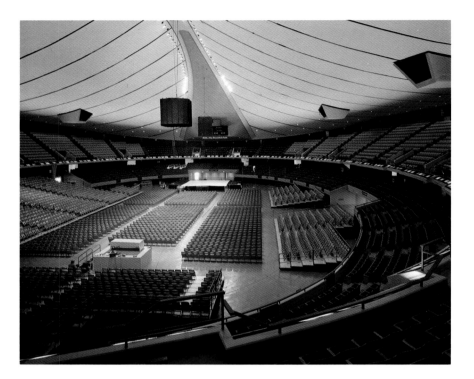

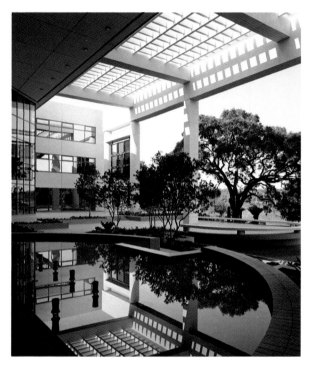

101

(above) From site selection through architectural and interior design, HNTB applied its talents to the Altamonte Springs, Florida headquarters of United Telephone Systems. Located on a 50-acre lakefront site, the 186,000 square-foot initial phase building was designed with energy efficiency and a pleasant working environment as top priorities. The initial phase was completed in 1982 with further expansion planned over the next decade.

(right) In keeping with the innovative musician after which the building is named, the Arnold Schoenberg Institute on the campus of the University of Southern California is composed of separate geometric forms and cantilevered planes grouped to form a two-level research, study and performance center. The unusual complex was designed by HNTB's Adrian Wilson Associates in Los Angeles. AWA was acquired by HNTB in 1976.

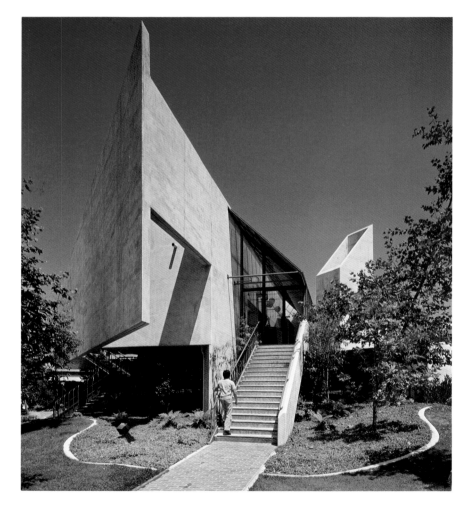

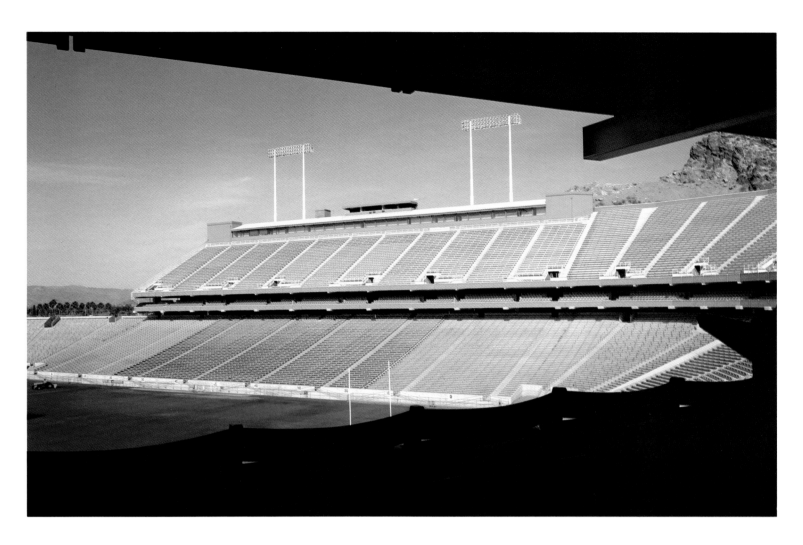

history in 1975 by becoming the firm's first architectural partner.

Now retired, Myers points out that both firms had much to gain by the merger:

> "In the years just prior to the merger, Kivett & Myers had been getting more and more clients nationwide. HNTB had offices in place all across the country: we could work with them to our advantage and theirs. And although HNTB had a small architectural section in place at the time of the merger, the acquisition instantly gave the firm a fully staffed, architectural services group that was known, proven, and came with forty-four years of reputation, good-will and clients."

HNTB partner Bill Love, FAIA, whose own architectural career began with Kivett & Myers, remembers watching now-retired Ralph Myers take up the challenge of making a home for architecture within HNTB:

> "Ralph Myers fought long and hard personally to convince — successfully — his partners that architects had to work and practice as architects. They couldn't try to practice architecture as engineers, so part of the first problem was how to get along with the systems that existed, the billings, the reporting, etc., that HNTB had developed, and fit those to a different kind of client."

When HNTB acquired Wadsworth, Jensen & Associates, of Phoenix, Arizona, in 1982 it gained both engineering and architectural capabilities in the Southwest. The additions designed for the Sun Devil Stadium at Arizona State University (top) were among the firm's notable projects prior to merger with HNTB.

HNTB's merger with Archonics, an Indianapolis-based architectural firm, in 1985 capped the first decade of the firm's venture into architecture. Archonics brought to the HNTB fold a talent for blending new and old. Such Indianapolis projects as the Eli Lilly corporate headquarters (below) and the 1916 Circle Theatre (with DVD&J). (right) required an eye for updating historic sites for modern uses. (bottom) Color, space and style were special considerations in Archonics' design of the St. Vincent Stress Center, Indianapolis, Indiana. The warm and peaceful 82-bed facility houses the Tri-County Mental Health office and units devoted to psychiatric care, chemical dependency, and hospice care.

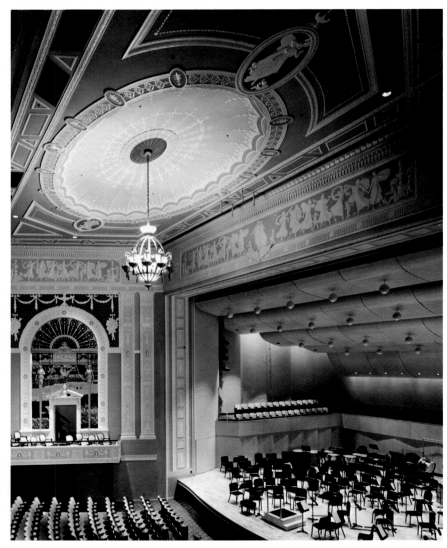

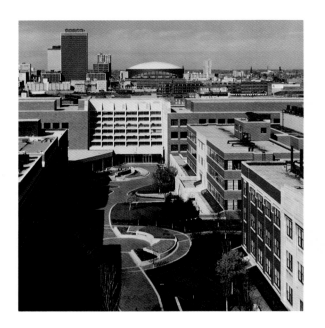

103

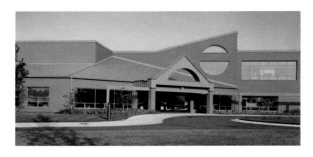

(facing page) HNTB's innovative masterplan for a 250-acre park along the White River in Indianapolis drew on the expertise of a team of world-renowned experts in waterfront and urban design. Included in the complex is a 750-foot observation tower, a major family entertainment center, a new home for the city's zoo, botanical gardens, as well as large outdoor public spaces for festivals, concerts, and celebrations.

For their part, the engineering partners accepted the difficult job of granting Myers and his architectural team the freedom they needed to make a go of it. For the first time, an HNTB partner was given a free hand to develop work all over the country, not just in an assigned geographic area. The going wasn't always easy. Myers faced the delicate task of working directly in the backyards of some partners who held their geographic turf close to their hearts. Surprisingly, only limited friction developed. Of course, the relative numbers of engineers to architects in the firm was also daunting from the start. Bill Love recalls:

> "HNTB had about 5 or 6 people on their architectural staff. Bill Meredith was the associate in charge of that group and we melded them into our operation and moved them physically to Ten Main Center (Kivett & Myers headquarters) .... As somebody laughingly said, 'They came to live in our house, but they own it!'"

Small in number, the architects nonetheless held — and hold — their own in HNTB's large practice. True to their flair for color and graphic design, the firm's architects brought to HNTB's marketing program a fresh and more aggressive look. HNTB's glossy, four-

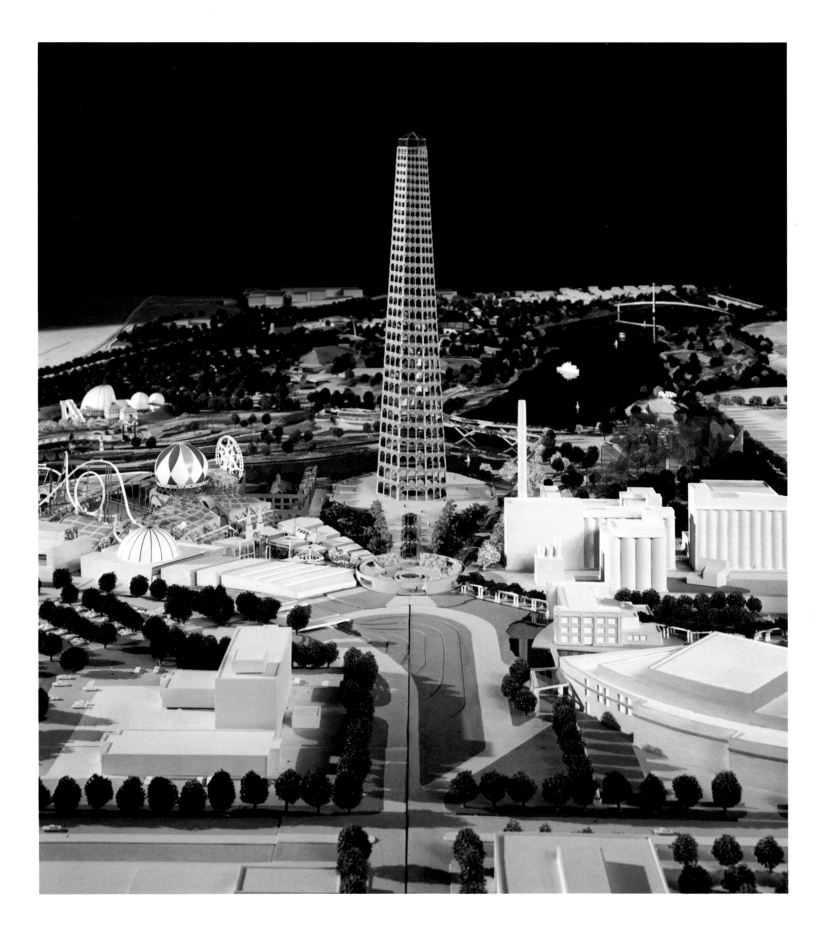

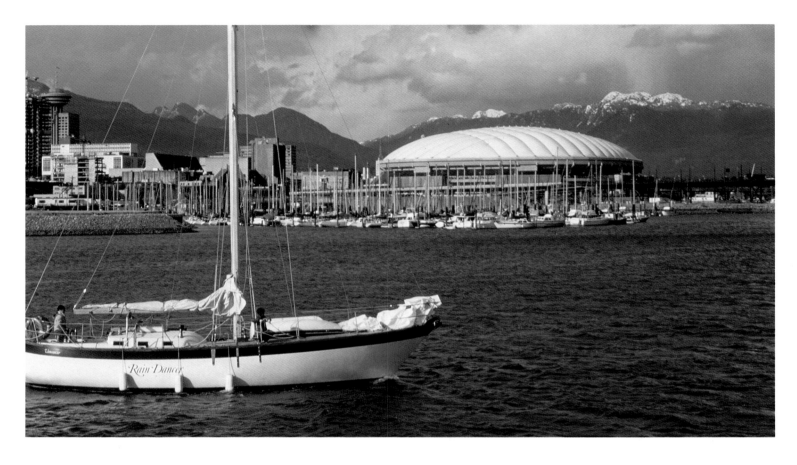

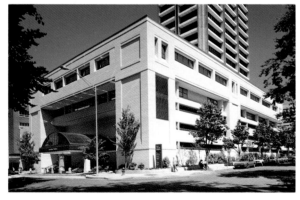

(above) HNTB used its special expertise in health facilities in designing a badly-needed surgical center for Saint Cabrini Hospital in downtown Seattle, Washington. The 21,000 square-foot Columbus Pavilion includes surgical suites, special procedure rooms, recovery rooms and a preoperative processing area.

(top) B.C. Place Stadium is the anchor structure of a redevelopment of a 200-acre industrial area in Vancouver, British Columbia. Designed as a multi-use facility, the 60,000 seat stadium is home to soccer and football teams. HNTB served as sports facilities design consultant to a local A/E firm for design through construction of the sleek, low profile stadium.

color perfect-bound brochure system was a direct result of the influence of Ralph Myers. Kivett & Myers also brought with it at the time of the merger a national reputation in the design of sports facilities. Their path-breaking design of the double-stadium Truman Sports Complex (in association with Charles Deaton, architect) in Kansas City in 1967 had established them as an early leader in the field. HNTB's high-profile sports architecture group today is a direct descendant of the Kivett & Myers house.

Having made a full-scale commitment to architecture through the Kivett & Myers merger, the partnership was open to bolstering their newest service line with additional talent. Less than two years after the acquisition of Kivett & Myers, HNTB accepted the opportunity to acquire Adrian Wilson Associates, an architectural firm based in Los Angeles, California. The firm had been founded in 1929, and by 1976 had worked on more than 4,000 projects around the world, including hospitals, convention centers, hotels, shopping centers, university facilities, and municipal buildings.

HNTB acquired Adrian Wilson Associates, says HNTB architectural partner Bill Love, "as much as anything because of what they were doing in the Far East." At the time of the merger in 1976, HNTB was actively exploring international markets. AWA was a particularly attractive acquisition because the firm boasted a strong overseas base. AWA had designed a number of major projects in Pacific Rim countries and over time had established branch offices in Korea, Japan, the Philippines and elsewhere. Soon after the merger, however, HNTB found that it could not take advantage of the numerous overseas offices of AWA, and decided to shut them down while maintaining and enhancing the Los Angeles operation. Today, the HNTB Los Angeles office, under the

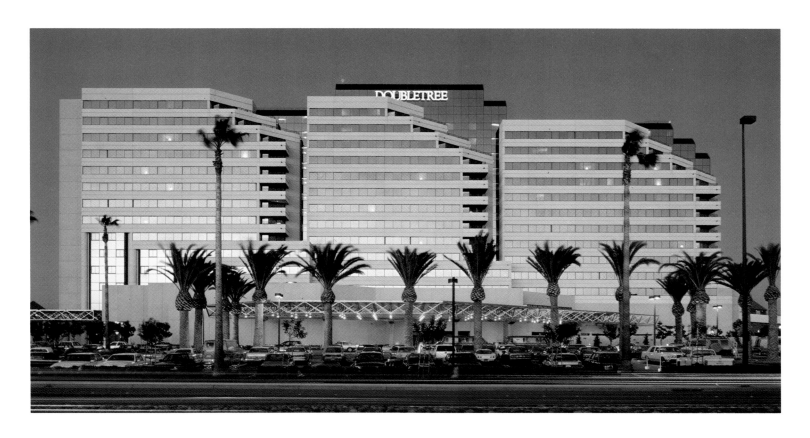

personal direction of HNTB architectural partner Bill Love, specializes in the design of major hotels, convention centers and other public assembly structures.

The decade following the acquisitions of Kivett & Myers and Adrian Wilson Associates were critical years for HNTB's architectural practice. There was a lot at stake. If the great experiment in integrating architecture and engineering into a multi-faceted design practice failed, HNTB's reputation, stability and bottom line might suffer. On the other hand, if the experiment proved successful, HNTB would have accomplished something that few peer firms had been able to do. Only time would tell.

Time did tell, and the story was a happy one for all concerned. Even with the pruning of AWA's operations to a single office in Los Angeles, HNTB's architectural service line grew ten-fold between 1975 and 1985. Contributing to the growth was the acquisition in 1982 of Wadsworth, Jensen & Associates, a Phoenix, Arizona architecture and engineering firm. WJA possessed recognized design strengths in several areas, including education facility design, sports pavilions, vehicle maintenance facilities and penal facilities. Architecture's growth during this period also saw two more architects rise to partnership rank — Bill Love in 1980 and Cary Goodman in 1985. Soon nearly a dozen HNTB offices boasted full-scale architectural departments.

As if to cap off that successful first decade of growth, HNTB accepted an invitation in 1985 to acquire another prestigious architectural firm: Archonics Design Partnership, an old and respected Indianapolis concern. Faced with decisions about whether and how much more to grow, Archonics had reached a critical juncture in the early 1980s. The firm decided to investigate the possibility of being acquired and gave a search firm the task of finding a suitable partner. HNTB was suggested. Long discussions

(top) The 16-story, 500-room Doubletree Hotel in the heart of Silicon Valley includes 35 suites and 15,000 square feet of meeting space. The hotel was master-planned as one component of the Santa Clara Trade and Conference Center.

106

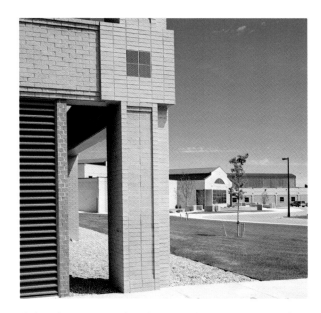

(above) Passive solar design takes advantage of Centennial Junior High School's southern exposure on a hillside overlooking the mountains around Casper, Wyoming.

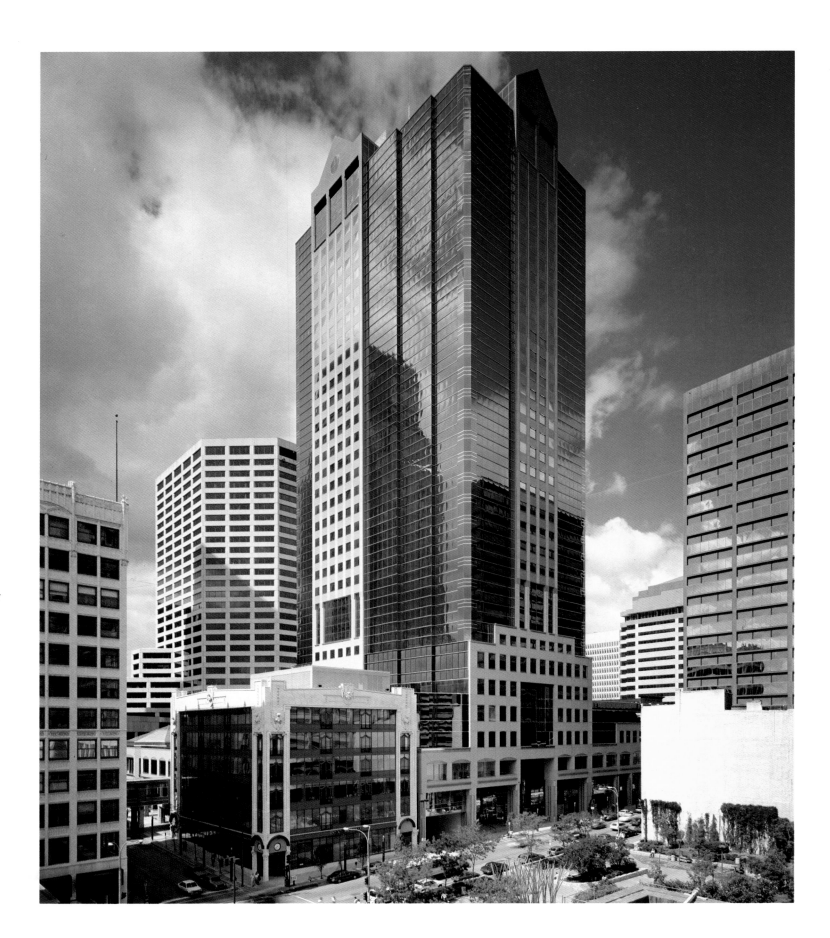

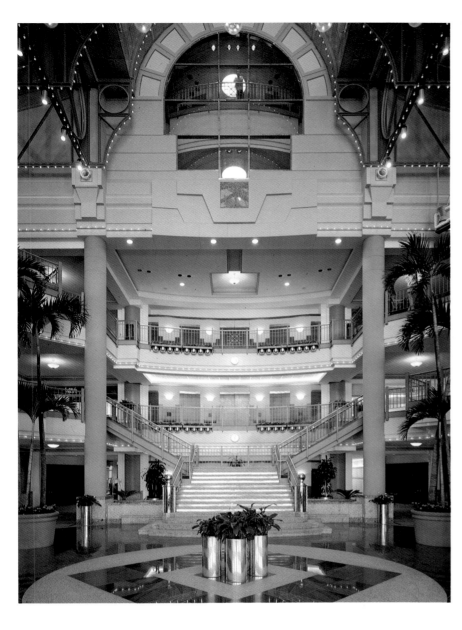

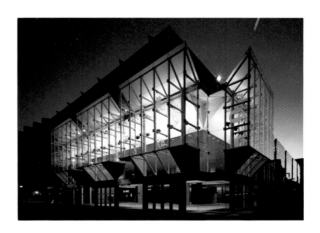

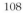

(facing page) In keeping with founder Ernest Howard's commitment to the quality of the built environment in his adopted hometown, HNTB has played a major role in the revitalization of downtown Kansas City. The 38-story AT&T Town Pavilion anchors a two-block complex of retail and office space which combines historic restoration of treasured landmarks with cutting-edge architectural design. (left) The grand lobby of the new AT&T Pavilion greets thousands of Kansas City office workers and shoppers every day.

(above) HNTB sought to create a feeling of openness in its recommendations for the renovation of the Baltimore Arena and Convention Center in Baltimore, Maryland. Expanded seating, relocation of the main entrance, and the creation of an outdoor plaza with a sports motif helped to update the 1962-built facility.

followed and a merger agreeable to all was designed. Archonics' small staff of architects joined HNTB's 12-year old Indianapolis office. Ewing Miller, FAIA, one of Archonics' principals and grandson of the firm's founder, became an HNTB associate.

Today, only 14 years after its introduction, HNTB's architecture service line is a source of constant pride to the firm. Already, architecture contributes approximately one-fourth to the firm's bottom line. In 1986, HNTB was named the sixth ranking architecture firm in the United States, based on annual fees, by *Building and Design* magazine. But the real "bottom line" success of HNTB's architecture experiment does not lie in its well-proved promises of financial gain for the firm. Instead, it is the successful transformation of one of the country's oldest and most respected civil engineering firms into HNTB, Architects, Engineers & Planners — with "Architects" actually heading the list — that resonates as a testament to HNTB's continuing ability to adapt and change with the times.

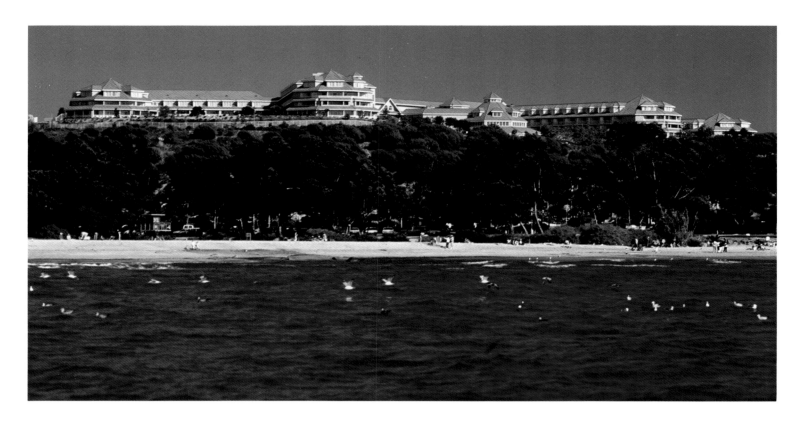

(top) Nestled above the Dana Point Yacht Harbor and Doheny State Park, the Dana Point Hotel luxury resort combines classic Victorian architectural style with modern conveniences. Every room in the 11-acre California resort offers an unobstructed view of the ocean.

109

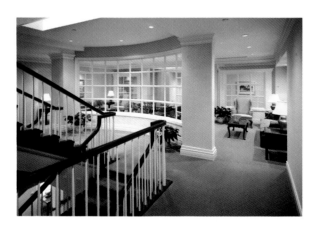

(above) As HNTB's architectural prowess grew during the mid-1970s so, too, did the firm's talents in interior design. A lively color scheme and a grand stairway connecting three floors give the offices of Kansas City law firm Shughart, Thomson & Kilroy an appealing, yet traditional, ambience which won the ABA Journal Award for design, 1986.

Important Building Blocks

The addition of architecture to HNTB's services was a high-profile, high-risk venture. As part of the partnership's strategy to diversify to cope with recessionary trends, architecture's almost exclusive emphasis on private sector projects was tailor-made to help the firm spread its "eggs" among different kinds of "baskets." Equally important, HNTB could now offer its clients an even more comprehensive range of services.

Extending that range of services, however, wasn't limited to architecture. In fact, HNTB had gotten its feet wet in the way of acquisitions more than a year before the Kivett & Myers merger when it acquired Henry B. Steeg & Associates of Indianapolis, an environmental engineering firm.

The company had been founded in 1939 by civil engineer and Purdue graduate Henry B. Steeg. Fraternity brother James Loer joined Steeg soon after. Following World War II, the small firm decided to take the plunge into the new field of sanitary engineering (now known as environmental engineering). Between 1945 and 1950, the company handled about 100 jobs, mostly sewer, sewage treatment, water supply, treatment or distribution. The firm's reputation in Indiana grew quickly and by 1960, when George Erganian took over as president, Steeg was the major environmental engineering firm in the state. By 1973, the company had handled more than 650 projects for more than 200 clients.

The idea of adding environmental engineering to HNTB's portfolio was appealing. The seeds of an environmental engineering service line in the firm had been sown in the 1960s when the national environmental movement was getting underway. Instead of fighting the environmentalists, HNTB had taken the initiative to incorporate the movement's legitimate concerns into project strategy. By the early 1970s, HNTB was well-versed in the

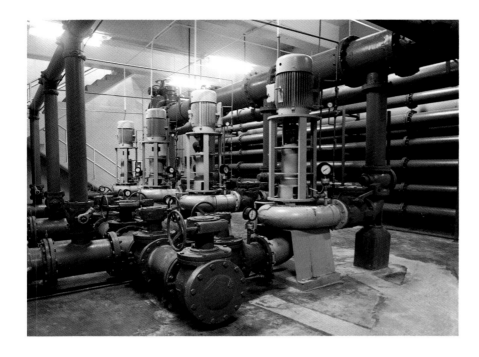

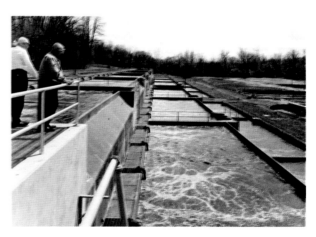

art and science of environmental impact studies, public hearings, and comprehensive planning.

The acquisition of Steeg took the process begun in the 1960s one step further. Instead of being one important sideline of a transportation project, the environment would be the main focus. Water treatment was especially high on the list of the government's environmental priorities, with special funds earmarked for secondary and tertiary water treatment. With the experience brought to the firm by Steeg, HNTB could make these areas a specialty. From there, the firm could expand into other kinds of environmental engineering projects.

On October 16, 1973, after more than a year of negotiations, Henry B. Steeg & Associates, Inc., joined the HNTB fold. The acquisition marked not only the formal beginning of HNTB's environmental engineering service line, but the first time that a man who had not come up through the ranks of the firm had been named to the partnership. As part of the merger agreement, Steeg president George Erganian became an HNTB partner, and Robert Coma (later to become a partner) and Don Ort became HNTB associates. Steeg's Indianapolis office became HNTB's base in Indiana.

George Erganian recalls that getting used to his new partners wasn't always easy:

> "In spite of all the warnings I had, I really wasn't prepared, completely prepared, for the type of hard-charging, business-like people I was dealing with."

Erganian, however, was quite satisfied with his decision to merge with HNTB. His reasoning echoes the same logic that had fueled HNTB's own decision to diversify:

> "We were looking to diversify because we recognized that if the government's environmental programs were cut back, the firm's position would be precarious. So I had had the concept for a long time that a merger or some method of diversifying the type of services we offered or our geographical areas of service would give

(right) In 1973 HNTB helped to bring the Florida Cities Water Company's wastewater treatment facilities near Sarasota up to new federal standards at a reasonable cost by designing a treatment process that required only expansions and modifications to the company's two existing plants.

(below right) Improved laboratory facilities were designed by HNTB as part of a rehabilitation and expansion of the wastewater treatment plant in Tipton, Indiana.

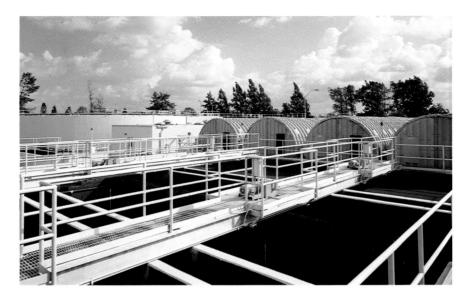

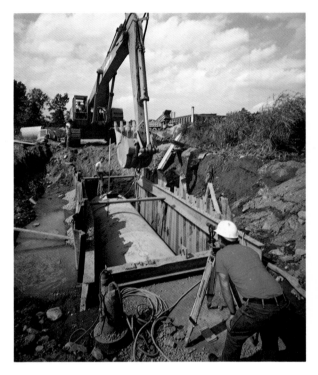

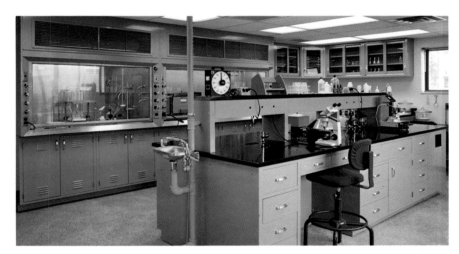

(above) A river crossing was just one of the challenges facing HNTB in 1976 when the firm was asked to design a new interceptor sewer for Worcester, Massachusetts. Replacing a system built in the 1920s, the pipe replacement and routing project carried a new 84-inch diameter interceptor across the Middle River to connect 177,000 residents and industries in Worcester to the Upper Blackstone Regional Wastewater Treatment Plant.

(facing page) Wastewater treatment plant expansion, Ft. Wayne, Indiana.

us a little better chance of surviving a downturn. As a result of our association with HNTB, we've picked up a good deal of work in the highway area and the architectural area, all of which supports the notion that diversification in one way or another is a good idea."

The "good idea" of diversification found HNTB shaking hands with the principals of Frankfurter & Associates, Inc. in 1974. Partner Ed Johnson in HNTB's Seattle office had been approached by a local engineering firm looking to be bought out. Frankfurter specialized in mechanical, electrical and chemical engineering for the paper and pulp industry. The firm had been established in 1958 by brothers Alroy E. and David R. Frankfurter. One of the brothers was ailing; the pair agreed that a merger with another company was the best way to secure their firm's future.

Frankfurter's specialty was further afield than that of Steeg from HNTB's traditional practice. On the other hand, Frankfurter came with a solid reputation and track record. HNTB was eager to add Frankfurter's proven talents to the firm's services. On June 1, 1974, the acquisition was consummated and Frankfurter & Associates, Inc. became Frankfurter, Inc., a wholly-owned subsidiary of HNTB.

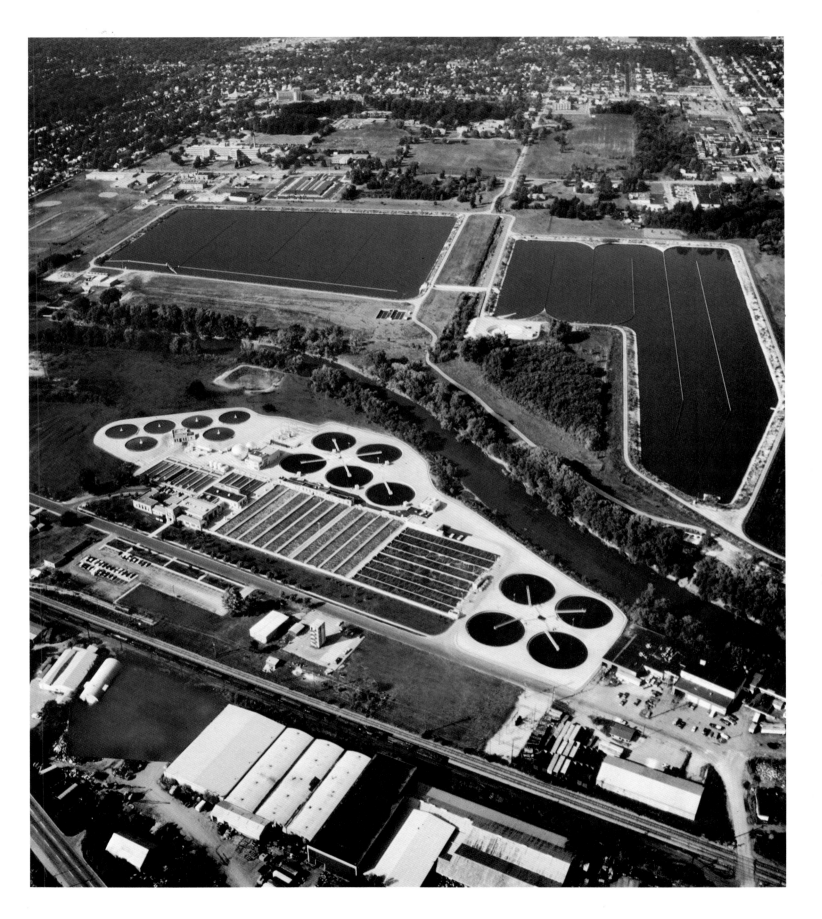

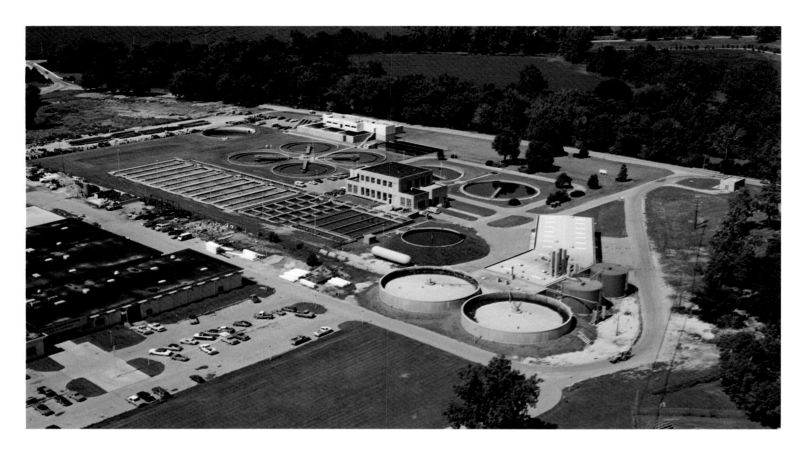

Steeg brought into the HNTB fold many long-time municipal clients. As the water and wastewater treatment needs of communities have grown over the years, HNTB has worked with local officials to design expanded and up-to-date facilities. In 1975, for example, the firm assisted Anderson, Indiana in a major expansion project at the town's Moss Island Road Wastewater Treatment Plant, (top).

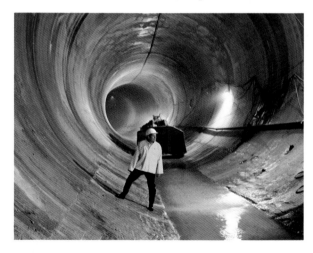

(above) HNTB designed a combined sewer overflow conveyance and storage tunnel for Milwaukee, Wisconsin as part of the city's $1.6 billion water pollution abatement program.

David Frankfurter remained at the helm. He and his staff, including partner-to-be Hugh Schall, moved into HNTB's Seattle headquarters.

The next addition of outside engineering expertise to HNTB's portfolio didn't take place until 1982. It was during these interim years that the merger with Kivett & Myers and the launching of the firm's architecture service line took place. Like the merger with Frankfurter & Associates in 1974, the 1982 acquisition of T.K. Dyer, Inc. was a direct result of well-established personal contact between an HNTB partner and the other firm's principals. As usual, the issue of "fit" was of paramount importance. Says HNTB partner Frank Hall:

> *"A lot of these acquisitions have just been the result of one partner pursuing it and then going back and selling it to the rest of the firm. It wasn't that the partnership sat down and said we ought to get into the rail and transit business. I met Tom Dyer, and I got to thinking about it, and I put together a proposal for the partnership."*

T.K. Dyer, Inc. had been established in 1963 by Thomas K. Dyer to provide general civil, structural, and rail transportation engineering services to railroads, transit agencies, and private clients. For Dyer, the merger was the end product of a long thinking process.

> *"I'd reached 60 and felt it was time to decide the future of the firm — what would happen after I left. I considered a purchase by key employees, but rejected it after some discussions and the realization that all of those key personnel were within five years of my own age. I'd also had several offers for the firm over the*

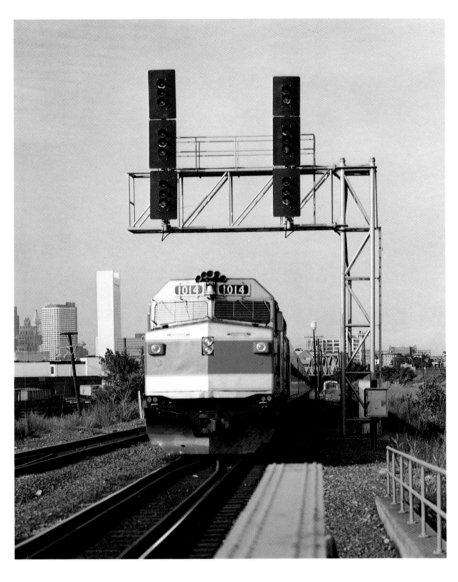

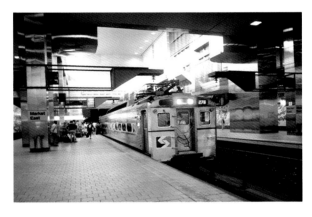

(left) The talents of T.K. Dyer, Inc., a railroad engineering firm acquired by HNTB in 1982, were applied to the reconstruction of the high-speed train corridor linking Boston with Washington, D.C. The addition of T.K. Dyer to the HNTB family expanded the firm's traditional services to railroads to include track and signal systems design.

(above) HNTB was involved in the revamping of Philadelphia's rail mass transit system in the mid-1980s. Here, the gleaming interior of the new Reading Terminal near city hall greets passengers of the SEPTA commuter rail system.

previous ten years, when I wasn't interested in selling, and those offers had educated me somewhat about what factors I should look at, how much the firm was worth."

Dyer knew what he was looking for in a purchaser.

"I wanted to see a financially strong, well-known firm with a good reputation and with a management that would be sensitive to feelings of TKD employees. The integrity of the acquirer's management was especially important, particularly of those handling the acquisition. I also wanted a purchase plan which would reward key people and provide employment contracts for them. Obviously, a satisfactory purchase price and a clear sense of the strong potential of the merger to benefit both firms were also important."

The T.K. Dyer acquisition gave HNTB in-house expertise in public transit and railway design. All of the principals and a majority of the employees had worked for railroads or transit authorities before coming to TKD. Their expertise has been put to use by HNTB on such projects as Washington, D.C.'s Metro transit

(right) HNTB has provided management services to the Arizona Department of Transportation for the design of I-10. The $900 million project carries 160,000 vehicles each day on a depressed roadway through the heart of the city.

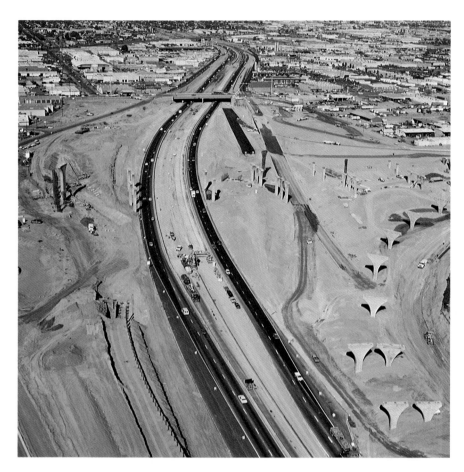

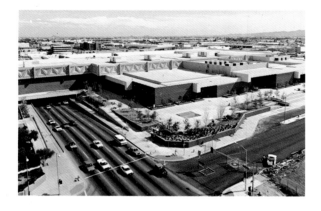

(above) The Phoenix Civic Plaza expansion employed both the architecture and engineering expertise of HNTB's Phoenix office.

115

system and Boston's complex Southwest Corridor. Thomas Dyer became an HNTB associate and remained president of T.K. Dyer, Inc. as part of the merger.

Acquisitions allowed HNTB not only to diversify into new fields, but also to open new branch offices — another important element of HNTB's diversification strategy. The acquisition of Steeg in 1973 had given the firm its first permanent base in Indiana. Nine years later, in 1982, the purchase of Wadsworth, Jensen & Associates in Phoenix, Arizona gave HNTB a permanent foothold in the previously untapped Southwest. HNTB had appeared on the local scene a year earlier with the establishment of a project office for the design of the $700 million Papago Freeway (I-10). The chance to acquire an established firm in the Phoenix area gave HNTB a permanent local home, in addition to more architectural and engineering muscle. The decision paid off; today, the Phoenix office is the third largest in HNTB.

Wadsworth, Jensen & Associates was founded in 1955 as the Engineering Corporation of America. In 1970, the firm expanded its services to include architecture and planning. At the same time it took the new name Wadsworth, Jensen & Associates. As part of the merger with HNTB in 1982, the principals of the firm — Roland Wadsworth, Jr., P.E. and Ross L. Jensen, A.I.A. — became HNTB associates. Ross Jensen notes that both firms clearly benefited from the acquisition. "The merger provided HNTB with a successful A/E firm of approximately 50 architects and engineers located in Phoenix and who had served the Southwest since 1955. WJA gained identity with a larger, established A/E firm whose resources

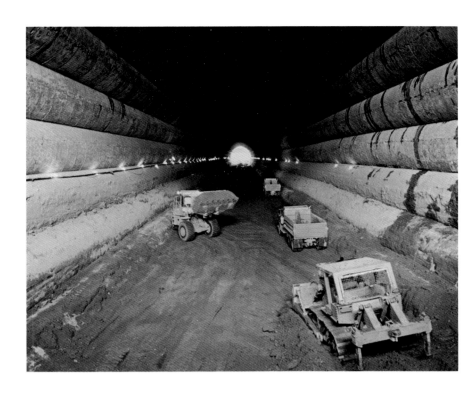

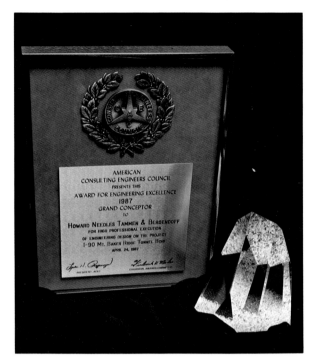

allowed much broader possibilities in project procurements both in size and diversity."

Like previous mergers between relatively large HNTB and small specialty firms, the period of adjustment following the formal merger "posed great potential and also many challenges," especially for WJA. Says Jensen:

> *"Going from a small, close-knit operation with a lot of employee-management 'intimacy' to one of larger scope and diversity was difficult. However, WJA was resilient and HNTB was tolerant and helpful."*

The most recent merger for HNTB has been the acquisition of five-year old ENECO Resources of Lexington, Kentucky in 1985, the same year that HNTB merged with Archonics of Indianapolis. This last acquisition has brought into the HNTB fold a young firm specializing in engineering and geotechnical services associated with the coal mining industry. Like the WJA acquisition in Arizona, the merger gave HNTB its first design office in Kentucky.

A Glance Backward

By the time HNTB acquired Archonics and ENECO in 1985, the worst of the recession of the 1970s was well in the past. Once again, HNTB had faced a tough period and come out ahead. In spite of a major economic downturn, in spite of the limited partnership experience of the men at its helm, and in spite of the risks involved in diversification, HNTB had not only survived the 1970s and 1980s, but turned the times to its advantage. Tough decisions about management and careful choices about diversification had paid off. Through an approach combining roughly equal parts of caution and boldness, HNTB had methodically transformed itself in little more than a decade into a dynamic and diversified organization with its eye on the future: HNTB, Architects, Engineers & Planners. ■

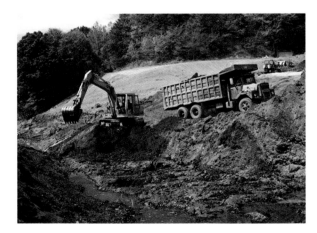

(above) 1985 acquisition of the Kentucky concern ENECO Resources, gave the firm special expertise in mining reclamation. One program at Buck Branch, Kentucky, involved rehabilitating a site which included nine open underground mine entrances, a coal refuse pile that was eroding into a stream, and a landslide which blocked a public road.

AFTERWORD
Today and Tomorrow

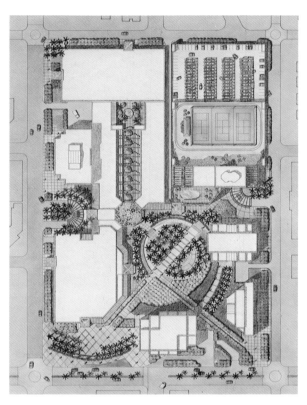

(above) The Arizona Center in Phoenix, Arizona displays HNTB's full architectural and engineering services. A mixed-use development of offices, hotel, retail, and restaurant facilities, the complex boasts a 25-story tower offering 500,000 square feet of new rentable space. A 1,700-car parking garage is located underground.

Today, only one of the 13 partners who came to the helm of HNTB before 1970 is still active: senior partner Charles Hennigan. His counterparts have all retired, one by one. A few others who became partners after 1970 have also come and gone: George Erganian, Bill Meredith, Ralph Myers. New partners, of course, have taken their places. Dan Spigai was elected in 1974. Frank Hall and Jack Cotton were named in 1978. Two years later, Bob Coma, Bill Love and Don Dupies joined the partnership. Jim Tuttle and Bob Miller were named in 1983. Hugh Schall was named in 1984. In 1985, Cary Goodman and Gordon Slaney were elected. Harvey Hammond joined in 1986, John Wight and Steve Goddard in 1987, and Dick Beckman in 1989.

This new generation of partners — HNTB's fourth — inherits a huge, multi-faceted practice spread among three dozen offices and carried out by a staff of more than 2,000 employees. What began three quarters of a century ago as a small partnership of bridge design specialists has become one of the country's largest and most successfully diversified architectural and engineering enterprises. Today, HNTB staff are as likely to be hard at work on perfecting the symmetry and graceful lines of a new building as on tackling the engineering challenges of a bridge or highway. From airports to water treatment plants to rapid transit projects, HNTB can rally an impressive team of staff experts from its network of offices to solve complex design problems that the firm's founders never dreamed of.

As the firm has changed, so too, the partnership which has led it. John Lyle Harrington, Ernest Howard, and Louis Ash were all respected engineers, devoted to the practice and advancement of their chosen profession. Their employees, and later partners, such as Henry Tammen, Enoch Needles, and R.N. Bergendoff, were likewise dedicated professionals. A love of bridge design was a shared bond among these talented men. But they also had more than bridges in common. They had a vision for the future, one that included building a permanent firm that could change with the times. As the nation's transportation needs evolved, these entrepreneurs boldly guided the firm into new arenas while at the same time taking care to preserve the firm's commitment to rigorous technical and business standards. The next two generations of partners continued both to guide and preserve, leading HNTB through periods of geographic expansion and dramatic growth and change. As the fourth generation of partners — two architects, two mechanical engineers, one environmental engineer, and 11 civil engineers — take up the reins of responsibility, they must decide anew how to balance the valued traditions of the past with the demands of the future. As Jack Cotton, current chairman of the Executive Committee, states, "Change today happens faster, is more expensive and places more demands on us. But HNTB has thrived on change, survived on change and will prosper on change."

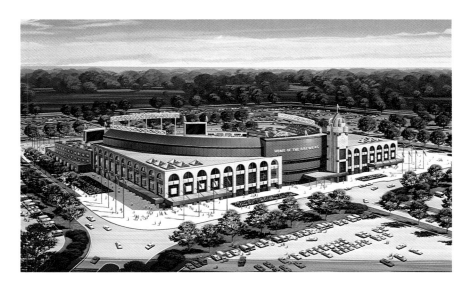

(left) Sports facilities design keeps HNTB's specialists busy. In Milwaukee, Wisconsin, HNTB has provided preliminary design services for a 48,000-seat multi-purpose stadium for the local major league franchise.

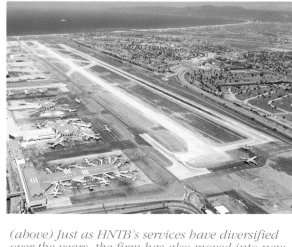

(above) Just as HNTB's services have diversified over the years, the firm has also moved into new geographic areas. HNTB has established itself on the West Coast through such projects as the firm's runway rehabilitation work at LAX International Airport, Los Angeles, California.

118

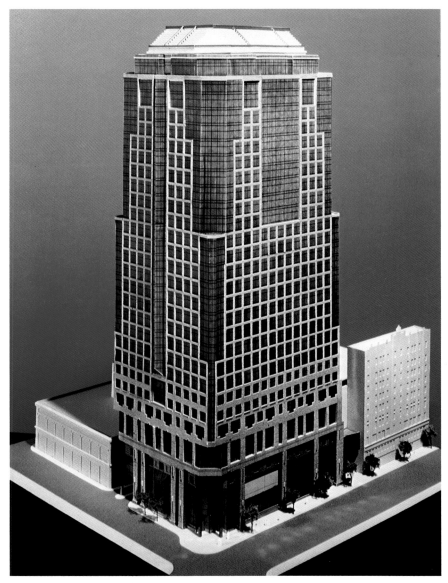

Architecture will continue to be an important growth area for HNTB, expanding into both new geographic areas and services. Projects such as the 30-story, 530,000-square foot office tower (left) in downtown Kansas City, Missouri, to be completed in 1991, enhance HNTB's image as a major national architecture firm.

(overleaf) Bridges, of course, remain a vital part of HNTB's practice three quarters of a century after the firm's founding. Opened in 1989, the concrete cable-stayed Dame Point Bridge crosses the St. John's River near Jacksonville, Florida, near the location where, 60 years earlier, a young civil engineer by the name of Enoch Needles started his career.

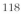

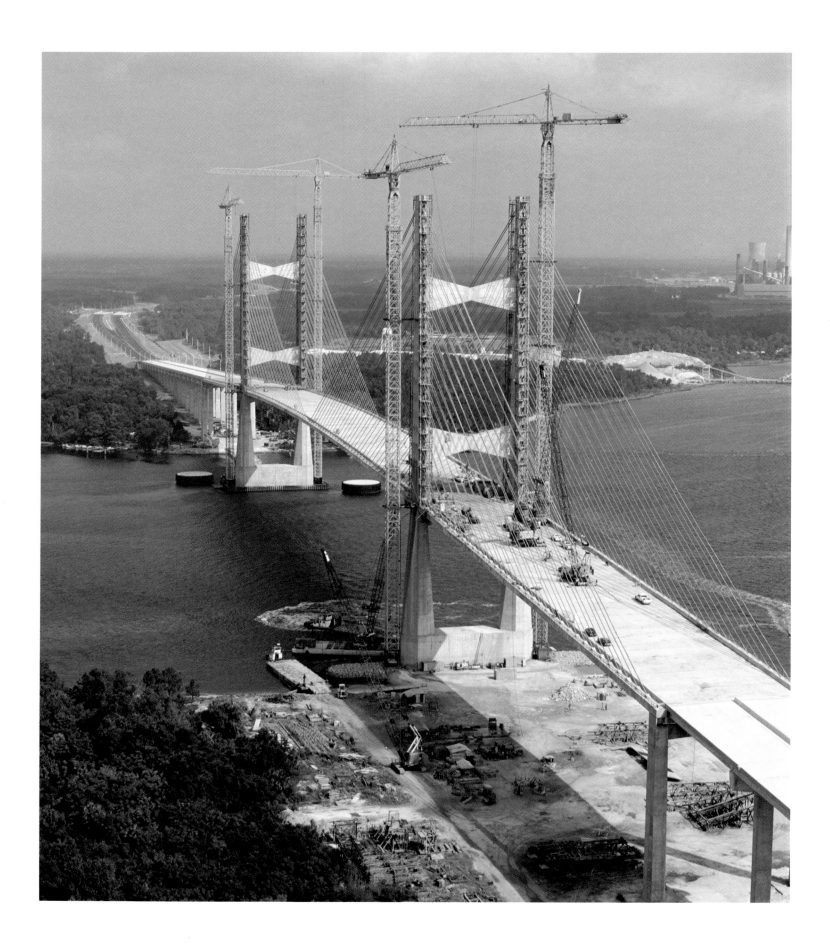

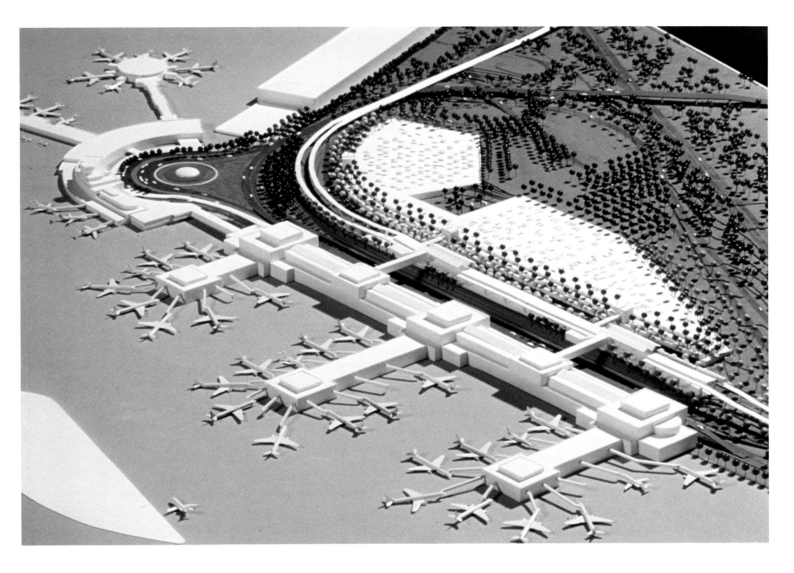

Forty-five years of airport planning and design experience position HNTB to help fill the increasing needs for new and expanded airport facilities across the country. The master plan for expansion of Washington National Airport (above) is an example of just one of a comprehensive array of architecture, engineering and planning services HNTB offers its airport clients.

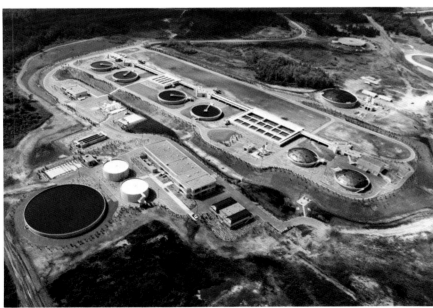

(left) HNTB frequently offers construction services to help clients see their plans become reality. For the Orlando Water Conserv I plant in Orlando, Florida, HNTB provided the city with assistance in dealing with the building contractor, obtaining construction permits, monitoring compliance, preparing a procedures manual, and coordinating efforts between city and design personnel.

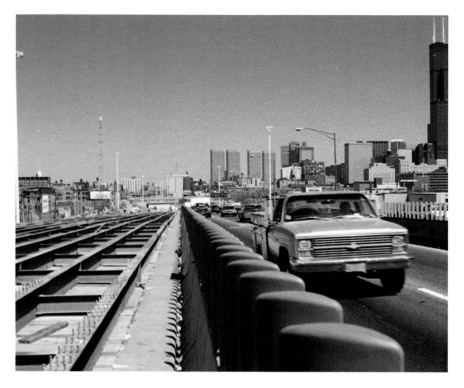

(right) Highway design will have to respond to overcrowding and wear of existing roadways. For example, more than 300,000 cars daily drive along Chicago's Dan Ryan Expressway (I-90/94) on what has been called the most heavily traveled road in the world. HNTB is providing construction services for one mile of a three-mile, $210 million reconstruction and widening of the route.

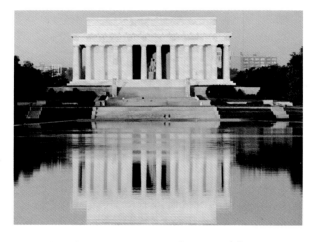

(above) A fitting assignment for one of the nation's oldest design firms, the renovation of the Lincoln and Jefferson Memorials will give HNTB an opportunity to make a special contribution to the nation's capitol. As part of a joint venture, HNTB will evaluate the condition of both landmarks and provide recommendations for preserving these national treasures.

What Lies Ahead

Among the challenges that this youngest generation of partners faces are new editions of old questions. Should the firm continue to grow? How much? In what directions? How can HNTB maintain its high standards and impart those standards to the next generation of partners and employees? What's the right mix of change and stability to ensure a sound future for the firm? Are annual fees alone the true measure of success, or is there greater reward in a small number of jobs very well done?

Answers to some of these questions will come readily. Others will merit the kind of lively and lengthy debate that flourishes in a partnership which prides itself on its diverse perspectives and personalities. A few things are already clear. For example, quality work and professional integrity will remain top priorities. Partners will continue to search for ways to balance the demands of modern management with a traditional commitment to hands-on responsibility for projects. As the partnership continues to grow in size, the pivotal associate level will gain in numbers and in importance. Current service lines will keep pace with new technological and design developments. New service lines will be explored. And the evolving global market will give the firm an opportunity to renew its interest in overseas work. "Most important to HNTB's future growth are ideas and a continuing infusion of individuals with vision," says Jack Cotton. "With ideas and shared vision there is no limit to what we can do."

Precisely what the future holds for HNTB, of course, is a question that only time will answer. It's also a story that must be left for the next generation to write. But for the men and women who will guide the firm in the years ahead, the possibilities are only as limited as their imagination and energy, enriched and empowered by a legacy of wisdom inherited from 75 years of success. ■

Partner Biographies

"… We older men have a deep and great pride in our profession which we are anxious to pass on to you. We do not want to preach to you. We want to help you, to ask you to love your work as we have learned to love ours."

Enoch Needles

Louis Russell Ash

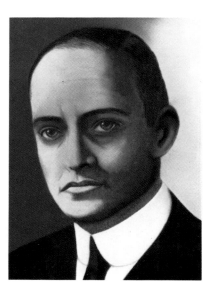

DOB: September 27, 1873
DOD: April 7, 1930
BIRTHPLACE: Union County, Kentucky
EDUCATION: University of Arkansas, B.C.E., 1893; University of Arkansas, B.E.E., 1894; University of Arkansas, C.E., 1902; University of Chicago, graduate work
JOINED HNTB: Harrington, Howard & Ash, 1914-1928; Ash-Howard-Needles & Tammen, 1928-1930
OTHER PROFESSIONAL EXPERIENCE: Mathematics Professor, Coe College, Cedar Rapids, Iowa, 1895-1901; Waddell & Hedrick, 1901-1907; I.G. Hedrick, 1907-1910; City Engineer, Kansas City, Missouri, 1910-1913; Waddell & Harrington, 1913-1914; City Manager, Wichita, Kansas, 1917-1919
PARTNERSHIP TENURE: 1914-1930
LEADERSHIP POSTS: Member, City Planning Commission, Kansas City, Missouri; Trustee, Park College, Parkville, Missouri; Director, Federal Trust Company, Kansas City, Missouri
SELECTED PROJECTS: Vicksburg Bridge, Vicksburg, Mississippi

John Lyle Harrington

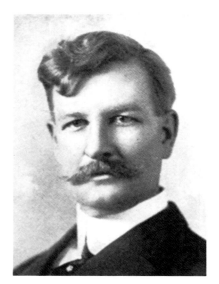

DOB: December 7, 1848
DOD: May 20, 1942
BIRTHPLACE: Lawrence, Kansas
EDUCATION: University of Kansas, B.S., A.B., C.E., with honors, 1895; McGill University, Montreal, Quebec, Canada, B.S. and M.S., 1906
JOINED HNTB: Harrington, Howard & Ash, 1914-1928
OTHER PROFESSIONAL EXPERIENCE: From 1895-1901: J.A.L. Waddell, Kansas City, Missouri; Elmira Bridge Company, Elmira, New York; Peycoyd Iron Works, Philadelphia, Pennsylvania; Keystone Bridge Works of Carnegie Steel Company, Pittsburgh, Pennsylvania; Bucyrus Company, South Milwaukee, Wisconsin; C.W. Hunt Company, New York, New York, 1901-1905; Locomotive and Machine Company, Montreal, Quebec, Canada, 1905-1906; Waddell & Harrington, 1907-1914; Harrington & Cortelyou, 1928-1942
PARTNERSHIP TENURE: 1914-1928
LEADERSHIP POSTS: President, ASME, 1923; Member, American Engineering Council, 1926-1932; Presidential appointee, Engineers Advisory Board of the Reconstruction Finance Corporation, 1932
SELECTED PROJECTS: Pond Creille Bridge, Sand Point, Idaho; Mississippi River Bridge at Louisiana, Missouri; Mississippi River Bridge at Cape Girardeau, Missouri; Colorado River Bridge at Blythe, California; Welland Canal Bridges, Ontario, Canada
SELECTED HONORS: Honorary Doctorate, Case School of Applied Science, 1930

Ernest Emmanuel Howard

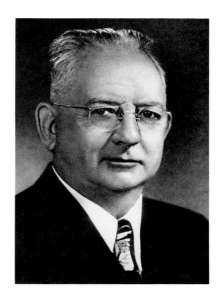

DOB: February 29, 1880
DOD: August 20, 1953
BIRTHPLACE: Toronto, Ontario, Canada
EDUCATION: University of Texas, Austin, Texas, B.S. and C.E., 1900
JOINED HNTB: Harrington, Howard & Ash, 1914-1928; Ash-Howard-Needles & Tammen, 1928-1940; Howard, Needles, Tammen & Bergendoff, 1941-1953
OTHER PROFESSIONAL EXPERIENCE: University of Texas, Instructor, Department of Civil Engineering, 1900-1901; Waddell & Hedrick, 1901-1907; Waddell & Harrington, 1907-1914; Corps of Engineers, U.S. Army, 1918-1919
PARTNERSHIP TENURE: 1914-1953
LEADERSHIP POSTS: President, Chamber of Commerce, Kansas City, Missouri; Chairman, Board of Directors, Kansas City University (now University of Missouri-Kansas City), 1930-1953; Chairman, American delegation, Third International Congress of the International Association of Bridge and Structural Engineers, 1948; President, ASCE, 1950
SELECTED PROJECTS: White House renovation, Washington, D.C.; Armour-Swift-Burlington Bridge, Kansas City, Missouri; River Don Bridge, Rostoff, Russia; Welland Canal Bridges, Ontario, Canada; Cuyahoga River Bridges, Ohio
SELECTED HONORS: Thomas Rowland Fitch Prize, ASCE, 1921; Doctor of Engineering, honoris causa, University of Nebraska, 1939; Doctor of Engineering, University of Missouri, 1951

Enoch Ray Needles

DOB: October 29, 1888
DOD: January 5, 1972
BIRTHPLACE: Brookfield, Missouri
EDUCATION: Missouri School of Mines, B.S.C.E., 1914; Missouri School of Mines, C.E., 1920
JOINED HNTB: Harrington, Howard & Ash, 1917-1928; Ash-Howard-Needles & Tammen, 1928-1940; Howard, Needles, Tammen & Bergendoff, 1940-1962
OTHER PROFESSIONAL EXPERIENCE: Kansas City Southern Railroad, 1915-1916; Kansas City Terminal Railroad, 1916-1917; Corps of Engineers, U.S. Army, 1942-1945
PARTNERSHIP TENURE: 1928-1962
LEADERSHIP POSTS: President, AICE, 1946; President, ARBA, 1949-1951; President, ASCE, 1955-1956; President, EJC, 1958-1959
SELECTED PROJECTS: Chesapeake & Delaware Canal Bridges, Delaware; Pulaski Skyway, New Jersey; Maine Turnpike; Delaware Memorial Bridge, Wilmington, Delaware; New Jersey Turnpike
SELECTED HONORS: Doctor of Engineering (honorary), Missouri School of Mines, 1937; Legion of Merit Award, U.S. Army, 1945; Designation of "Needles Room" at ARBA (now ARBTA) headquarters in Washington, D.C., 1965

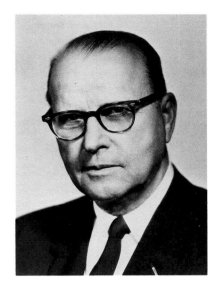

Henry Casper Tammen

DOB: November 15, 1884
DOD: July 7, 1961
BIRTHPLACE: Yankton, South Dakota
EDUCATION: University of California, 1906
JOINED HNTB: Waddell & Harrington, 1908-1914; Harrington, Howard & Ash, 1914-1928; Ash-Howard-Needles & Tammen, 1928-1940; Howard, Needles, Tammen & Bergendoff, 1941-1949
OTHER PROFESSIONAL EXPERIENCE: Western Pacific Railroad, 1906-1908
PARTNERSHIP TENURE: 1928-1949
LEADERSHIP POSTS: Councilor, AICE, 1946-1949
SELECTED PROJECTS: Welland Canal Bridges, Ontario, Canada; Harlem River (lift span), Triborough Bridge, New York, New York; Old Lyme-Old Saybrook Bridge, Connecticut; Delaware Memorial Bridge, Wilmington, Delaware; Edison Bridge, Perth Amboy, New Jersey

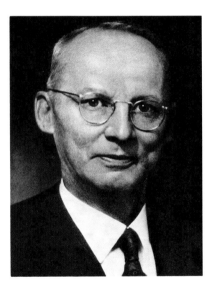

Ruben Nathaniel Bergendoff

DOB: January 4, 1899
DOD: November 14, 1976
BIRTHPLACE: Newman Grove, Nebraska
EDUCATION: Augustana College, Rock Island, Illinois, one year; University of Pennsylvania, B.S.C.E., 1921
JOINED HNTB: Harrington, Howard & Ash, 1922-1928; Ash-Howard-Needles & Tammen, 1928-1940; Howard, Needles, Tammen & Bergendoff, 1941-1968
OTHER PROFESSIONAL EXPERIENCE: North Carolina State Highway Department, 1921-1922
PARTNERSHIP TENURE: 1940-1968
LEADERSHIP POSTS: President, Rotary Club, Kansas City, Missouri; Member, Board of Trustees, Midwest Research Institute
SELECTED PROJECTS: South Omaha Bridge, Omaha, Nebraska; Broadway and Paseo Bridges, Kansas City, Missouri; Kansas City Freeway Sytem; Toledo Expressway System; Mississippi River Bridge at Dubuque, Iowa; Florida Turnpike
SELECTED HONORS: Life Member, ASCE; Thomas Rowland Fitch Award (co-winner), ASCE, 1950; Distinguished Service in Engineering Award, University of Missouri, 1957

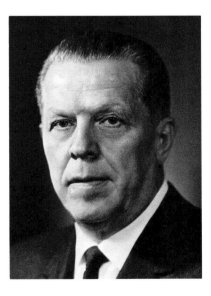

Theodore Jessup Cambern

DOB: September 29, 1901
DOD: May 2, 1979
BIRTHPLACE: Erie, Kansas
EDUCATION: University of Kansas, B.S.C.E., 1925
JOINED HNTB: 1925
OTHER PROFESSIONAL EXPERIENCE: Harrington & Cortelyou, 1928-1940
PARTNERSHIP TENURE: 1950-1966
SELECTED PROJECTS: Mississippi River Bridge, Helena, Arkansas; Calcasieu River Bridge, Lake Charles, Louisiana; Shreveport Expressway System, Shreveport, Louisiana; Dallas-Ft. Worth Turnpike; Duluth-Superior Bridge, Duluth, Minnesota

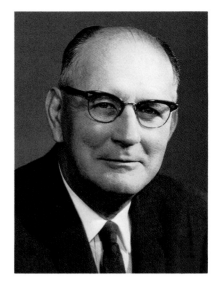

James Powers Exum

DOB: October 11, 1900
DOD: December 22, 1977
BIRTHPLACE: Mobeetie, Texas
EDUCATION: University of Texas, B.S.C.E., 1922
JOINED HNTB: Harrington, Howard & Ash, 1922-1924, 1925-1928; Ash-Howard-Needles & Tammen, 1928-1932; Howard, Needles, Tammen & Bergendoff, 1948-1965
OTHER PROFESSIONAL EXPERIENCE: Bridge Division, Texas Highway Department, 1924-1925, 1932-1948
PARTNERSHIP TENURE: 1950-1965
LEADERSHIP POSTS: President, AICE, 1960; State Bridge Engineer, Texas
SELECTED PROJECTS: Maine Turnpike, extension; New Jersey Turnpike, extension; Woodrow Wilson Memorial Bridge, Washington, D.C.; Silas N. Pearman Bridge, Charleston, South Carolina
SELECTED HONORS: Distinguished Graduate Award, University of Texas, 1965

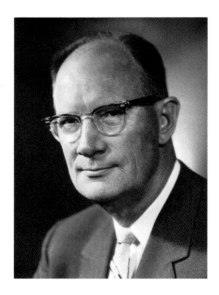

125

Ellis E. Paul

DOB: August 6, 1900
DOD: July 1, 1984
BIRTHPLACE: Kansas City, Missouri
EDUCATION: University of Kansas, B.S.C.E., 1922; University of Kansas, C.E., 1931
JOINED HNTB: 1922
OTHER PROFESSIONAL EXPERIENCE: U.S. Air Corps, 1942-1945
PARTNERSHIP TENURE: 1950-1965
LEADERSHIP POSTS: U.S. Representative, International Congress on Lighting
SELECTED PROJECTS: Burlington-Bristol Bridge, Burlington, New Jersey; Harlem River Bridge, New York, New York; Bronx Kills Bridge, New York, New York; Delaware Memorial Bridge, Wilmington, Delaware; Massachusetts Turnpike

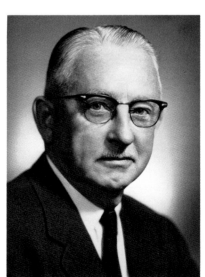

Josef Sorkin

DOB: April 14, 1906

BIRTHPLACE: Tchernigove, Russia

EDUCATION: University of Nebraska, B.S.C.E., 1929

JOINED HNTB: 1939

OTHER PROFESSIONAL EXPERIENCE: Nebraska State Highway Department, 1929-1934; Montana State Highway Commission, 1934-1935; Central Nebraska Public Power and Irrigation District, 1935-1938

PARTNERSHIP TENURE: 1950-1969

LEADERSHIP POSTS: Chairman, HNTB Executive Committee, 1969; President, Kansas City Section, ASCE; Board of Trustees, University of Nebraska Foundation

SELECTED PROJECTS: Potomac River Bridge (14th Street), Washington, D.C.; Missouri River Bridge, Leavenworth, Kansas; Kansas Turnpike (Kansas City to Oklahoma border); Mississippi River Bridge (Burlington Railroad), Quincy, Illinois; Rio-Niteroi Bridge over Guanabara Bay, Brazil

SELECTED HONORS: Grand Conceptor, Rio-Niteroi Bridge, Brazil; First Prize, AISC, Niobara River Bridge, Valentine, Nebraska, 1932 (accorded listing in "The National Register of Historic Places" 1988); Thomas Rowland Fitch Prize (co-winner), ASCE, 1950; Honorary and Life Member, ASCE, 1987

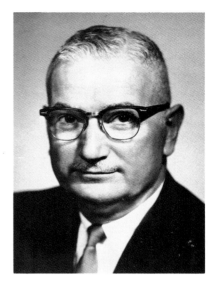

Elmer Knowles Timby

DOB: December 19, 1905

BIRTHPLACE: Salt Lake City, Utah

EDUCATION: Ohio State University, B.S.C.E., 1928; Ohio State University, C.E., 1933

JOINED HNTB: Ash-Howard-Needles & Tammen, 1938, 1939, summers; Howard, Needles, Tammen & Bergendoff, 1941-1943, 1949-1968

OTHER PROFESSIONAL EXPERIENCE: Princeton University, Civil Engineering Department, 1929-1949 (Chairman, 1946-1949); U.S. Navy, 1943-1946, Design & Control, floating dry docks in advance areas; Consultant on design, Golden Gate & San Francisco, Oakland Bridges

PARTNERSHIP TENURE: 1950-1968

LEADERSHIP POSTS: Vice President and representative at United Nations, IABSE, 1966-1969, 1972-1980; Chairman, Committee on Federal Procurement of Architect/Engineer Services, 1968-1970; Vice President, ARTBA, 1968; Bureau of Public Roads Commission on Long Span Bridges; GSA Commission on Selection of A/E Consultants

SELECTED PROJECTS: Delaware Memorial Bridge, Wilmington, Delaware; West Virginia Turnpike; Miami International Airport, Miami, Florida; Shirley Highway Improvement, Alexandria, Virginia; Introduction of electronic computation to highway and structural design

SELECTED HONORS: Engineer of the Year in Private Practice, NSPE, 1971; Friedman Professional Recognition Award, ASCE, 1971; Past Presidents' Award for Public Service in Engineering, ACEC, 1980; Honorary Member, ASCE; Past President, Engineering Division, ARTBA

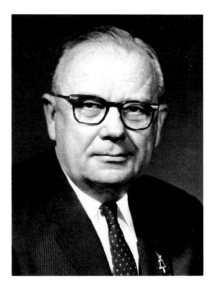

Carl Lee Erb, Jr.

DOB: September 11, 1913

DOD: December 5, 1971

BIRTHPLACE: Lincoln, Nebraska

EDUCATION: University of Nebraska, B.S.C.E., 1935

JOINED HNTB: 1941

OTHER PROFESSIONAL EXPERIENCE: Chicago, Burlington and Quincy Railroad, 1935-1937; Central Nebraska Public Power and Irrigation District

PARTNERSHIP TENURE: 1957-1971

LEADERSHIP POSTS: President, AICE, 1970

SELECTED PROJECTS: Maine Turnpike; Denver-Boulder Turnpike, Colorado; Cleveland Expressway System, Cuyahoga County; Ohio Freeway System; Detroit-Superior Bridge Rehabilitation, Cleveland, Ohio

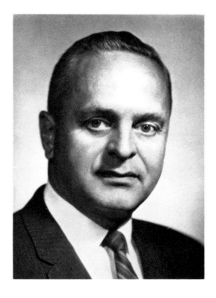

Carl H. Peterson

DOB: June 1, 1913
BIRTHPLACE: Brooklyn, New York
EDUCATION: Louisiana State University, B.S.C.E., 1938
JOINED HNTB: 1939
OTHER PROFESSIONAL EXPERIENCE: Louisiana Highway Department, 1938-1939; Fraser-Brace Engineering Company, St. Louis, Missouri, 1941-1942; Corps of Engineers, U.S. Army, 1942-1946
PARTNERSHIP TENURE: 1962-1967
SELECTED PROJECTS: Delaware Memorial Bridge, Wilmington, Delaware; New Jersey Turnpike; West Virginia Turnpike; Florida Turnpike; Miami International Airport

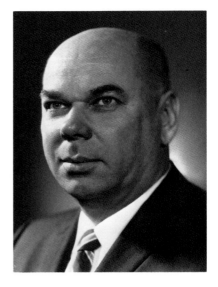

Frank E. Bleistein

DOB: February 2, 1915
DOD: April 20, 1969
BIRTHPLACE: Kansas City, Missouri
EDUCATION: University of Kansas, B.S.C.E., 1936
JOINED HNTB: 1946
OTHER PROFESSIONAL EXPERIENCE: Kansas Highway Department, 1936-1937; Chicago, Rock Island and Pacific Railway Company, 1937-1941; Ed. H. Honnen Construction Company, Colorado Springs, Colorado, 1941-1943; Civil Engineer Corps, U.S. Navy, 1943-1946
PARTNERSHIP TENURE: 1964-1969
SELECTED PROJECTS: Hood Canal Floating Bridge, Seattle, Washington; I-5 Freeway, Seattle, Washington; Milwaukee Road Railroad Bridge, Hastings, Minnesota

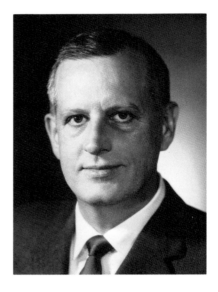

H. Christopher Lamberton, Jr.

DOB: February 28, 1918
BIRTHPLACE: Kansas City, Missouri
EDUCATION: University of Kansas, B.S.C.E., 1942; New York University, M.S.C.E., 1949
JOINED HNTB: 1946
OTHER PROFESSIONAL EXPERIENCE: Burns & McDonnell Engineering Company, Kansas City, Missouri, 1940-1941; Panhandle Eastern Pipe Line Company, Kansas City, Missouri, 1939-1940; Blaw-Knox Company, Pittsburgh, Pennsylvania, 1942-1944; U.S. Marine Corps, 1944-1946
PARTNERSHIP TENURE: 1964-1981
LEADERSHIP POSTS: Chairman, Aerospace Transport Division, ASCE, 1967-1968; Chairman, Committee on Direct Connecting Ramps, ITE, 1968; Chairman, HNTB Executive Committee, 1972
SELECTED PROJECTS: Hartsfield-Atlanta International Airport; Miami International Airport; Second Delaware Memorial Bridge, Wilmington, Delaware; Rio-Niteroi Bridge, Brazil; Delaware Turnpike
SELECTED HONORS: Design in Steel, American Institute of Steel Construction, 1965; Excellence, Outstanding Design, Public Works Construction

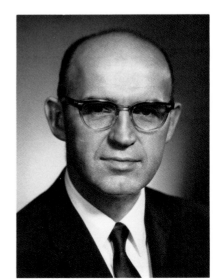

James Francis Finn

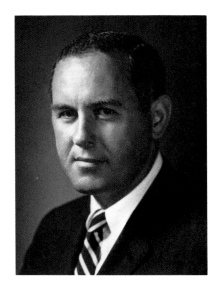

DOB: July 11, 1924

BIRTHPLACE: Jersey City, New Jersey

EDUCATION: St. Peter's College, Jersey City, New Jersey, 1942; Stevens Institute of Technology, 1946-1949; Newark College of Engineering, B.S.C.E., 1953

JOINED HNTB: 1956

OTHER PROFESSIONAL EXPERIENCE: Corps of Engineers, U.S. Army, 1943-1946; New Jersey Department of Conservation and Economic Development, 1949-1956

PARTNERSHIP TENURE: 1965-1987

LEADERSHIP POSTS: Chairman, HNTB Executive Committee, 1973-1974; Administrative Contact Partner, HNTB, 1976-1986

SELECTED PROJECTS: New Jersey Turnpike; I-287, New Jersey; Route 24 Freeway, New Jersey; I-280, Harrison, New Jersey; Route 15 Freeway, New Jersey

SELECTED HONORS: Fellow, ACEC; Fellow, ASCE

Paul Lowe Heineman

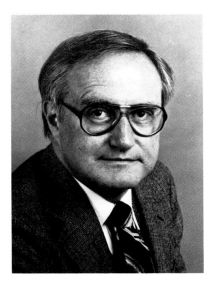

DOB: October 24, 1924

BIRTHPLACE: Omaha, Nebraska

EDUCATION: University of Omaha, 1942; Iowa State University, Ames, Iowa, B.S.C.E., 1945; Iowa State University, Ames, Iowa, M.S., 1948

JOINED HNTB: 1948

OTHER PROFESSIONAL EXPERIENCE: Civil Engineer Corps, U.S. Navy, 1945-1946; Iowa State University, Instructor, Department of Theoretical and Applied Mechanics, 1946-1948

PARTNERSHIP TENURE: 1965-1987

LEADERSHIP POSTS: Chairman, HNTB Executive Committee, 1979-1980; Treasurer, Director and Executive Committee, The Road Information Program, 1983-1988

SELECTED PROJECTS: Mobile River Bridges, Mobile, Alabama; Missouri River Bridge, Sioux City, Iowa; I-70 and I-670, Kansas City, Kansas; Missouri River Bridges, Burlington Northern Railroad, Sioux City, Iowa and Rulo, Nebraska; Interstate Routes 235 and 380, Des Moines and Cedar Rapids, Iowa

SELECTED HONORS: Professional Achievement Citation in Engineering, Iowa State University, 1988; Fellow, ACEC; Life Fellow, ASCE

128

Joseph Henry Looper

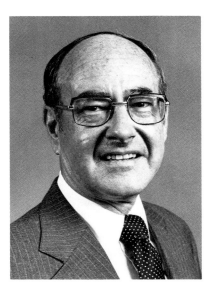

DOB: March 1, 1926

BIRTHPLACE: Lovell, Wyoming

EDUCATION: University of Colorado, Boulder, Colorado, B.S.C.E., 1945

JOINED HNTB: 1954

OTHER PROFESSIONAL EXPERIENCE: U.S. Navy, 1943-1946, 1952-1954; Bureau of Public Roads, Washington, D.C., 1946-1952

PARTNERSHIP TENURE: 1965-1980

LEADERSHIP POSTS: Twice Chairman, HNTB Partnership and Executive Committee; President, Rotary Club of Milwaukee Northwest, 1970-1971; Governor, District 627, Rotary International, 1986-1987

SELECTED PROJECTS: Sunshine State Parkway, Florida; Milwaukee Harbor Bridge, Milwaukee, Wisconsin; Marquette Interchange, Milwaukee, Wisconsin; Crosstown Expressway, Chicago, Illinois; I-70, Glenwood Canyon, Colorado

SELECTED HONORS: Engineer of the Year, Engineers and Scientists of Milwaukee, 1969; Captain, Civil Engineer Corps, U.S.N.R.(ret)

Robert Oyloe Drange

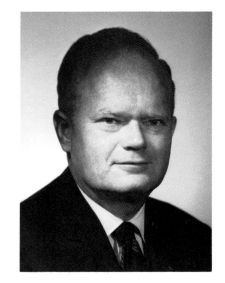

DOB: March 14, 1924

BIRTHPLACE: Watertown, South Dakota

EDUCATION: South Dakota School of Mines & Technology, 1942-1943; Iowa State University, B.S.C.E., 1945

JOINED HNTB: 1948

OTHER PROFESSIONAL EXPERIENCE: Civil Engineer Corps, U.S. Navy, 1943-1946, 1952-1954; Rust Engineering Company, 1946-1948

PARTNERSHIP TENURE: 1966-1977

LEADERSHIP POSTS: President, Philadelphia Section, ASCE; President, Planning and Design Division, ARTBA; Chairman, Committee for Federal Architectural-Engineering Services; Vice President, ARTBA

SELECTED PROJECTS: Omaha Expressway System; Kansas Turnpike; Charleston, West Virginia Freeway System; West Virginia Turnpike; Kansas City Stadium, Arena and Convention Center Study

SELECTED HONORS: Guy Kelcey Award, ARTBA; *Who's Who in America — 40th Edition*; Life Fellow, ASCE, ACEC

Donald Edward Harper

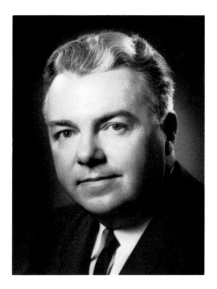

DOB: May 16, 1922

BIRTHPLACE: Kansas City, Missouri

EDUCATION: Junior College of Kansas City; University of Illinois, B.S.C.E., 1943

JOINED HNTB: 1948

PRIOR PROFESSIONAL EXPERIENCE: Curtiss-Wright Corporation, St. Louis, Missouri, 1943-1944; U.S. Navy, 1944-1946; Black & Veatch, Kansas City, Missouri, 1946-1948

PARTNERSHIP TENURE: 1966-1971

LEADERSHIP POSTS: Chairman, Engineering Committee of IBTTA, three years; Vice President, HNTB International, Inc., 1971-1975

SELECTED PROJECTS: Dallas-Fort Worth Turnpike, Texas; Dallas North Tollway, Texas; San Luis Pass Bridge, Galveston, Texas; Mississippi River Bridge, Helena, Arkansas; Lake Charles Bypass, Louisiana

SELECTED HONORS: Bronze Star Medal, World War II; Life Member, Fellow, ASCE

129

Bernard Henry Rottinghaus

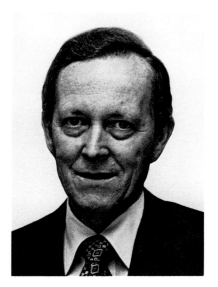

DOB: January 26, 1922

BIRTHPLACE: Corning, Kansas

EDUCATION: Kansas State University, B.S.M.E., 1948

JOINED HNTB: 1949

OTHER PROFESSIONAL EXPERIENCE: U.S. Navy Air Corps, 1942-1945

PARTNERSHIP TENURE: 1966-1978

LEADERSHIP POSTS: Board of Directors, Nemaha Valley Community Hospital, 1982-1986; Chairman, TRB Committee A2A02, 1970-1979; Chairman, ASHTO Committee (Transit), 1973

SELECTED PROJECTS: Capitol Approach Interchange, St. Paul, Minnesota; I-35, Duluth, Minnesota; I-75, Dayton, Ohio; Hiawatha Avenue Interchange Bridge, Minneapolis, Minnesota; Cedar Avenue Bridge, Minneapolis, Minnesota

SELECTED HONORS: Service Award, TRB, 1979; ASCE Life Member

Gerard Francis Fox

DOB: January 9, 1923

BIRTHPLACE: New York City, New York

EDUCATION: Cornell University, B.C.E. with distinction, 1948; Polytechnic Institute of Brooklyn, graduate work, 1948-1952; Columbia University, graduate work, 1955-1958

JOINED HNTB: 1948

OTHER PROFESSIONAL EXPERIENCE: U.S. Air Force, 1942-1946; Columbia University, Adjunct Professor of Civil Engineering & Engineering Mechanics, 1967-1988

PARTNERSHIP TENURE: 1967-1988

LEADERSHIP POSTS: Vice President, IABSE, 1979-1987; Chairman, Structural Division, ASCE, 1967; Vice Chairman, Structural Stability Research Council, 1986-1989

SELECTED PROJECTS: Rio-Niteroi Bridge, Brazil; Penang Bridge, Malaysia; Dame Point Bridge, Jacksonville, Florida; Newark Bay Bridge, New Jersey; Metro Transit System, Washington, D.C.

SELECTED HONORS: National Academy of Engineering, 1976; Ernest E. Howard Award, ASCE, 1980; John A. Roebling Medal, International Bridge Conference, 1987

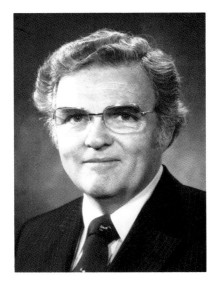

William Mahler Wachter

DOB: April 17, 1917

BIRTHPLACE: Greensboro, North Carolina

EDUCATION: Oregon State University, B.S.C.E., 1939; University of Iowa, M.S.C.E., 1941

JOINED HNTB: 1956-1957, 1963-1982

OTHER PROFESSIONAL EXPERIENCE: Corps of Engineers, U.S. Army, 1942-1946; University of Hawaii, 1948-1956, 1959-1963; Superintendent of Public Works, Hawaii, 1957-1959; Territorial Highway Engineer, Hawaii, 1957-1959; Hawaii, Governor's Cabinet, 1957-1959

PARTNERSHIP TENURE: 1967-1982

LEADERSHIP POSTS: Chairman, Board of Harbor Commissioners, Hawaii, 1957-1959; Chairman, Hawaii Water Authority, Hawaii, 1957-1961; Dean-Engineering, Vice President-Administration, University of Hawaii, 1959-1963

SELECTED PROJECTS: I-695, Boston, Massachusetts; Massachusetts Route 2 Location Study, Massachusetts; Massachusetts Turnpike; Iran Toll Road; East-West Center, at University of Hawaii

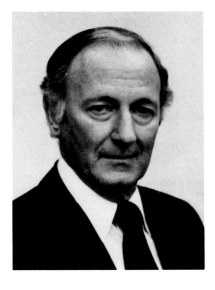

Browning Crow

DOB: May 25, 1923

BIRTHPLACE: Kansas City, Missouri

EDUCATION: University of Missouri, B.A., 1944; University of Missouri, B.S.C.E., 1948

JOINED HNTB: 1948

OTHER PROFESSIONAL EXPERIENCE: U.S. Navy, 1943-1946

PARTNERSHIP TENURE: 1968-1987

LEADERSHIP POSTS: First Chairman of PSC, 1985-1986

SELECTED PROJECTS: Denver-Boulder Turnpike, Colorado; Ohio Turnpike; Transportation Research Center, Ohio; I-71 Freeway, Cleveland, Ohio; I-271 Freeway, Cuyahoga County, Ohio

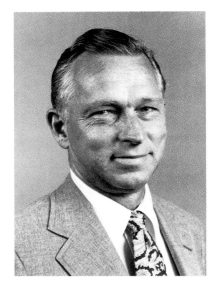

Charles Thomas Hennigan

DOB: December 18, 1930
BIRTHPLACE: Brooklyn, New York
EDUCATION: City College of New York, B.S.C.E., 1954
JOINED HNTB: 1954
PARTNERSHIP TENURE: 1969-Present
LEADERSHIP POSTS: Chairman of the Partnership, 1981-1983
SELECTED PROJECTS: New Jersey Turnpike; I-84 Interchange, Waterbury, Connecticut; Virginia Beach-Norfolk Expressway, Virginia; Capitol Beltway, Washington, D.C.; East-West Expressway, Orlando, Florida

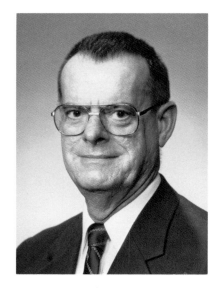

Edgar Burton Johnson

DOB: March 1, 1923
BIRTHPLACE: Kansas City, Kansas
EDUCATION: Kansas State University, B.S.C.E. with honors, 1947
JOINED HNTB: 1951
OTHER PROFESSIONAL EXPERIENCE: Kansas State University, Instructor, Civil Engineering Department, 1947-1949; Finney & Turnipseed, Topeka, Kansas, 1949-1951
PARTNERSHIP TENURE: 1970-1985
SELECTED PROJECTS: Kansas Turnpike; Mt. Baker Ridge Tunnel, Seattle, Washington; I-5 Seattle Freeway; Factoria/South Bellevue Interchanges (I-90); Penang Bridge, Malaysia
SELECTED HONORS: ASCE John O. Bickel Award, 1987; ENR Award for Chief Joseph Dam Project, 1980; ENR Award for I-90 Tunnel, 1986; Grand Conceptor, I-90 Tunnel, Seattle, Washington

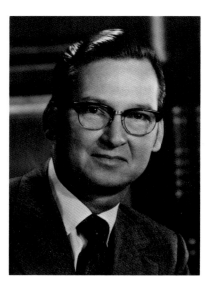

131

Daniel Joseph Watkins

DOB: December 18, 1923
BIRTHPLACE: Albia, Iowa
EDUCATION: Albia Junior College, 1940-1942; Iowa State University, B.S.C.E., 1947
JOINED HNTB: 1947
OTHER PROFESSIONAL EXPERIENCE: U.S. Navy, 1943-1946
PARTNERSHIP TENURE: 1970-1988
LEADERSHIP POSTS: Chairman, Board of Directors, Carondelet Health Corporation, 1986, 1987; Chairman, Chamber of Commerce, Kansas City, Missouri, 1982-1983; Chairman, Board of Regents, Rockhurst College, Kansas City, Missouri, 1987, 1988
SELECTED PROJECTS: Grand/Main Plan, Kansas City, Missouri; Dallas North Tollway, Dallas, Texas; Jesse H. Jones Memorial Bridge, Houston, Texas; Wornall Road Bridge, Kansas City, Missouri; H. Roe Bartle Convention Center, Kansas City, Missouri
SELECTED HONORS: "Councilman of the Year," Prairie Village, Kansas, 1970; "Professional Achievement Citation in Engineering" from Iowa State University, 1984; 1987 Civic Citation Award by the National Conference of Christians and Jews, Greater Kansas City Region; recipient, Marston Medal from Iowa State University, 1989

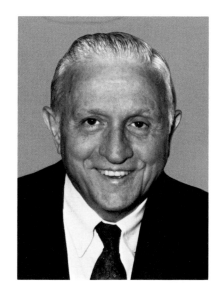

George Krikor Erganian

DOB: September 11, 1917
BIRTHPLACE: San Francisco, California
EDUCATION: City College of New York, 1936; Purdue University, B.S.C.E., 1943; Purdue University, M.S.C.E., 1947
JOINED HNTB: 1973
OTHER PROFESSIONAL EXPERIENCE: Tennessee Valley Authority, 1943-1944; Indiana State Board of Health, 1947-1951; Henry B. Steeg & Associates, Indianapolis, Indiana, 1951-1973
PARTNERSHIP TENURE: 1973-1981
LEADERSHIP POSTS: President, Henry D. Steeg and Associates, 1961-1973; President, Indiana Water Pollution Control Association, 1955, 1961; Member, Construction Grants Advisory Group to the EPA, 1981-1985; Commissioner from the State of Indiana to the Midwest Compact for Low-Level Nuclear Waste Disposal, 1982-1986
SELECTED PROJECTS: Sanitary Disposal Wastewater Projects, Richmond, Indiana; Environmental Projects, Anderson, Indiana; Wastewater Projects, Fort Wayne, Indiana; Water and Wastewater Projects, Lafayette, Indiana; Wastewater Treatment, Evansville, Indiana
SELECTED HONORS: Arthur Sidney Bedell Award, Water Pollution Control Federation, 1963; Honorary Membership, AWWA, 1984; "Sagamore-of-the-Wabash" (Governor Otis R. Bowen, 1981, and Governor Robert D. Orr, 1986)

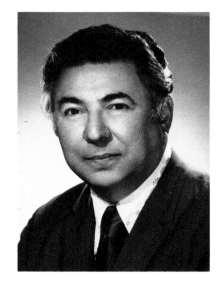

Daniel John Spigai

DOB: March 4, 1933
BIRTHPLACE: Bronx, New York
EDUCATION: Manhattan College, B.S.C.E., 1954
JOINED HNTB: 1957
OTHER PROFESSIONAL EXPERIENCE: New York Central Railroad, 1954-1955; U.S. Army, 1955-1957
NAMED ASSOCIATE: 1971
PARTNERSHIP TENURE: 1974-Present
LEADERSHIP POSTS: Chairman, ARTBA, 1988; Chairman, HNTB Partnership, 1986-1987; Board of Directors, St. Mary's Conference, 1988
SELECTED PROJECTS: Route 15 Improvement, New Jersey; 1969 Turnpike Widening, New Jersey; Buffalo International Airport; Baltimore-Washington International Airport; Washington National Airport

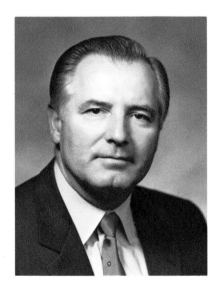

132

Ralph E. Myers

DOB: November 30, 1917
BIRTHPLACE: Kansas City, Missouri
EDUCATION: University of Illinois, B.S., Architecture
JOINED HNTB: 1975
OTHER PROFESSIONAL EXPERIENCE: Clarence E. Kivett, Architect, 1940-1941; Finley Engineering College, 1940-1941; North American Aviation, 1941-1945; Kivett & Myers, 1945-1974
PARTNERSHIP TENURE: 1975-1982
LEADERSHIP POSTS: Founding Member, Board of Directors, The Southgate Bank, 1956-1988; Director, Kansas City Chapter of AIA, 8 years; Partner, Kivett & Myers, 1945-1974
SELECTED PROJECTS: Kansas City International Airport, Kansas City, Missouri; Harry S Truman Sports Complex, Kansas City, Missouri; Missouri Public Service Building, Lee's Summit, Missouri; Doubletree Hotel, Monterey, California; Missouri State Office Building, Kansas City, Missouri
SELECTED HONORS: Plym Prize, 1942 Airport Design & 1951 Architectural Design; LeBrun Competition, 1950, Railroad Station; Brunner Fellowship, Research Grant to produce movie, "Architecture, USA," 1954-1955; Fellow, AIA

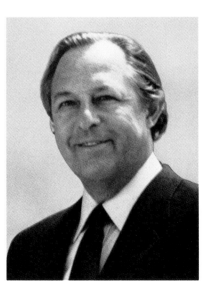

John LeGrand Cotton

DOB: May 29, 1930
BIRTHPLACE: Davenport, Iowa
EDUCATION: University of Virginia, 1948-1949; University of Notre Dame, B.S.C.E., 1951
JOINED HNTB: 1954
OTHER PROFESSIONAL EXPERIENCE: U.S. Navy, 1951-1954
NAMED ASSOCIATE: 1974
PARTNERSHIP TENURE: 1978-Present
LEADERSHIP POSTS: Chairman, HNTB Executive Committee, 1988-Present; Construction Industry President's Forum
SELECTED PROJECTS: West Bank Expressway, Louisiana; Mississippi River Bridge at Natchez; I-220 Shreveport, Louisiana; I-49 North-South Expressway, Louisiana; I-75, Dayton, Ohio

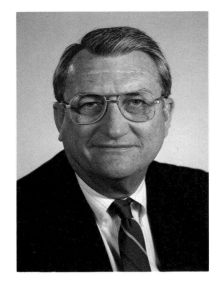

Francis Xavier Hall

DOB: October 2, 1930
BIRTHPLACE: North Bergen, New Jersey
EDUCATION: New Jersey Institute of Technology, B.S.C.E., 1952; Rensselaer Polytechnic Institute, M.C.E., 1955
JOINED HNTB: 1955
OTHER PROFESSIONAL EXPERIENCE: Lockheed Aircraft Corporation, 1952; E.I. DuPont DeNemours, Inc., 1952; Corps of Engineers, U.S. Army, 1952-1954
NAMED ASSOCIATE: 1973
PARTNERSHIP TENURE: 1978-Present
LEADERSHIP POSTS: Chairman, Thomas K. Dyer, Inc., 1982-Present; President, Engineers Club of Boston, 1985-1988; Vice President, SAME, 1982-1983
SELECTED PROJECTS: Southwest Corridor Project — Section III, Boston, Massachusetts; Massachusetts Turnpike; Ninth Street Bridge & Approaches, Richmond, Virginia; Second Delaware Memorial Bridge, Wilmington, Delaware; Shirley Highway Improvements, Alexandria, Virginia

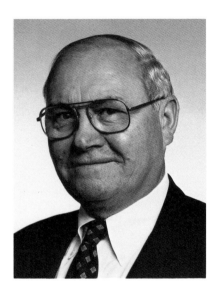

133

Robert Stephen Coma

DOB: December 23, 1936
BIRTHPLACE: McKeesport, Pennsylvania
EDUCATION: Rose-Hulman Institute of Technology, B.S.C.E., 1959
JOINED HNTB: 1973
OTHER PROFESSIONAL EXPERIENCE: Henry B. Steeg & Associates, 1961-1973; Indiana State Highway Commission, 1959-1961
NAMED ASSOCIATE: 1973
PARTNERSHIP TENURE: 1980-Present
LEADERSHIP POSTS: Administrative Contact Partner, 1986-Present; Rose-Hulman Consulting Engineering Council, 1979-Present; Carmel Clay School Board, 1976-1984
SELECTED PROJECTS: City of Carmel, Indiana Civic Square; Hoosier Dome Joint Venture, Indianapolis, Indiana; Water and Wastewater Projects, Anderson, Indiana

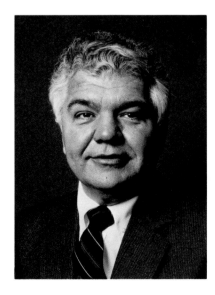

Donald Albert Dupies

DOB: April 17, 1934

BIRTHPLACE: Waukegan, Illinois

EDUCATION: Marquette University, B.C.E., 1957

JOINED HNTB: 1959

OTHER PROFESSIONAL EXPERIENCE: Corps of Engineers, U.S. Army, 1957-1959

NAMED ASSOCIATE: 1974

PARTNERSHIP TENURE: 1980-Present

LEADERSHIP POSTS: Director, ASCE Board of Directors, 1983-1985; Chairman, ASCE Committee on Public Communication, 1986-1989; Chairman, HNTB Professional Services Committee, 1986-Present

SELECTED PROJECTS: Crosstown Interceptor/Inline Pump Station, Milwaukee, Wisconsin; Program Management Services-MWPAP, Milwaukee, Wisconsin; Downtown Freeways/Directional Interchanges, Milwaukee, Wisconsin; Major Bridge/Highway Improvements, Green Bay, Wisconsin; 27th Street Viaduct Replacement, Milwaukee, Wisconsin

SELECTED HONORS: Professional Achievement Award, 1985; Marquette University College of Engineering; Engineers Joint Council; *Who's Who in Engineering, 3rd Edition*; Marquis, *Who's Who in the Midwest, 16th Edition*; Veterans Administration Commendation, 1982

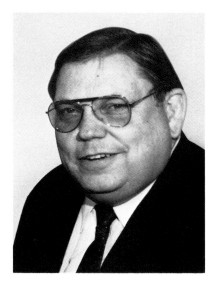

William Love

DOB: September 27, 1932

BIRTHPLACE: Des Moines, Iowa

EDUCATION: Iowa State University, Bachelor of Architecture, 1955

JOINED HNTB: 1975

OTHER PROFESSIONAL EXPERIENCE: U.S. Air Force, 1955-1957; Kivett & Myers, Kansas City, Missouri, 1957-1970, 1975; Patty Berkebile, Nelson, Love, 1970-1974; Love Architects, 1974-1975

NAMED ASSOCIATE: 1977

PARTNERSHIP TENURE: 1980-Present

LEADERSHIP POSTS: Chairman, AIA National Documents Committee, 1988-1989; President, Kansas City Chapter, AIA, 1979; Chairman, Construction Industry Affairs Convention, Kansas City, Missouri, 1973-1974

SELECTED PROJECTS: Truman Sports Complex, Kansas City, Missouri; Dana Point Resort Hotel, Dana Point, California; Palm Springs Convention Center, Palm Springs, California; Hilton Hotel, Irvine, California; Doubletree Hotel/Techmart Complex, Santa Clara, California

SELECTED HONORS: Fellow, AIA, 1987; Tau Sigma Delta, Architectural Honorary, 1954; President's Award, Kansas City Chapter AIA, 1974, 1977, 1983

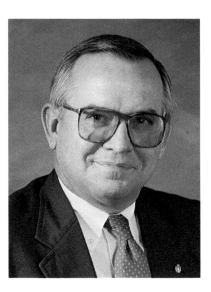

134

William Clyde Meredith

DOB: May 21, 1929

BIRTHPLACE: Omaha, Nebraska

EDUCATION: University of Nebraska, B.S.C.E., 1952

JOINED HNTB: 1952

OTHER PROFESSIONAL EXPERIENCE: U.S. Navy Air Force, 1946-1949; Corps of Engineers, U.S. Army, 1951

NAMED ASSOCIATE: 1972

PARTNERSHIP TENURE: 1981-1984

SELECTED PROJECTS: Kansas City Federal Office Building; Statehouse Underground Garage, Columbus, Ohio; Truman Medical Center Construction Management, Kansas City, Missouri; Phoenix Civic Center Expansion; San Diego Convention Center Project Management

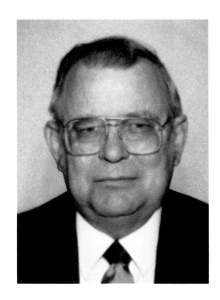

Robert D. Miller

DOB: November 27, 1937
BIRTHPLACE: Jackson, Ohio
EDUCATION: University of Colorado, B.S.C.E., 1961
JOINED HNTB: 1963
OTHER PROFESSIONAL EXPERIENCE: Bureau of Public Roads, Denver, Colorado, 1959-1962
NAMED ASSOCIATE: 1979
PARTNERSHIP TENURE: 1983-Present
LEADERSHIP POSTS: Board of Directors, American Segmental Bridge Institute; Chairman, ADOT Highway Development Group, Organizational Development Study; Member, CALTRANS Consultant Engineers Advisory Task Force; Member, City of Phoenix Revenue Resources Committee; Chairman, Bridge and Tunnel Service Group; Board Member, Phoenix Community Alliance
SELECTED PROJECTS: I-10 West Papago/Inner Loop, Phoenix, Arizona; Sky Harbor Airport Master Plan, Phoenix, Arizona; Lake Roosevelt Bridge, Arizona; Santa Clara County, California, Transportation Program; Orange County, California, Transportation Corridors
SELECTED HONORS: *Engineering News-Record Magazine*, "Those Who Made Marks in 1987"

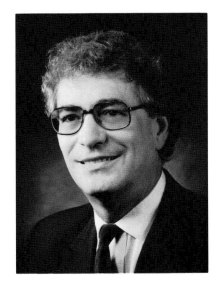

James L. Tuttle, Jr.

DOB: January 15, 1942
BIRTHPLACE: Mobile, Alabama
EDUCATION: Louisiana Tech University, 1960; Mississippi State University, B.S.C.E., 1963
JOINED HNTB: 1963
NAMED ASSOCIATE: 1980
PARTNERSHIP TENURE: 1983-Present
LEADERSHIP POSTS: Chairman, Aviation Service Group
SELECTED PROJECTS: Hartsfield-Atlanta International Airport; Miami International Airport; Florida Turnpike
SELECTED HONORS: Engineer of the Year in Construction, Georgia, 1979; "Marksman of the Year," *Engineering-News Record*, 1980

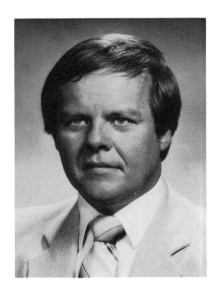

Hugh Elwood Schall

DOB: May 15, 1941
BIRTHPLACE: Pittsburgh, Pennsylvania
EDUCATION: U.S. Naval Academy, B.S., Engineering, 1963; Golden Gate University, San Francisco, California, M.B.A., 1977
JOINED HNTB: 1976
OTHER PROFESSIONAL EXPERIENCE: U.S. Navy, 1963-1970; Crown Zellerbach Corporation, Antioch, California, 1970-1974; Fibreboard Corporation, Vernon, California, 1974-1976
NAMED ASSOCIATE: 1980
PARTNERSHIP TENURE: 1984-Present
LEADERSHIP POSTS: Chairman, Secondary Fibers Committee, TAPPI
SELECTED PROJECTS: Washington State Convention and Trade Center, Seattle, Washington; Trident Submarine Base, Kings Bay, Georgia; Honolulu Municipal Complex, Honolulu, Hawaii; Illumi-Nations, EPCOT Center, Orlando, Florida; U.S. Naval Station, Puget Sound, Everett Homeport, Everett, Washington
SELECTED HONORS: ACEC First Honor Award for Gray's Harbor Jet Array System

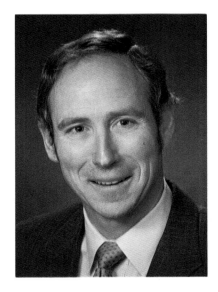

Cary Conrad Goodman

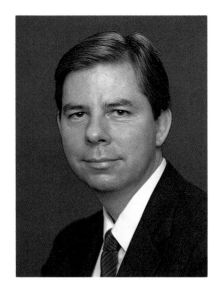

DOB: November 8, 1943
BIRTHPLACE: Kansas City, Missouri
EDUCATION: Trinity University, San Antonio, Texas, B.S., 1966, Major in Construction Technology; University of Texas, Austin, Texas, Bachelor of Architecture, with honors, 1970
JOINED HNTB: 1978
OTHER PROFESSIONAL EXPERIENCE: Urban Architects, 1970-1972; Seligson Associates, 1972-1974; Abend Singleton Associates, 1974-1976; Cary Goodman & Associates, 1976-1978
NAMED ASSOCIATE: 1980
PARTNERSHIP TENURE: 1985-Present
LEADERSHIP POSTS: Member, Board of Trustees, Kansas City Museum, 1987-Present; Member, Board of Directors, Friends of Art, Nelson-Atkins Museum of Art, 1988-Present; Member, Board of Directors, Downtown Council, Kansas City, Missouri, 1984-Present
SELECTED PROJECTS: AT&T Town Pavilion, Kansas City, Missouri; United Telecom, Corporate Offices, Fairway, Kansas; Employers Reinsurance, Corporate Offices, Overland Park, Kansas; North Supply Office Building, Industrial Airport, Kansas; White River Park Master Plan, Indianapolis, Indiana
SELECTED HONORS: Visiting Design Critic, University of Kansas and Kansas State University; Invited participant in Design for Urban Spaces, Cooper-Hewitt Museum

Gordon Holt Slaney, Jr.

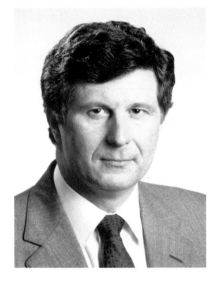

DOB: April 18, 1943
BIRTHPLACE: Brockton, Massachusetts
EDUCATION: Northeastern University, B.S.C.E., 1966; Northeastern University, M.S.C.E., 1973
JOINED HNTB: 1966
NAMED ASSOCIATE: 1980
PARTNERSHIP TENURE: 1985-Present
LEADERSHIP POSTS: Board of Directors, ACEC of New England, 1987-Present
SELECTED PROJECTS: Central Artery/Third Harbor Tunnel, EIS, Boston, Massachusetts; Central Artery North Area Project, Boston, Massachusetts; South Station Transportation Center, Boston, Massachusetts; Boston Harbor Program Management, Boston, Massachusetts; Pittsfield Wastewater Treatment Facility, New Hampshire
SELECTED HONORS: Boston Society of Civil Engineers, Construction Technical Award, 1985

136

Harvey K. Hammond, Jr.

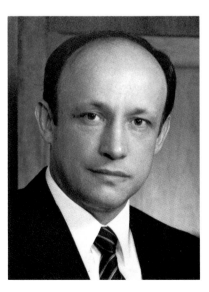

DOB: July 14, 1942
BIRTHPLACE: Mauston, Wisconsin
EDUCATION: University of Wisconsin-Platteville, B.S.C.E., 1966
JOINED HNTB: 1966
NAMED ASSOCIATE: 1979
PARTNERSHIP TENURE: 1986-Present
LEADERSHIP POSTS: American Public Works Association, Wisconsin Chapter, Director 1986-1989; President, Transportation Development Association of Wisconsin, 1989; Member, Greater Milwaukee Committee, 1988-Present; ITE, Wisconsin Chapter President 1976; District IV Chairman 1977; Hunter Business District Board of Directors 1988-Present; Chairman, HNTB Transportation Service Group; Chairman, ITE Committee, GA-33; Executive Director, Metro 2020. 1989-Present
SELCTED PROJECTS: Major highway projects, Wisconsin; Lakeview (1,500 acre) Corporate Park, Wisconsin; Computerized Traffic Control System, Racine, Wisconsin
SELECTED HONORS: ASCE — Wisconsin Section; Wisconsin Young Civil Engineer of the Year, 1976

Stephen Gartin Goddard

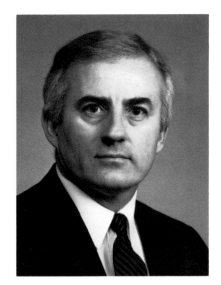

DOB: October 13, 1941

BIRTHPLACE: Greensburg, Indiana

EDUCATION: Purdue University, B.S.M.E., 1963; University of South California, M.S.M.E., 1968

JOINED HNTB: 1973

OTHER PROFESSIONAL EXPERIENCE: U.S. Air Force, Space and Missile Systems Organization, 1965-1968; Thiokol Chemical Corporation, Brigham City, Utah, 1969-1973

NAMED ASSOCIATE: 1979

PARTNERSHIP TENURE: 1987-Present

LEADERSHIP POSTS: Board Member, Consulting Engineers of Indiana, Inc., 1987-1989; Chairman, Environmental Engineering Service Group, 1989; Board of Directors and Executive Committe Member, Consulting Engineers of Indiana, 1987-1989

SELECTED PROJECTS: Indianapolis International Airport Runway 4R-22L, Indianapolis, Indiana; In-system Combined Sewer Overflow Control Project, Evansville, Indiana; Municipal and Industrial Wastewater Treatment Projects, Indiana

John Welles Wight, Jr.

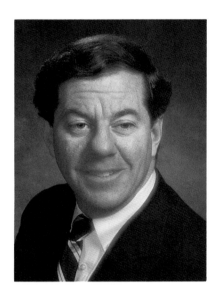

DOB: June 27, 1943

BIRTHPLACE: Summit, New Jersey

EDUCATION: Cornell University, B.S.C.E., 1967; Cornell University, M.S.C.E., 1968

JOINED HNTB: 1968

NAMED ASSOCIATE: 1982

PARTNERSHIP TENURE: 1987-Present

LEADERSHIP POSTS: Member, Executive Committee, Houston Northwest Chamber of Commerce, 1986-1988; Board Member, Texas Good Roads & Transportation, 1988-Present

SELECTED PROJECTS: Governor Alfred E. Driscoll Expressway, New Jersey; Tehran Bandar-e-Shapur Motorway, Iran; Jesse H. Jones Memorial Bridge, Texas; Southwest Freeway/Transitway, Texas; Austin Outer Parkway, Texas

137

Richard Dean Beckman

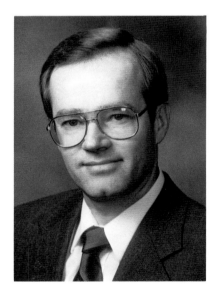

DOB: October 18, 1940

BIRTHPLACE: Montevideo, Minnesota

EDUCATION: South Dakota State University, B.S.C.E., 1962; Michigan State University, M.S.C.E., 1963

JOINED HNTB: 1967

OTHER PROFESSIONAL EXPERIENCE: U.S. Air Force, 1964-1967

NAMED ASSOCIATE: 1977

PARTNERSHIP TENURE: 1989-Present

LEADERSHIP POSTS: APWA, Minnesota Chapter, Director, 1984-1986

SELECTED PROJECTS: Hennepin Avenue Suspension Bridge, Minneapolis, Minnesota; Lake Street/Marshall Avenue Bridge, Minneapolis-St. Paul, Minnesota; I-35E/I-494 Interchange, Dakota County, Minnesota; I-394/County Road 18 Interchange, Minneapolis, Minnesota; Minneapolis-St. Paul International Airport Planning, Minnesota